ATHEROSCLEROSIS

ANNALS OF THE NEW YORK ACADEMY OF SCIENCES
Volume 454
October 15, 1985

ATHEROSCLEROSIS

Edited by K. T. Lee

The New York Academy of Sciences
New York, New York
1985

Cover: The cover shows a scanning electron micrograph of the luminal surface of a coronary artery in a hypercholesterolemic pigeon (see page 94).

Library of Congress Cataloging in Publication Data

Main entry under title:

Atherosclerosis.

(Annals of the New York Academy of Sciences, ISSN 0077-8923; v. 454)
Papers presented at the Saratoga Springs Conference on Atherosclerosis held on August 8–12, 1984; sponsored by the Dept. of Pathology at Albany Medical College.
Includes bibliographies and index.
1. Atherosclerosis—Congresses. I. Lee, K. T. II. Saratoga Springs Conference on Atherosclerosis (1984). III. Albany Medical College. Dept. of Pathology. IV. Series. [DNLM: 1. Arteriosclerosis—congresses. W1 AN626YL v. 454 / WG 550 A8672 1984]
Q11.N5 vol. 454 500 s 85-18927
[RC692] [616.1'36]
ISBN 0-89766-303-9
ISBN 0-89766-304-7 (pbk.)

SP
Printed in the United States of America
ISBN 0–89766–303–9 (cloth)
ISBN 0–89766–304–7 (paper)
ISSN 0077–8923

ANNALS OF THE NEW YORK ACADEMY OF SCIENCES

Volume 454
October 15, 1985

ATHEROSCLEROSIS[a]

Editor and Conference Chairman

K. T. LEE

Organizing Committee

ROBERT W. WISSLER,
WILBUR A. THOMAS,
FUJIO NUMANO,
GARDNER C. MCMILLAN, and
K. T. LEE

CONTENTS

[a]The papers in this volume were presented at the Saratoga Springs Conference on Atherosclerosis, which was held on August 8–12, 1984, sponsored by the Department of Pathology at Albany Medical College.

Part III. Matrix
Chair: Herbert C. Stary

Part IV. Macrophages
Chair: Henry C. McGill

Part V. Prostaglandins; Cyclic Nucleotides
Chair: Gerald S. Berenson

Part VI. Thrombotic Process
Chair: Seymour Glagov

Part VII. Lipoprotein Receptors
Chair: Peter M. Alaupovic

Part VIII. Lipoproteins

Chair: PAUL S. ROHEIM

Part IX. Growth Factors

Chair: COLIN J. SCHWARTZ

Part X. Endothelial Cells

Chair: ABEL L. ROBERTSON

Part XI. Cell Population Kinetics
Chair: JACK C. GEER

Part XII. New Directions
Chair: K. T. LEE

Financial assistance was received from:

- JAPAN ARTERIOSCLEROSIS RESEARCH FOUNDATION
- THE NEW YORK ACADEMY OF SCIENCES

- AMERICAN CYANAMID CO.
- AYERST LABORATORIES RESEARCH, INC.
- BRISTOL MYERS CO.
- BURROUGHS WELLCOME CO.
- E.I. DU PONT DE NEMOURS & CO.
- EISAI PHARMACEUTICAL CO., JAPAN
- HOFFMANN–LA ROCHE, INC.
- MCNEIL PHARMACEUTICAL
- MERCK SHARP & DOHME RESEARCH LABORATORIES
- NEW ENGLAND NUCLEAR
- NORWICH EATON PHARMACEUTICALS, INC.
- PARK DAVIS COMPANY
- THE PFIZER FOUNDATION, INC.
- A.H. ROBBINS CO.
- G.D. SEARLE CO.
- STERLING WINTHROP RESEARCH INSTITUTE
- THE UPJOHN COMPANY

Introductory Remarks

K. T. LEE

Department of Pathology
Albany Medical College
Albany, New York 12208

I wish to take this opportunity to thank the people who made this conference possible: The Organizing Committee consisting of Robert W. Wissler, Wilbur A. Thomas, Fujio Numano, and Gardner C. McMillan; Ms. Elizabeth Dougherty, who handled all the correspondence and registration of the participants; Ms. Maureen Phillips and her staff at Skidmore College, who helped make our stay at this beautiful campus so comfortable and enjoyable; and needless to say, all of the speakers, discussants, chairmen, and participants. I should also extend my sincere thanks to all organizations and pharmaceutical companies who have made generous contributions to help meet our financial obligation, and finally, to the New York Academy of Sciences which graciously agreed to publish this proceeding as one of their *Annals*.

Atherosclerosis research is in the midst of a rapid transition from relying primarily on classical biochemistry, physiology, and pathology into a new era of utilization of the approaches of cellular and subcellular pathobiology, molecular biology, membrane biology, modern genetics, and the remarkable tools of immunochemistry. As this occurs, research related to atherosclerosis is becoming increasingly complex, and the information explosion is immense. Approximately two years ago, some members of the Organizing Committee conceived an idea of having a conference to bring together leading scientists in various disciplines of atherosclerosis research to explore the current status and to attempt to put together a comprehensive picture of the atherosclerotic process.

I do hope that this conference will provide a forum for putting new developments and achievements into focus and encourage an active interaction of various disciplines to achieve the goal of understanding atherosclerosis.

PART I. OVERVIEW

Nature and Definitions of Atherosclerosis

GARDNER C. McMILLAN

Division of Heart and Vascular Diseases
National Heart, Lung, and Blood Institute
Bethesda, Maryland 20205

The past decade has seen the application of cellular and molecular biology to research on atherosclerosis. The results have created an explosion of information and far more insight into the mechanisms producing this disorder than one would have thought possible ten years ago. On the one hand, the circulating products of cells, such as lipoproteins, have been described in intimate molecular structure, and the details of structure have been related to cellular metabolic function and to the homeostasis of their systemic levels. On the other hand, the details of cellular functions and the intracellular and extracellular metabolic pathways for substances and reactions in the arterial wall, relevant to plaque building, have also been elucidated in a remarkable way.

I have had the opportunity this year to attend three conferences which, each in its own way, displayed the impact of cellular and molecular biology on research and its potential to illuminate atherogenesis. One was the Lofland Conference on arterial wall metabolism; the second was the M.D. Anderson Conference of cellular proliferation and differentiation; and the third was the international conference on the biology of the vascular endothelial cell, held recently at the Massachusetts Institute of Technology. The ability to separate, measure, and characterize proteins with great precision; the ability to grow cell lines and isolate clones in culture; the use of co-culture; the use of microchemistry and tracer chemistry of great sensitivity and specificity; and the methodology of molecular genetics dominated the papers at these conferences. As much as these methods have taught us in the past few years, I think we all believe that we shall learn vastly more from them in the near future.

Most of the metabolic and molecular work with lipoproteins and apoproteins has used specimens from humans and is directly relevant to man. So, too, is the work on cell surface receptors and on the genome that has explored human genetic variants of apoproteins and receptors. Nearly all the rest of our current pathogenetic studies at the cellular and molecular levels are based upon highly artificial model systems that may be prismatic in their simplicity, but are of unestablished biological relevance for human atherosclerosis. Many of the phenomena observed in these surrogate experimental systems will no doubt prove to be relevant, but others are from systems so artificial that one is tempted to dismiss them out of hand as without meaning for atherosclerosis. However, that is not to say that such information is without value, but rather that its relevance may lie elsewhere.

It is my belief that the next decade of work must begin to examine the question of biological relevance at the same time as it continues to expand our information base. Cellular and molecular events will need to be tried in the context of tissues, and tissue events will need to be tried in the setting of the animal model—preferably the nonhuman primate models which share so many proteins with us. Finally, and to the extent possible, the findings from the cellular and molecular systems will have to be assessed for relevance with human atherosclerosis and its various forms and expressions. The opportunities to study human atherogenesis with pathogenetic experiments are obviously limited, but the opportunities for observational studies are extensive. The human disease will need to be reexamined descriptively to establish the qualitative and quantitative occurrence of phenomena observed in the experimental systems if we are to understand their relevance or significance for the disorder in humans.

It is these considerations that lead me to present here some aspects of the nature and characteristics of human atherosclerosis. There is nothing novel about what I shall show. In any case, not many novel observations have been made on the human lesion in the past decade or two. Nevertheless, the material represents a kind of definition of atherosclerosis and it has complete relevance.

First, let us look back to the coining of the words, "arteriosclerosis," and "'atherosclerosis," by J.F. Lobstein, in 1833, and by Felix Marchand, in 1904, respectively. These are shown in slides copied from their papers. Their ideas are those of gross pathology. Over the years, definitions have been elaborated further. A Canadian pathologist, the late James Paterson, chaired a WHO working group some years ago that developed a more elaborate descriptive classification and definition which combined gross and microscopic features, and which was capable, within its terms of reference, of encompassing the variety of plaques that may be seen.[1] However, it is not a match for our present-day knowledge of pathogenesis and it is seldom used today, although it is a relatively recent and officially sanctioned classification. One or more revised definitions, that express better our ideas of pathogenesis, will require more penetrating studies of the human lesion than we have at present.

Let me refresh you about some of the aspects of human lesions that will need to be accommodated in such definitions. They represent changes which research in molecular and cellular biology must address. Vascular changes occur in infancy and childhood that manifest intimal thickening with excess cellularity, proteoglycan matrix accumulation, and fibrous matrix formation. Some contain fat, others do not. By age 15 to 20 or 25 years, occasional, large, and eccentric plaques that contain a necrotic lipid core and have a fibrous cap may be found. They appear as transitional lesions developing into adult atherosclerosis. We are unsure to what degree and how such childhood changes may relate to adult disease, and we know nothing about the circumstances that bring about the cellular proliferation and differentiation to secrete so much matrix. They must, however, be part of our definition and classification.

Turning to lesions in the adult, we find a variety too great to illustrate here. Some emphasize lipid accumulation, others matrix secretion, but all are space-occupying and show evidence of cellular proliferation and infiltration. There is often evidence of thrombotic processes and of cellular necrosis or atrophy. Many show features that imply episodic development, and secondary degenerative changes are common. Such variations need accommodation within any definition. However, it is desirable to move from a simple illustration to a pathogenetic context, and that requires us to consider cellular proliferation, differentiation, and the molecular composition and flux in the plaques.

Cells in plaques inhabit an environment partly of their own making and partly imposed upon them by substances from the blood and the products of other cells. It is an arena vastly more complex than cell culture models. Its complexity can be studied in whole tissue (three-dimensional) preparations of plaques from adults.

Perhaps, the most impressive aspects of such plaques are the intracellular lipid and the bulk of non-fibrous and fibrous matrix surrounding the cells. Presumably, the smooth muscle cells differentiate to secrete matrix, thus isolating and suspending themselves in intercellular material. Presumably, the monocyte/macrophages, which can also secrete sulfated proteoglycan matrix, migrate through the matrix or are engulfed by it while they express their capacity to accumulate lipid. Presumably, the matrix modulates proliferative behavior, complexes lipid, and influences migration and other cell behaviors. Such changes must also be part of our definition. However, when we turn to the cellular biology of such changes in humans, we find that we know very little compared to what we know from model systems. Consequently, we lack data for comparison of those systems with plaques.

The aortic endothelium in humans is often different from that seen in animals or in culture. Its most characteristic abnormalities are loss of regular pattern and the frequent presence of giant multinuclear forms.[2] I suppose, one may speculate that any of the pathological processes that may lead to multinucleate giant cell formation, including viral infection, could be candidates to explain these appearances. Nothing is known about any accompanying functional derangements or whether such abnormal endothelial cells have a role in atherogenesis.

Lesions in humans have a very variable time course. They may be progressive, episodic, stationary, or regressive. A few years ago, Dr. Michael DeBakey published a number of angiograms taken on two or more occasions, sometimes many years apart, in the same patients, that illustrate this point.[3]

Clearly, in the human condition, pathogenetic processes at the cell and tissue level can persist or, although previously active, they can cease. We know nothing of the responsible mechanisms, although we do know that reduction of a dominant risk factor such as smoking, hypertension, or hypercholesteremia reduces the clinical consequences of atherosclerosis. The variations in atherogenesis over time must be a component in our definition.

One may mention some other features. The lesions are focal; they have preferred sites of occurrence,[3] and sites where they are seldom found; lesion location and progression is often typical enough to produce a number of syndromes of clinical interest. There is a sex difference in the severity of coronary atherosclerosis, but not in the extent of aortic atherosclerosis; the sex difference is abolished by diabetes mellitus.

These various features, perhaps extended somewhat in scope, can form the basis for one or more definitions. The process of definition would need to encompass childhood and adult phenomena, a great variety of changes including secondary ones (a distinction that may not be simple to draw), peculiarities of location, variability of time course, biochemical composition, and other features. Such a definition, essentially descriptive in nature, has value and can serve in important ways to guide and validate the relevance of research into mechanisms.

However, one wonders if we may stand at the threshold of definitions with more significance for pathogenesis and for pathogenetic classification. We can now think seriously about atherosclerosis in terms of cell proliferation and cell differentation. I use the word "differentiation" simply to mean that cells differ in structure or function from their previous state, and that they express much more or less of some normal characteristic or that they may express some novel characteristics.

We have grown accustomed to the idea that proliferation is an essential component of the definition of plaques and perhaps even to the idea of an arrest of proliferation. It is less common to think of the definition of plaques in terms of cellular differentiation—differentiation to migrate, to express receptors, to participate in cell-cell interactions, or to form matrix. Much of what has been shown here of human lesions can be encompassed within the ebb and flow of cellular differentiation as a response to primary etiological stimuli, such as hyperlipidemia, hypertension, or other injurious circumstances.

It has become necessary to test human lesions, as far as this may be possible, with the probes that we apply to our surrogate cellular systems. I believe two valuable ends will be gained. One will be the screening of information derived from cellular and molecular biology for its relevance to human atherosclerosis. The other, together with refined descriptive and etiological associations, can provide a new class of definitions for atherosclerosis based on fundamental pathogenetic mechanisms.

REFERENCES

1. WORLD HEALTH ORGANIZATION. 1958. Classification of Atherosclerotic Lesions Technical Report. No. 143.
2. REPIN, V. S., V. V. DOLGOV, O. E. ZAIKINA, I. D. NOVIKOV, A. S. ANTONOV, M. A. NIKOLAEVA & V. N. SMIRNOV. 1984. Heterogeneity of endothelium in human aorta. A quantitative analysis by scanning electron microscopy. Atherosclerosis **50:** 35–52.
3. DEBAKEY, M. E. 1978. Patterns of atherosclerosis and rates of progression. *In* Atherosclerosis Reviews, vol. 3. R. Paoletti & A. M. Gotto, Jr., Eds.: 1–56. Raven Press. New York.

Macrophage Foam Cells in the Coronary Artery Intima of Human Infants[a]

HERBERT C. STARY

Department of Pathology
Louisiana State University Medical Center
New Orleans, Louisiana 70112

We studied the coronary arteries of human infants that died within the first five years of life, and obtained data on incidence, extent, location, and fate of macrophages and macrophage foam cells in the intima. This work is part of our continuing study of the evolution of atherosclerosis in young people, which now includes 900 cases which died at an age between full-term birth and 29 years, in the period 1979 to 1984. The arteries are being analyzed by various techniques. In about 300 of the total 900 cases, the interval between death and autopsy was short enough (generally ten hours or less) to make them suitable for high-resolution light microscopy and electron microscopy. The coronary arteries of these 300 cases were, therefore, fixed by perfusion with 3% glutaraldehyde under a pressure of 100 mm Hg. The 55 cases reported here are those among the 300 that were within the first five years of life. Thirty of the infants were female and twenty-five were male. We confined our studies of the perfusion-fixed coronary arteries to a segment that consisted of the left main branch, the left main bifurcation, and the proximal 15 mm of the left anterior descending branch because atherosclerotic lesions develop in this segment most often.

After perfusion, we removed this segment from the heart unopened, and cut it into five consecutive tube-like portions, each measuring from three to four mm in length, and embedded each upright in Maraglas. From each, we cut 1-μm cross sections with glass knives. The high resolution of morphological detail that is possible in 1-μm sections allowed us to identify macrophages and macrophage foam cells by light microscopy, and to study large areas. Cell identification and counting was with a Nikon NCG 60× objective and an eyepiece grid. We used the electron microscope to check light microscopic quantitations, and to confirm macrophage and macrophage foam cell identity vis-à-vis smooth muscle cells. Some intimal cells we could not classify by light or by electron microscopy. We believe, however, that we correctly identified the majority. We obtained morphometric data from 1-μm cross sections by projecting them on a horizontal board and by digitizing the outlines of structures with the cursor of a Graf pen. We obtained the areas of the media, glycosaminoglycan-rich intima, musculoelastic intima, and total intima and, at four equidistant points around the circumference, the thickness of these layers. Incisions with which we had marked the coronary segments before we embedded them, indicated the relation of the thickest part of the intima (eccentric intima thickening) to the flow divider and to anterior and posterior walls of the artery.

Structure of Coronary Artery Intima of Infants

The intima had two distinct patterns, both present in every infant coronary artery from the first month of life on.

[a]This work was supported by the National Institutes of Health, grant no. HL–22739.

The first pattern, also known as diffuse intima thickening (diffuse thickening), encompassed three-quarters of the coronary artery circumference. Here the intima was of moderate and relatively uniform thickness.

Eccentric intima thickening (eccentric thickening), also known as cushion, pad, or bolster, was the second pattern. It extended over the remaining one-quarter to one-third of the coronary circumference, always located more or less opposite the flow divider wall as an eccentric crescent, which attained, at its middle, several times the thickness of diffuse thickening.

Both the diffusely and the eccentrically thick intima patterns consisted of two main layers which differed in density of intimal smooth muscle cells and in the nature of the extracellular matrix. The upper (luminal) layer was rich in glycosaminoglycan (GAG) matrix (which sometimes formed pools) and poor in smooth muscle cells and elastic fibers. The underlying (musculoelastic) intima layer was poor in GAG, but rich in intimal smooth muscle cells and elastic fibers which were in a dense and orderly arrangement.

Diffuse thickening extended from the coronary ostium through the length of the proximal coronary artery and beyond the limits of the segment we studied. Eccentric thickening was more limited. It extended from the main branch, just proximal to the main left bifurcation, into the left anterior descending branch, just distal to the bifurcation. When eccentric thickening disappeared, diffuse thickening encompassed all of the coronary circumference.

Frequency and Location of Macrophage Foam Cells in Infant Intima

The intima of 19 of the 55 infants had macrophage foam cells within the limits of the coronary artery segment we studied. Of 28 infants aged between full-term birth and seven months, 14 (50%) had macrophage foam cells in coronary artery intima. Subsequently, in older infants, macrophage foam cell incidence declined. Of the 27 infants older than seven months, only five (18%) had macrophage foam cells in coronary artery intima.

When macrophage foam cells were present, they usually occurred in both intima patterns. In some cases they were present only in eccentric thickening. When the quantity of macrophage foam cells present around the coronary artery circumference was uneven, eccentric thickening contained the larger number.

Macrophage foam cells were usually distributed as widely spaced isolated cells, but several infants had, in addition, macrophage foam cells clustered as groups of cells. Both the thinly spaced and the clustered macrophage foam cells occurred in the upper layer of the intima, and here, the glycosaminoglycan-rich matrix pools were their preferred spot.

Macrophages without lipid droplet inclusions occurred both in the intima of infants that also had macrophage foam cells and in the intima of infants that had none. Macrophages without inclusions were thinly dispersed in the upper intima layer as isolated cells. They were not arranged as clusters of cells. Their overall number varied somewhat from one case to the next.

Cause of Macrophage Foam Cells in Infant Intima

We do not have, so far, adequate data on the nature of the diet received by individual infants in our study, or on their blood lipids. It is possible that the presence or absence of macrophage foam cells in the coronary intima of infants could be explained by the composition of the food that the individual infants received. The decrease in macrophage foam cells after the first year or so, could be explained by the customary changes in diet as infants mature.

Serum triglyceride levels have been reported to be higher, and cholesterol levels lower, in infants in the first year of life than in older preschool children. It has also been reported that infants in the first year of life that were breast-fed had higher serum cholesterol levels than those that received a formula diet. Although we do not know which of the infants were breast-fed and which received a formula diet, we do know that the majority received a formula diet.

Origin of Macrophage Foam Cells in Infant Intima

While the scanning and electron-microscopic data of many investigators strongly suggest that monocytes transmigrate the endothelium to populate the intima as macrophage foam cells, we have evidence that macrophage foam cells can also increase by proliferating locally in the intima. We reported mitotic macrophage foam cells in the experimental intimal lesions of monkeys.[1] Recently we also identified mitotic macrophage foam cells in the coronary artery fatty streak of a 25 year-old man. Villaschi and Spagnoli[2] used radioautography to study human fibroatheromatous plaques and found that cells with the features of monocytes and macrophage foam cells had been labeled with tritiated thymidine.

After the first seven months, cases with macrophage foam cells in the intima became infrequent. Macrophages without droplets were always present, however. It is likely that these macrophages represent a resident population that can become foam cells and that can divide on demand.

Fate of Macrophage Foam Cells in Infant Intima

The decline, after the first seven months, in cases with macrophage foam cells suggests that macrophage foam cells present earlier were removed, and that resident macrophages did not form foam cells much for several years after the first year. We have no evidence that macrophage foam cells were removed from the intima by transmigration through the endothelium, but we did see dead macrophage foam cells in the intima. We, therefore, assume that macrophage foam cells disappear from the intima because they die. Remnants of the dead cells did not accumulate in the intima of infants; presumably, the rate of accumulation did not overwhelm the capacity for clearance of debris.

In experiments with monkeys, in which lipid-rich food caused massive macrophage foam cell accumulations in the intima, macrophage foam cells died when the dietary stimulus was removed. The time interval between diet change and disappearance from the intima of most macrophage foam cells was four to six months,[3] indicating that this was the life span of macrophage foam cells in monkeys. If infant macrophage foam cells have a similar life span, then it can be presumed that the stimulus that caused them, ceased or diminished early in the first year of life.

Relation of the Macrophage Foam Cells of Infant Intima to the Fatty Streak and Atheroma of Older Children and Adults

Macrophage foam cells of infants predominated in eccentric thickening, a location in which fatty streaks predominated in older children, and the only location in which atheromas developed in some older children, adolescents, and young adults. This correspondence in location is apparent from data that come from our total sample of cases extending to 29 years. In spite of this similarity in location, it is unlikely that the macrophage foam cells of infant intima are the early stage of fatty streaks and atheromas. The absence of continuity (as seen in the foam-cell-poor interval after the first seven months of life) speaks against it.

When cases with macrophage foam cells in coronary intima again became frequent in the second half of the first decade, macrophage foam cells were a component of grossly visible fatty streak lesions. In fatty streaks, lipid droplets were accumulated in both macrophages and in the structural intimal smooth muscle cells. In addition, extracellular lipid and debris particles were thinly scattered among the lipid-laden cells. Fatty streaks located in eccentric thickening had features revealing them as transitional stages to atheromas. Atheromas were lesions with massive extracellular lipid accumulations (necrotic cores). In fatty streaks and in atheromas, smooth muscle cells with lipid droplets usually numerically predominated over macrophage foam cells.

The process of lesion expansion included accumulation of lipid droplets in more smooth muscle cells. Since these were longer-lived and were, apparently, more resistant to injury than macrophages, they became the numerically dominant cell type that was laden with lipid droplets.

Still, macrophages appear to be the first line of defense in the intima, being the first to accumulate and digest lipid droplets. It is likely that, by reason of their capacity for rapid intracellular degradation and rapid cell turnover (rapid immigration, rapid proliferation, short life span), macrophages account for most lipid uptake and degradation even in lesions in which they are numerically inferior.

REFERENCES

1. STARY, H. C. & M. R. MALINOW. 1982. Ultrastructure of experimental coronary artery atherosclerosis in cynomolgus macaques. Atherosclerosis **43:** 151–175.
2. VILLASCHI, S. & L. G. SPAGNOLI. 1983. Autoradiographic and ultrastructural studies on the human fibro-atheromatous plaque. Atherosclerosis **48:** 95–100.
3. STARY, H. C., D. A. EGGEN & J. P. STRONG. 1977. The Mechanism of Atherosclerosis Regression. *In* Atherosclerosis IV. G. Schettler *et al.*, Eds.: 394–404. Springer-Verlag. Berlin, Heidelberg, New York.

A New Way to Look at Atherosclerotic Involvement of the Artery Wall and the Functional Effects[a]

ROBERT W. WISSLER, DRAGOSLAVA VESSELINOVITCH,
HARRY R. DAVIS, PAUL HENRI LAMBERT,[b]
AND MANUELA BEKERMEIER

The Specialized Center of Research on Atherosclerosis
and
Department of Pathology
The University of Chicago
Chicago, Illinois 60637

[b]*WHO Immunology Research and Training Centre*
and
WHO Transfusion Centre
Hospital Cantonal
Geneva, Switzerland

INTRODUCTION

There have been immense advances during the past two decades in our understanding of the pathogenesis of atherosclerosis. These have been derived mainly from modern epidemiologic studies[1–3] and intensified clinical-pathological investigations,[4,5] as well as improved animal model research[6–9] and pioneering cellular pathobiological[10–13] and molecular biochemical studies.[14,15] Very little attention has been paid to the *configuration* of the lesions or to the degree of involvement of the media or to the correlated functional effects resulting from configurational variations which are often observed. Lesion components are now being measured carefully in a number of laboratories[16–18] and hemodynamic effects are receiving increasing attention,[19,20] but we know of only one paper in which the configuration of atherosclerotic lesions and the extent of involvement of the arterial media have been emphasized and interpreted in relation to functional effects. In an astute analysis, Roberts noted that human atherosclerotic lesions in medium-sized (muscular) arteries may be concentric or eccentric.[4]

THE EXPERIMENTAL MODEL: CONTRASTS WHICH LED TO THIS DISCOVERY

Many animal models of human atherosclerosis have been developed,[6] but only a few have fulfilled the need to reproduce faithfully the advanced human plaque[7,8] and to

[a]This manuscript is the result of studies carried out with the support of grant no. HL–15062, which provides partial funding for the Specialized Center of Research on Atherosclerosis at the University of Chicago.

reproduce many of its important effects. FIGURE 1 presents some of these models in diagrammatic form. It is evident that there are many variations in the way in which each of these models affects the artery and the host. In addition to remarkable variations in lesion components, especially at the cellular and matrix levels, these models present many other variables which almost certainly influence their usefulness for certain types of studies. Although, in a sense, all models of human disease are useful, they must all be used with caution and with as complete an understanding as possible of the similarities to and differences from human disease.

Almost all animal models of human atherosclerosis which have been established and utilized have, as their principal etiologic agent, chronic hyperlipidemia. TABLE 1 presents a list of some of the major justifications for the use of this approach for animal models of atherosclerosis.

How do the plaques produced in primate models compare with the human disease? Recently, we have had the opportunity to study more thoroughly the lesions in homozygous familial hyperlipidemia (FH) patients dying in their early teens, and to compare their histopathological features and the quantitative evaluation of their plaque components with those found in individuals with severe disease, with relatively slightly elevated serum lipids, and who die in their seventh decade or older. We have,

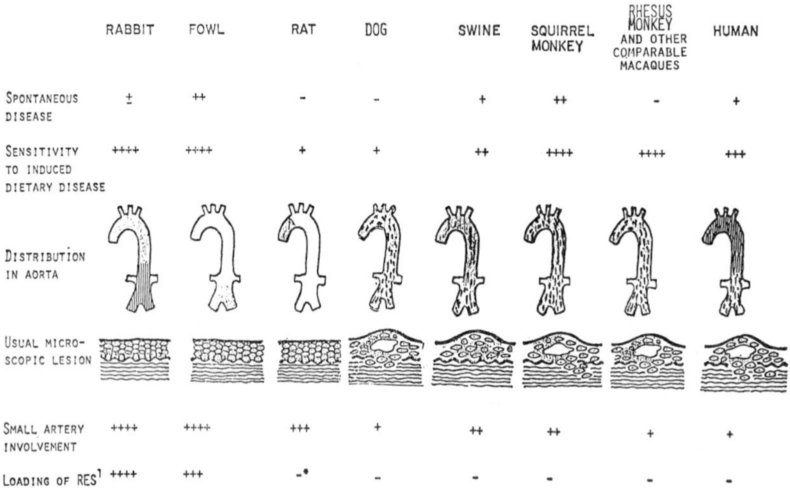

FIGURE 1. This is a diagrammatic representation of some of the most notable variables in the responses of commonly used animal models of atherosclerosis which have been studied and reported. It should be noted that the heading "FOWL" is meant to include pigeons, as well as the cockerel, and to a certain extent other fowl models, such as the Japanese Quail. The gross topography part of the diagram includes some lesions (parallel lines), which, generally speaking, are diffuse and less severe than those indicated by fine stippling or focal plaques. The microscopic part of the diagram represents an attempt to differentiate between foam cell lesions (i.e., little round circles) and predominantly smooth muscle cell lesions (i.e., ellipsoid), with some of them frequently showing the necrotic centers of true atheromata.

[1]RES = Reticuloendothelial System

*Possible +++ with combined Na cholate, thiouracil, and high fat & cholesterol feeding. Raised lesions with either coconut oil and cholesterol rich ration or with thiouracil or other thyroid ablation & high fat & cholesterol rich ration to produce sustained serum cholesterol over 700 mg %.

TABLE 1. Justification of Use of Hyperlipidemic Models for Atherosclerosis Research

1. Many of the hyperlipidemic models (dog, swine, selected primates) have lesion components similar to human atherosclerosis.
2. Other proposed models without hyperlipidemia generally do not result in a chronic lesion with morphologic and biochemical similarity to the human disease.
3. Thus far, human populations have not been reported with low serum lipids and a high incidence of advanced atherosclerosis.
4. Accelerated plaques in humans (FH, etc.) closely resemble slowly developing lesions in humans.
5. Accelerated plaques resulting from chronic hyperlipidemia in many animal models closely resemble slowly developing lesions in humans and in FH.

also, compared these morphometric analyses of human atherosclerotic plaques with those from rhesus monkeys who are autopsied after two years of severe hyperlipoproteinemia. It has become apparent that these lesions are equivalent in appearance and components, as well as in a qualitative sense. These equivalent lesions, developing in widely different time frames with very high or only modestly elevated blood lipids, demonstrate that time is not the major determinant of lesion composition.

These comparative studies have increased our reliance on the rhesus model and its resulting lesions[6–8] because of their similarity to human disease. FIGURE 2 emphasizes and illustrates that general principle of "equivalence."

Out of that formulation and our interest in establishing whether cynomolgus and rhesus models are equivalent and comparable, has come a series of four experiments in our laboratory which has yielded data on this question. In this study, stretching across five years,[21–23] we have had ample opportunity to compare the arterial responses of cynomolgus macaques (*M. fascicularis*) with those of rhesus macaques (*M. mulatta*) under a variety of experimental conditions of time intervals involved and type of atherogenic ration used. While some of the detailed data from the most recent of these four experiments are still being gathered, the purpose of this report is to document some of the rather unexpected findings that we have observed in this study.

TABLE 2 summarizes these findings in general terms. It indicates that circulating immune complexes are present in the cynomolgus monkey serum, especially when animals are fed an atherogenic ration. In contrast, the rhesus serum shows little, if any, elevation of these complexes above background, and no detectable rise when the atherogenic ration is fed. The table also indicates that there are definite contrasts between the arterial lesions of the two species. In general, the rhesus atheromatous lesions are eccentric, mostly intimal, and accompanied by little arterial dilatation after one year of feeding the most atherogenic ration we have used in our studies (FIGURE 3). The cynomolgus lesions, on the other hand, are very different. In most of the numerous standard samples from the coronary arteries which we have examined and measured quantitatively by means of the computer-assisted morphometric methods described previously,[16–18] we have found that most of the atheromatous lesions involve the arterial wall concentrically. They, frequently, are most active in the media where a large population of foam cells is present, extending into the adventitia, with little recognizable media remaining (FIGURE 4). Furthermore, accompanying this pattern of concentric transmural involvement of the artery wall, there is evidence of much more dilatation of the diseased artery, as reflected by an increase in the circumference of the external elastic lamina (EEL), than we usually observe in the most severe of the rhesus coronary artery lesions.

Some of the data resulting from the immune complex determinations are given in

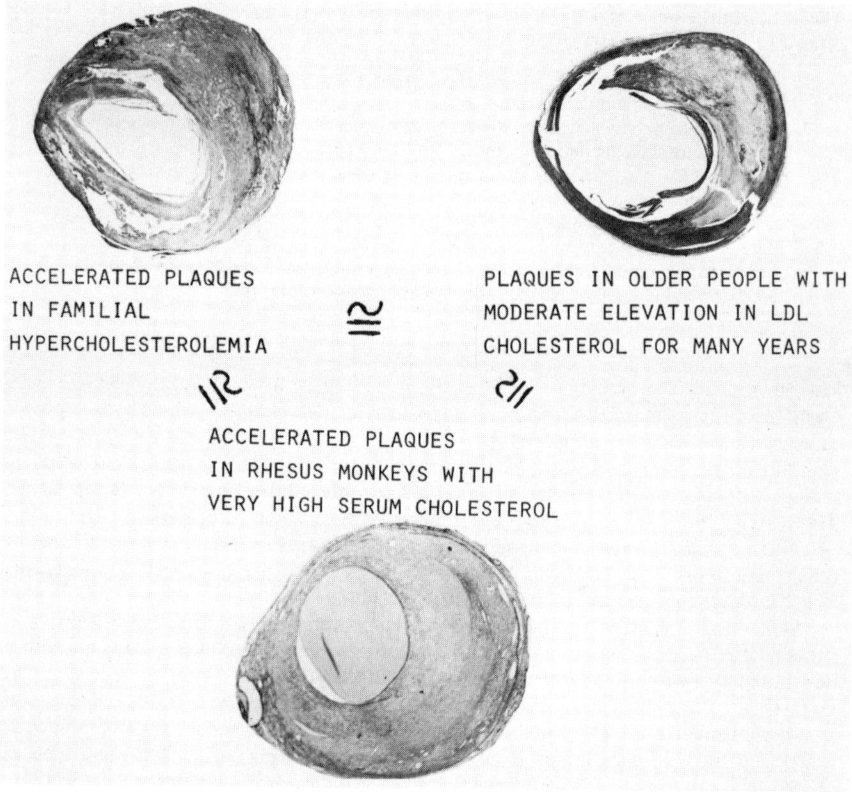

FIGURE 2. This diagram of equivalence is designed to indicate that, in their advanced form, the lesion components' size and the relative proportions of the components of the advanced plaques are similar, whether one is evaluating the lesions in a 14 year-old girl with homozygous familial hypercholesterolemia,[a] a 75 year-old man who dies with a blood cholesterol level of 240 mg %, or a rhesus monkey with a 2-year history of hypercholesterolemia resulting from a high cholesterol diet combined with a high intake of coconut oil and butter. Note the similar features of the eccentric lesions which demonstrate fibrous plaques, abundant collagen, and necrotic centers in all instances.

FIGURE 5. The values for the rhesus are considered to be background by one of us who has had extensive experience working with these methods, while the values for the cynomolgus are consistently elevated when they are fed the atherogenic ration. Although the data are not yet complete, additional determinations on the baseline sera from these same cynomolgus monkeys also show definite elevations.

Microscopic sections of unopened pressure-perfused muscular arteries are easily

[a]Material obtained through the courtesy of Professor H.C. Seftel, Head of the Lipid Disorders Clinic, Johannesburg Hospital and University of the Witwatersrand, and of Dr. P. King, Principal Pathologist and Senior Lecturer, Department of Pathology, South African Institute of Medical Research and University of the Witwatersrand, Johannesburg.

TABLE 2. Rhesus and Cynomolgus Lesions Produced Simultaneously with Identical Experimental Design

		Rhesus	Cynomolgus
Immune complex in serum	PEG ppt.[a]	−	+ +
	Clq Bind.	±	+ + +
	Congl. Bind.	−	+ + +
Lesion configuration		Eccentric	Concentric
Medial and adventitial involvement		+	+ + +
Artery dilatation		+	+ + +

[a]PEG ppt. = Polyethylene Glycol ppt.
Clq Bind. = Complement Factor 1 q Binding
Congl. Bind. = Conglutinin Binding

classified as showing eccentric or concentric lesions when the printouts of the morphometric analyses are examined. TABLE 3 summarizes the average results of two experiments in which this assessment was made by two independent observers. Interobserver agreement was excellent using relatively simple guidelines. Lesions were classified as concentric when more than three-quarters of the arterial circumference was involved in the transmural process. They were recorded as eccentric lesions when at least half of the circumference of the artery was free of medial lesions. Using this

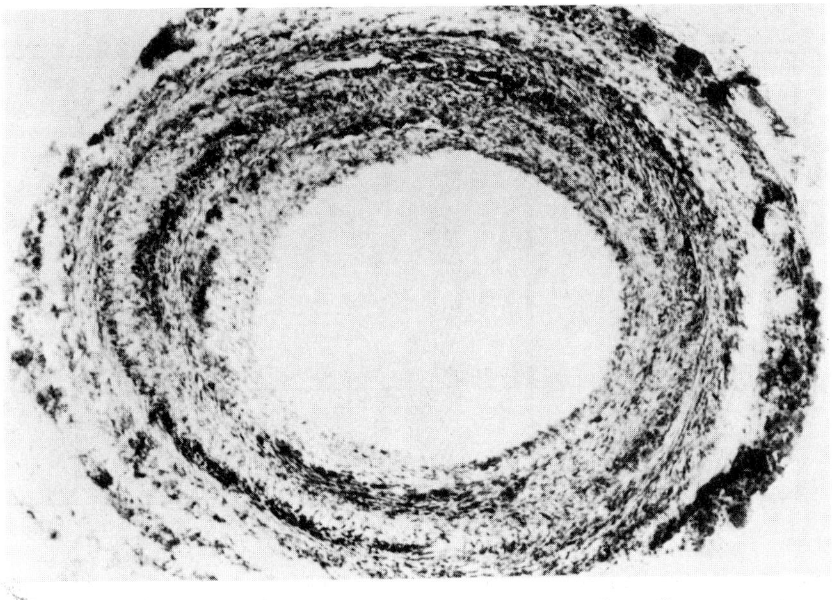

FIGURE 3. A typical cynomolgus monkey's proximal left anterior descending coronary artery lesion after twelve months' feeding of a high cholesterol diet, rich in coconut oil and butter fat. Note the severe destructive medial involvement and extensive adventitial foam cell infiltration, in addition to the concentric intimal cell prolification and lipid deposition. Oil red 0 fat stain. (Republished from R.W. Wissler and D. Vesselinovitch. Periodica Angiologica **5:** 178 (1984), with permission of the publishers.)

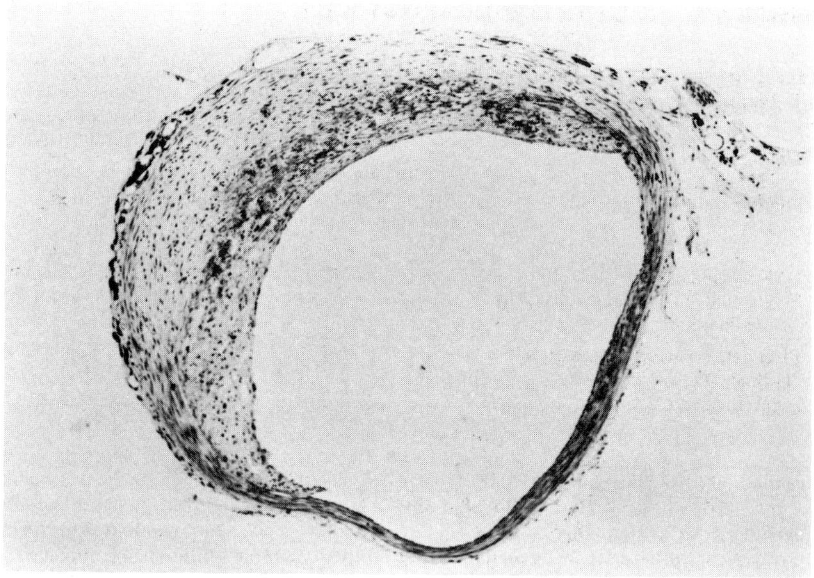

FIGURE 4. This lesion is representative of the eccentric coronary artery lesions seen after one year of feeding a diet high in coconut oil, butter oil, and cholesterol. It is a well localized, largely intimal, and mixed fibrous and fatty plaque with both intracellular and extracellular lipid. Oil red 0 fat stain. (Republished from R.W. Wissler and D. Vesselinovitch. Periodica Angiologica **5:** 178 (1984), with permission of the publishers.)

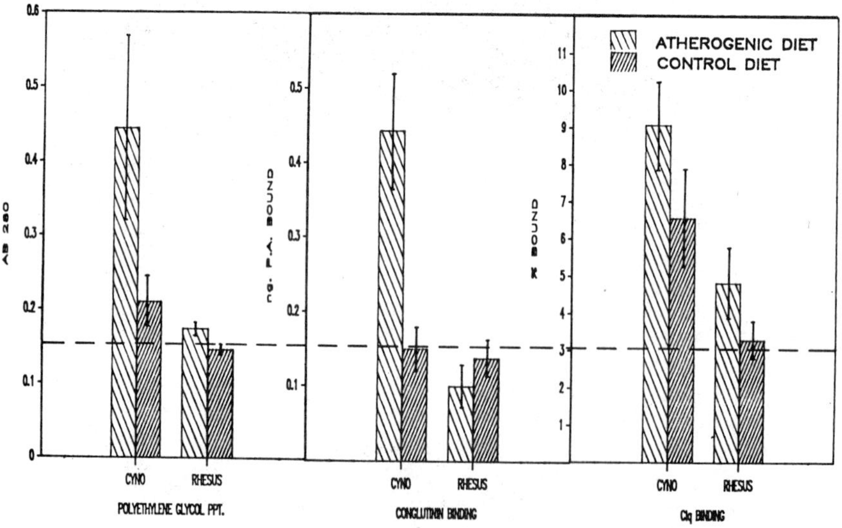

FIGURE 5. Circulating Immune Complexes: This bar graph reflects the results of determining the circulating immune complexes in the cynomolgus and rhesus monkeys at the termination of one experiment in which the two species were fed the same diets, atherogenic and control, simultaneously for the same length of time. The quantitative results (Mean ± Standard Error of the Mean) show a striking similarity no matter which method we used. The baseline which is drawn in (dashed line) represents the usual "cutoff point" for nonspecific background values. In general, the results show a remarkable contrast between the two species. This is somewhat greater in the hyperlipidemic animals, which are fed the atherogenic diet.

TABLE 3. Classification of the Coronary Artery Lesions from Rhesus and Cynomolgus Monkeys

	Total Number of Sections Examined	Average of Two Experiments	
		Eccentric	Concentric
[a]Rhesus Lesions	81	91%	9%
[a]Cynomolgus Lesions	63	25%	75%

[a]All animals used for this analysis were fed a peanut oil and cholesterol rich ration for 12 months prior to autopsy. The classification of the lesions was made from digitizer generated images of cross sections of the coronary arteries prepared for histopathological examination and projected for morphometry of the principal lesion components.

system and combining the results from two studies, the cynomolgus monkeys showed a 75% incidence of concentric lesions, while the rhesus monkeys showed 91% eccentric lesions. In addition, the cynomolgus coronary arteries showed a progressive dilatation of the EEL as the disease progressed,[21] presumably due to the weakening of the media of the artery wall, which is essentially destroyed by the concentric transmural lesions.

As these studies continued, Dr. Vesselinovitch and I found that when the hyperlipidemia is corrected by means of diet or drug therapy, although much of the stainable lipid disappears from the lesion and the necrotic centers become much smaller, the lumens did not enlarge, presumably because the damaged media undergoes scarring and contraction in a concentric pattern.

Dr. Harry R. Davis and I, with the help of Dr. Vesselinovitch, have made a rather comprehensive study of the pathogenesis of cynomolgus atherosclerosis and rhesus atherosclerosis with time, in animals fed the same atherogenic ration simultaneously.[24–26] TABLE 4 shows a number of contrasts between the reactions of these species to a high cholesterol diet, rich in coconut oil and butter. These are divided into differences in the responses of blood lipids and lipoproteins; reticuloendothelial (RES) function, including circulating lipophages, xanthomata, and hepatic RES storage; aortic chemis-

TABLE 4. Contrast of Rhesus and Cynomolgus Response Induced by Identical Diet Fed for Same Length of Time

Response	Rhesus	Cynomolgus
Serum Cholesterol Elevation	+ + +	+ + + +
Serum Triglyceride Elevation	0	+ +
Lipoprotein α/β Shift	+ + +	+ + + +
β-VLDL Presence	+	+ + +
HDL-Cholesterol Decrease	0	+ + +
Circulating Lipophages	+	+ +
RES Lipid Storage	+	+ + + +
Xanthomata	+ +	+ + + +
Aorta Chemistry:		
Cholesterol	+ +	+ + + +
Triglyceride	+ +	+ + + +
DNA	+ +	+ +
Apo B	+ +	+ + + +
Monocyte Derived Macrophages in Arterial Lesions	+	+ + + +
Arterial Lysosomal Enzyme Activities	+	+ + + +
Arterial Cholesteryl Ester Synthesis	+	+ + +
Arterial Cell Proliferation	+ + + +	+ +

TABLE 5. Analysis of Myocardial Infarct Research Unit (MIRU) Autopsies for Types of Coronary Artery Lesions at Points of Severe Stenosis

Categories of Specimens	Cases	Artery Sections With Severe Stenosis
Total	59	242
Total with Eccentric Only (E)	28 (48%)	80 (33%)
Total with Concentric Only (C)	4 (7%)	10 (4%)
Total with Eccentric & Concentric (E & C)	27 (45%)	152 (63%)
		106 E
		46 C
Total Sections with E		186 (77%)
Total Sections with C		56 (23%)

try and cell population data; lysosomal enzyme activity and cholesteryl ester synthesis; as well as measurement of cellular proliferation in the arterial lesions.

HUMAN LESIONS—HOW DO THEY COMPARE?

The next step in this investigation was to evaluate the occurrence of these two configurations of atherosclerotic coronary lesions in 59 human autopsy cases in which there was a clear-cut history of ischemic heart disease, and in which 242 points of severe stenosis of the proximal coronary arteries were examined for lesion configuration and involvement of the media. TABLES 5 and 6 present the results of this part of the study. It is evident that the two types of lesions were found in these severely diseased coronary arteries. Of the 59 cases studied, only four had solely concentric lesions. Of the total of 59 cases examined, there were a number of cases, 28 in all, which had only eccentric lesions. Almost an equal number of cases showed both eccentric and concentric lesions, so that of the 242 sections taken through the areas of most severe stenosis, 186, or about 80%, were eccentric (FIGURE 6) and 56, or about 20%, were concentric (FIGURE 7).

It is evident from further study of these sections (TABLE 6), that many more of the sections from the human cases which showed concentric lesions also demonstrated thrombosis. Forty-one percent of these lesions exhibited evidence of old or recent thrombosis, whereas only 9% of the eccentric lesions were complicated by thrombosis.

This finding and the general configuration of concentric transmural coronary lesions raise some interesting questions regarding the functional effects of concentric and eccentric lesions. As has been emphasized by Buja and Willerson,[5] as well as Buja and co-workers,[27] who have reviewed the mechanisms which may trigger coronary spasm, the reaction of spasm requires a reasonable amount of healthy contractile arterial media for it to occur. This suggests that eccentric lesions, even when they are quite large, are much more likely to support arterial spasm, whereas concentric

TABLE 6. The Thrombotic Process in Eccentric and Concentric Lesions in Humans

	With Thrombi		Without Thrombi	
Type of Lesion	No. of Sections	%	No. of Sections	%
Eccentric	17	9	167	91
Concentric	19	41	27	59

transmural lesions may not. These major functional associations of eccentric and concentric lesions are tabulated in TABLE 7. They may have a strong influence on a number of the most substantial clinical consequences of advanced atherosclerosis.

DISCUSSION AND SUMMARY

Insofar as our studies have gone, they indicate that there are remarkable differences in response between macaque species fed identical atherogenic rations for

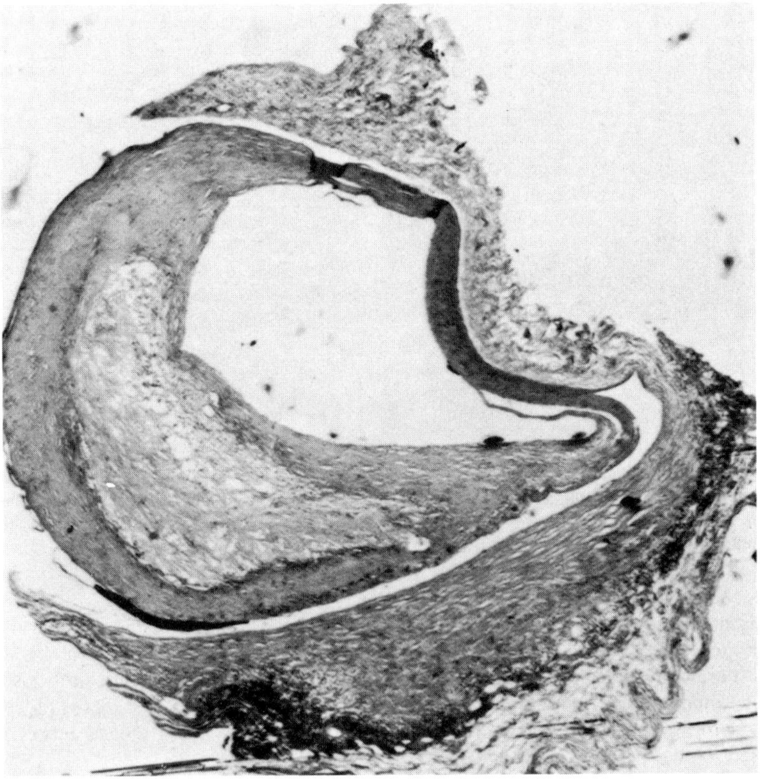

FIGURE 6. This lesion, which comes from the left anterior descending coronary artery of a 55 year-old female who suffered from severe atherosclerotic ischemic heart disease, shows a typical eccentric plaque with little involvement of the intima.

the same length of time and under identical conditions (TABLE 8). These seem to be related to the presence or absence of circulating immune complexes and may have a strong influence on configuration of the arterial lesions (FIGURE 5). If immune complexes are present in sufficient quantities throughout atherogenesis, the lesions appear to be largely *concentric* and *transmural* and to involve the media and adventitia, as well as the intima.

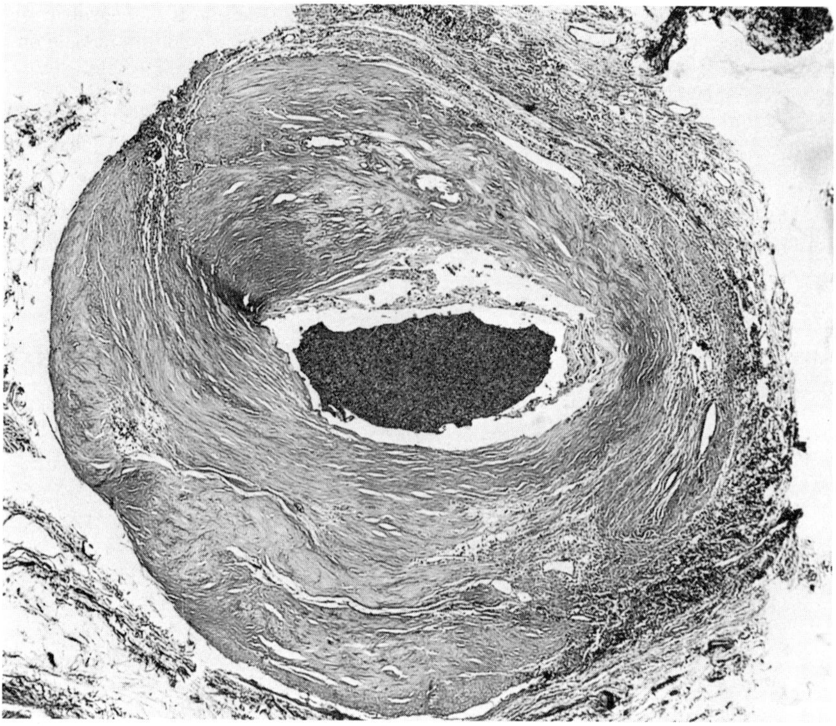

FIGURE 7. This left circumflex artery from a 70 year-old male demonstrates the features of one type of concentric lesion found at areas of severe stenosis of the coronary arteries. Its lumen is partially filled with the residue of a barium gelatin mixture used to perform the postmortem arteriogram. Some concentric lesions which we studied showed multiple lipid filled necrotic areas and more adventitial inflammatory reaction.

TABLE 7 also suggests that this reaction of the medium-size muscular artery during atherogenesis may lead to more dilatation of the artery as the media is weakened, so that there may be less potential for spasm and more potential for thrombosis. The development of effective regression with lumen expansion, as the lipid leaves the lesion, may be limited by the scarring and collagenization, and constrictive contraction of the injured media.

In fact, there is documented evidence that the cynomolgus lesions do not undergo

TABLE 7. Major Functional Associations of Eccentric and Concentric Lesions

	Arterial Dilatation	Potential For Spasm	Potential for Thrombosis	Effective Regression (Lumen Expands)
Eccentric Lesions (Rhesus Monkeys)	−	+	±(?)	+
Concentric Lesions (Cynomolgus Monkeys)	+	±(?)	+	−

the same degree of effective regression[21,28,29] in terms of lumen expansion, as we, and others, have observed in rhesus monkeys.[30–32] The successful regression studies carried out by Malinow and co-workers[33] in cynomolgus monkeys, using either cholestyramine or alfalfa saponins, are probably largely a function of very skillful use of the model. They employed a relatively brief and relatively mild induction period, and achieved excellent regression of lesions.

The configuration of the coronary artery atherosclerotic lesions, which develop when the endothelium is intact and no immune complexes are circulating, generally follows the rules which have been worked out by careful hemodynamic studies.[34,35] In general, on curving surfaces the progressive atheromatous coronary lesions are eccentric,[4] develop in predictable areas,[36] and tend to be more related to areas of low shear and departures from unidirectional linear flow.[37,38]

When immune complexes are present, the hemodynamically determined pattern, which usually controls the eccentric configuration of the coronary artery plaque, gives way to a much more general plaque pattern characteristic of endothelial injury by immunologically triggered inflammation.[39–42]

TABLE 8. Summary of Immune Complex Effects on Pathogenesis of Atherosclerosis in Primates

1. Remarkable differences in response between species of macaque monkeys fed identical atherogenic rations include:
   A. Predominantly concentric lesions in some, and almost all eccentric lesions in others.
   B. More medial involvement in some, mostly intimal in others.
   C. Circulating immune complexes in some species, little in others.
   D. Other contrasts in lipid–lipoprotein and arterial-cellular responses.
2. Experimental transmural concentric lesions in some species are accompanied by more arterial dilatation and less effective lesion regression (arterial lumen restoration) in these species.
3. The same morphological contrasts (A & B) in advanced human atherosclerotic lesions are correlated with a high incidence of thrombosis in the concentric lesions.

Thus far, there has been very little published work on the cellular pathobiology of *arterial* endothelial injury and arterial smooth muscle cell injury produced by immune complexes even though this has been a highly prized model for the study of experimental atherosclerosis superimposed upon serum sickness or other immunological injury in the rabbit.[43–46] This form of atheroarteritis is probably at least partially responsible for the unusual configuration of the lesions in the cynomolgus monkey where immune complex renal disease has been repeatedly demonstrated. It may, unfortunately, alter the pathogenesis and configuration of lesions in a number of other monkey models.[47–50] Although each of these studies emphasizes the renal lesions of immune complex origin, the results suggest that the circulating antigen combined with antibody is likely to be involved in the formation of a different type of atheroarteritis vascular lesion, namely a concentric and transmural arterial lesion.

This type of immunologically induced inflammatory lesion in the arteries of rabbits has been extensively studied ever since Rich and Gregory first reported it in 1943,[51] followed by a publication from this laboratory confirming the phenomenon in 1946.[52] Because of the illuminating studies led by Germuth,[53] Dixon,[54] and others,[55] it has become the prototype of immune complex arteritis. As has already been mentioned, the model has also been used extensively by the experimental pathologists at Cornell to produce a special type of atheroarteritis in rabbits.[43–46]

Unfortunately, the modern methods of studying endothelium to detect immunological injury have apparently not been applied to the arterial endothelium in animals subjected to the serum sickness insult. Obviously, the focal nature of the lesions makes such a systematic study difficult, if not impossible. Fortunately, we are now entering an era in which the detection of antigen and antibody in the lesions of experimental and human atheroarteritis should help establish an important immunological contribution to the pathogenesis of some lesions.

ACKNOWLEDGMENTS

This study was aided by the technical help of Laura Harris, Timothy Bridenstine, and Blanche Berger. The manuscript was prepared with the skillful assistance of Gertrud Friedman for which we are very grateful. Gordon Bowie also provided valuable photographic assistance.

REFERENCES

1. DAWBER, T. R. 1980. The Framingham Study. The Epidemiology of Atherosclerotic Disease. Harvard Univ. Press. Cambridge, Mass.
2. KEYS, A. 1975. Coronary heart disease—the global picture. Atherosclerosis **22:** 149–192.
3. BLACKBURN, H. 1979. Conference on the health effects of blood lipids: Optimal distributions for populations. Workshop Report: Epidemiological Section. Preventive Medicine **8:** 612–678.
4. ROBERTS, W. C. 1975. The coronary arteries in coronary heart disease. Morphologic observations. Pathobiol. Annu. **5:** 249–282.
5. BUJA, L. M. & J. T. WILLERSON. 1981. Clinicopathologic correlates of acute ischemic heart disease syndromes. Am. J. Cardiol. **47:** 343–356.
6. WISSLER, R. W. & D. VESSELINOVITCH. 1978. Evaluation of animal models for the study of the pathogenesis of atherosclerosis. *In* International Symposium State of Prevention and Therapy in Human Arteriosclerosis and in Animal Models. W. H. Hauss, R. W. Wissler & R. Lehmann, Eds.: 13–29. Westdeutscher-Verlag. Opladen, W. Germany.
7. STRONG, J. P. 1976. Atherosclerosis in Primates. Prim. Med., vol. 9. Karger. Basel.
8. WISSLER, R. W. & D. VESSELINOVITCH. 1977. Atherosclerosis in nonhuman primates. *In* Advances in Veterinary Science and Comparative Medicine, vol. 21. C. A. Bradley, C. E. Cornelius & C. F. Simpson, Eds.: 351–420. Academic Press. New York.
9. WATANABE, Y. 1980. Serial inbreeding of rabbits with hereditary hyperlipidemia (WHHL-rabbit). Incidence and development of atherosclerosis and xanthoma. Atherosclerosis **36:** 261–268.
10. WISSLER, R. W. 1979. The emerging cellular pathobiology of atherosclerosis. Artery **5:** 409–423.
11. ROSS, R. 1981. Atherosclerosis: A problem of the biology of arterial wall cells and their interactions with blood components. Arteriosclerosis **1:** 293–311.
12. WISSLER, R. W. 1984. The pathobiology of the atherosclerotic plaque in the mid-1980's. *In* Regression of Atherosclerotic Lesions: Experimental Studies and Observations in Humans. M. R. Malinow & V. H. Blaton, Eds.: 5–20. Plenum Press. N.Y.
13. STEINBERG, D. 1983. Lipoproteins and atherosclerosis: A look back and a look ahead. Arteriosclerosis **3:** 283–301.
14. GOLDSTEIN, J. L. & M. S. BROWN. 1977. The low density lipoprotein pathway and its relation to atherosclerosis. Annu. Rev. Biochem. **46:** 897–930.
15. MAHLEY, R. W. 1982. Atherogenic hyperlipoproteinemia. The cellular and molecular biology of plasma lipoproteins altered by dietary fat and cholesterol. Med. Clin. North Am. **66:** 375–402.
16. WISSLER, R. W., D. VESSELINOVITCH, T. J. SCHAFFNER & S. GLAGOV. 1980. Quantitating rhesus monkey atherosclerosis progression and regression with time. *In* Atherosclerosis,

vol. V. A. M. Gotto, Jr., L. C. Smith & B. Allen, Eds.: 757–761. Springer-Verlag. New York.

17. BOND, M. G., J. K. SAWYER, B. C. BULLOCK, W. BARNES & R. BALL. 1983. Animal studies of atherosclerosis progression and regression. *In* Clinical Diagnosis of Atherosclerosis. Quantitative Methods of Evaluation. M. G. Bond, W. Insull, Jr., S. Glagov, A. B. Chandler & J. F. Cornhill, Eds.: 435–451. Springer-Verlag. New York.
18. GLAGOV, S., J. GRANDE, D. VESSELINOVITCH & C. K. ZARINS. 1981. Quantitation of cells and fibers in histologic sections of arterial walls. Advantages of contour tracing on a digitizing plate. *In* Connective Tissues in Arterial and Pulmonary Disease. T. McDonald & A. B. Chandler, Eds.: 57–93. Springer-Verlag. New York.
19. GLAGOV, S., C. K. ZARINS, K. E. TAYLOR, R. A. BOMBERGER & D. P. GIDDENS. 1983. Evidence that high flow velocity and endothelial disruption are not the principal factors in experimental plaque localization. *In* Fluid Dynamics as a Localizing Factor for Atherosclerosis. G. Schettler, R. M. Nerem, H. Schmid-Schönbein, H. Mörl & C. Diehm, Eds.: 208–211. Springer-Verlag. Berlin.
20. REIDY, M. A. & D. E. BOWYER. 1977. Scanning electron microscopy of arteries. The morphology of aortic endothelium in hemodynamically stressed areas associated with branches. Atherosclerosis **26:** 181–194.
21. VESSELINOVITCH, D. & R. W. WISSLER. 1982. Correlation of types of induced lesions with regression of coronary atherosclerosis in two species of macaques. *In* Lipoproteins and Coronary Atherosclerosis. G. Noseda, C. Fragiacomo, R. Fumagalli & R. Paoletti, Eds.: 401–406. Elsevier. Amsterdam.
22. WISSLER, R. W. & D. VESSELINOVITCH. 1983. Atherosclerosis—Relationship to coronary blood flow. Am. J. Cardiol. **52:** 2A–7A.
23. WISSLER, R. W. & D. VESSELINOVITCH. 1984. New concepts of factors involved in the natural history and regression of atherosclerosis. Periodica Angiologica **5:** 178–187.
24. DAVIS, H. R. & R. W. WISSLER. 1984. Apoprotein B quantitation in rhesus and cynomolgus monkey atherosclerotic lesions. Atherosclerosis **50:** 241–252.
25. DAVIS, H. R., D. VESSELINOVITCH & R. W. WISSLER. 1984. Reticuloendothelial system response to hyperlipidemia in rhesus and cynomolgus monkeys. J. Leukocyte Biol. **36:** 63–80.
26. DAVIS, H. R., D. VESSELINOVITCH & R. W. WISSLER. 1984. Histochemical detection and quantification of macrophages in rhesus and cynomolgus monkey atherosclerotic lesions. J. Histochem. Cytochem. **32:** 1319–1327.
27. BUJA, L. M., L. D. HILLIS, C. S. PETTY & J. T. WILLERSON. 1981. The role of coronary arterial spasm in ischemic heart disease, Arch. Pathol. Lab. Med. **105:** 221–226.
28. HOLLANDER, W., B. KIRKPATRICK, B. PADDOCK, J. COLOMBO, M. NAGRAJ & S. PRUSTY. 1979. Studies on the progression and regression of coronary and peripheral atherosclerosis in the cynomolgus monkey. Exp. Mol. Pathol. **30:** 55–73.
29. ARMSTRONG, M. L. & M. C. MEGAN. 1974. Responses of two macaque species to atherogenic diet and its withdrawal. *In* Atherosclerosis, vol. III. G. Schettler & A. Weizel, Eds.: 336–338. Springer-Verlag. Berlin.
30. ARMSTRONG, M. L., E. D. WARNER & W. E. CONNOR. 1970. Regression of coronary atheromatosis in rhesus monkeys. Circ. Res. **27:** 59–67.
31. VESSELINOVITCH, D., R. W. WISSLER, R. HUGHES & J. BORENSZTAJN. 1976. Reversal of advanced atherosclerosis in rhesus monkeys. I. Light microscopic studies. Atherosclerosis. **23:** 155–176.
32. CLARKSON, T. B., M. G. BOND, B. C. BULLOCK & C. A. MARZETTA. 1981. A study of atherosclerosis regression in Macaca mulatta. IV. Changes in coronary arteries from animals with atherosclerosis induced for 19 months and then regressed for 24 or 48 months at plasma cholesterol concentrations of 300 or 200 mg/dl. Exp. Mol. Pathol. **34:** 345–368.
33. MALINOW, M. R., P. MCLAUGHLIN, H. K. NAITO, L. A. LEWIS & W. P. MCNULTY. 1978. Effect of alfalfa meal on shrinkage (regression) of atherosclerotic plaques during cholesterol feeding in monkeys. Atherosclerosis **30:** 27–43.
34. NAUMANN, A. & H. SCHMID-SCHÖNBEIN. 1983. A fluid-dynamicist's and a physiologist's look at arterial flow and arteriosclerosis. *In* Fluid Dynamics as a Localizing Factor for

Atherosclerosis. G. Schettler, R. M. Nerem, H. Schmid-Schönbein, H. Mörl & C. Diehm, Eds.: 9–25. Springer-Verlag. Berlin.
35. NEREM, R. M. & M. J. LEVESQUE. 1983. The case for fluid dynamics as a localizing factor in atherogenesis. *In* Fluid Dynamics as a Localizing Factor for Atherosclerosis. G. Schettler, R. M. Nerem, H. Schmid-Schönbein, H. Mörl & C. Diehm, Eds.: 26–37. Springer-Verlag. Berlin.
36. SVINDLAND, A. 1983. The localization of sudanophilic and fibrous plaques in the main left coronary bifurcation. Atherosclerosis **48:** 139–145.
37. KU, D. N. & D. P. GIDDENS. 1983. Pulsatile flow in a model carotid bifurcation. Arteriosclerosis **3:** 31–39.
38. ZARINS, C. K., D. P. GIDDENS, B. K. BHARADVAJ, V. S. SOTTIURAI, R. F. MABON & S. GLAGOV. 1983. Carotid bifurcation atherosclerosis. Quantitative correlation of plaque localization with flow velocity profiles and wall shear stress. Circ. Res. **53:** 502–514.
39. RYAN, S. & W. RYAN. 1983. Endothelial cells and inflammation. Clin. Lab. Med. **3:** 577–599.
40. YAMAGUCHI, H., H. TAKEUCHI & C. H. TORIKATA. 1978. Studies on morphological changes of arteries by administration of soluble immune complexes to low calcium diet bred guinea pigs—Special reference to the morphological pathogenesis of arteritis. Exp. Pathol. **15:** 361–369.
41. ACCINNI, L. & F. J. DIXON. 1979. Degenerative vascular disease and myocardial infarction in mice with lupus-like syndrome. Am. J. Pathol. **96:** 477–492.
42. KONDO, Y., Y. NIWA, J. TAKIZAWA, B. AKIKUSA, M. SANO & H. SHIGEMATSU. 1979. Accelerated serum sickness in the rabbit. IV. Characteristic endarteritis in the pulmonary artery. Lab. Invest. **41:** 119–127.
43. MINICK, C. R., G. E. MURPHY & W. C. CAMPBELL. 1966. Experimental induction of atherosclerosis by the synergy of allergic injury to arteries and lipid rich diet. 1. Effect of repeated injection of horse serum in rabbits fed dietary cholesterol supplement. J. Exp. Med. **124:** 635–651.
44. MINICK, C. R. & G. E. MURPHY. 1973. Experimental induction of atheroarteriosclerosis by the synergy of allergic injury to arteries and lipid rich diet. II. Effect of repeatedly injected foreign protein in rabbits fed a lipid-rich, cholesterol-poor diet. Am. J. Pathol. **73:** 265–300.
45. ALONSO, D. R., P. K. STAREK & C. R. MINICK. 1977. Studies on the pathogenesis of atheroarteriosclerosis induced in rabbit cardiac allografts by the synergy of graft rejection and hypercholesterolemia. Am. J. Pathol. **87:** 415–442.
46. MINICK, C. R., D. R. ALONSO & L. RANKIN. 1977. Immunologic arterial injury in atherogenesis. Prog. Biochem. Pharmacol. **14:** 225–233.
47. POSKITT, T. R., H. P. FORTWENGLER, JR., J. C. BOBROW & G. J. ROTH. 1974. Naturally occurring immune-complex glomerulonephritis in monkeys (*Macaca irus*). I. Light, immunofluorescence, and electron microscopic studies. Am. J. Pathol. **76:** 145–164.
48. GIDDENS, W. E., JR., J. T. BOYCE, G. A. BLAKLEY & W. R. MORTON. 1981. Renal disease in the pigtailed macaque (*Macaca nemestrina*). Vet. Pathol. **18** (Suppl. 6): 70–81.
49. BOYCE, J. T., W. E. GIDDENS, JR. & R. SEIFERT. 1981. Spontaneous mesangioproliferative glomerulonephritis in pigtailed macaques (*Macaca nemestrina*). Vet. Pathol. **18** (Suppl. 6): 82–88.
50. STILLS, H. F., JR. & B. C. BULLOCK. 1981. Renal disease in squirrel monkeys (*Saimiri sciureus*). Vet. Pathol. **18** (Suppl. 6): 38–44.
51. RICH, A. R. & J. E. GREGORY. 1943. The experimental demonstration that periarteritis nodosa is a manifestation of hypersensitivity. Bull. Johns Hopkins Hosp. **72:** 65–88.
52. HOPPS, H. C. & R. W. WISSLER. 1946. The experimental production of generalized arteritis and periarteritis (periarteritis nodosa). J. Lab. Clin. Med. **31:** 939–957.
53. GERMUTH, F. G., JR. & R. H. HEPTINSTALL. 1957. The development of arterial lesions following prolonged sensitization to bovine gamma globulin. Bull. Johns Hopkins Hosp. **100:** 58–70.
54. DIXON, F. J., J. J. VAZQUEZ, W. O. WEIGLE & C. G. COCHRANE. 1958. Pathogenesis of serum sickness. Arch. Pathol. **65:** 18–28.
55. ALERCON-SEGOVIA, D. & A. L. BROWN. 1964. Classification and etiologic aspects of necrotizing angiitis. An analytic approach to a confused subject with a critical review of the evidence for hypersensitivity in polyarteritis nodosa. Mayo Clin. Proc. **39:** 205–222.

Effects of Synthetic Glycosides on Cholesterol Absorption[a]

M. RENE MALINOW

Laboratory of Cardiovascular Diseases
Oregon Regional Primate Research Center
Beaverton, Oregon 97006
and
Department of Medicine
Oregon Health Sciences University
Portland, Oregon 97201

The glycosides contained in an extract of alfalfa meal, operationally named alfalfa saponins,[1] prevent the hypercholesterolemia expected in monkeys given high-cholesterol diets,[2–4] as well as preventing the development of atherosclerosis in cholesterol-fed rabbits.[5] They also induce regression of atherosclerosis in cholesterol-fed monkeys.[4] Although the mechanism of these effects has not been totally unraveled, it is likely that it involves lowered intestinal absorption of cholesterol[3,6,7] and increased fecal excretion of neutral steroids and bile acids.[3] Because of the complex nature of the alfalfa extract, which contains more than thirty different saponins, peptides, carbohydrates, and pigments, and probably other unidentified material,[1] I deemed it important to study glycosides with chemically defined structures. Consequently, a small series of glycosides was synthesized. This series contained the aglycone tigogenin, present in digitonin saponins,[8] which prevents hypercholesterolemia in monkeys,[9] or diosgenin, a spirostane derivative closely related to tigogenin. Subsequently, I studied the effects of these glycosides on intestinal absorption of cholesterol in rats.

MATERIALS AND METHODS

Chemicals

Tigogenin (5α, 20α, 22α, 25α spirosten-3β-ol) and diosgenin (Δ5, 20α, 22α, 25α spirosten-3β-ol) were obtained from Steraloids (Wilton, NH). The β-D(+) glucose pentaacetate and D-cellobiose octoacetate were purchased from Sigma (St. Louis, MO) and K & K Laboratories (Plainview, NY), respectively.

Hydrobromic acid and stannic chloride were obtained from Matheson, Coleman, and Bell (Norwood, OH). Synthesis of predominantly β anomers of tigogenin glucoside, tigogenin cellobioside, diosgenin glucoside, and diosgenin cellobioside was accomplished either by adapting the Koenigs-Knorr reaction[10] modified by Rosevear *et al.*,[11] or the method of Hanessian and Banoub.[12] Purity of the resulting compounds was estimated at around 90% in silica gel on thin-layer chromatography plates (LK5DF, Whatman Chemical Separation, Inc., Clifton, NJ), developed in methylene chloride:methanol:water (83:15:2:2,vol/vol), and visualized with a phosphomolibdic acid alcoholic solution.

[a]Publication no. 1351 of the Oregon Regional Primate Research Center was supported by grants RR-00163 and HL-16587 from the National Institutes of Health.

Alfalfa saponins, used as positive controls, were kindly prepared by A.L. Livingston and G.O. Kohler (Western Regional Research Center, U.S. Department of Agriculture, Berkeley, CA) according to the method of Malinow *et al.*[13] The [1,2-^{3}H(N)]cholesterol (s.a. 55 Ci/mmol) from New England Nuclear (Boston, MA) was purified by thin-layer chromatography before use.

Animals

Male adult Sprague-Dawley rats were used. The method, which has been already described for estimation of intestinal absorption of cholesterol,[6] was slightly modified; only its main features are presented here. For one week before the experiment, rats receiving drinking water *ad libitum* were meal fed, between 0800 h and 1000 h, a semi-purified ration consisting of casein (26%), sucrose (46%), safflower oil (2%), alphacel (19.5%), Hegsted IV salt mix (ICN Nutritional Biochemicals, Plainville, NY; 4%), vitamins OWP (ICN Nutritional Biochemicals; 2%), crystalline vitamin D_3 (10 μg/100 g), and DL-methionine (0.5%).[14] Intestinal absorption of cholesterol was calculated as the difference between an oral 2-mg dose of radioactive cholesterol, given through a gastric tube after completion of the morning meal, and the excretion of labeled neutral steroids during a subsequent 72-h period of feces collection. Drinking water and food were provided *ad libitum* during the 72-h period.

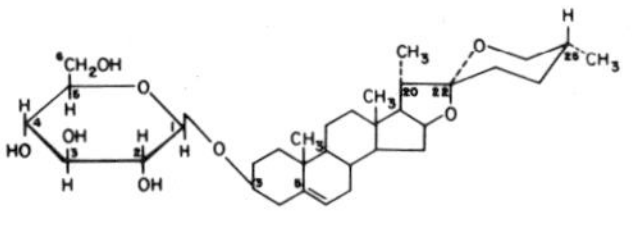

Diosgenin Glucoside

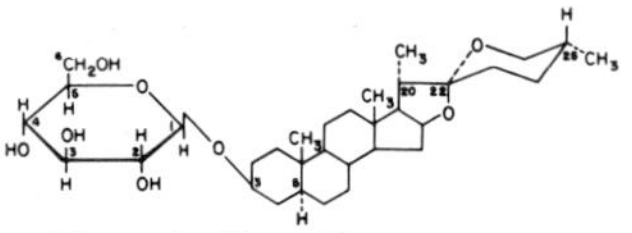

Tigogenin Glucoside

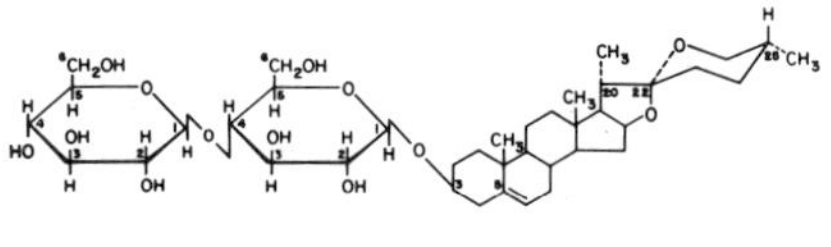

Diosgenin Cellobioside

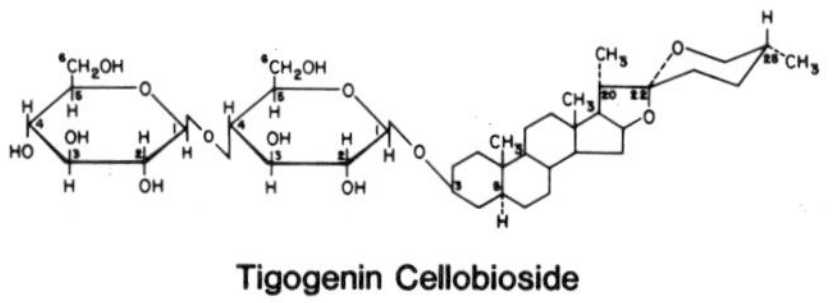

Tigogenin Cellobioside

FIGURE 1. Proposed structures of synthetic glycosides (β anomers).

Animals were stratified and assigned to the different groups according to a strictly random procedure. The synthetic glycosides, as well as alfalfa saponins, were suspended in water with cellulose as the dispersing agent; control rats received only cellulose.

RESULTS AND DISCUSSION

The proposed structures of the members of the series are shown in FIGURE 1. TABLE 1 indicates that synthetic glycosides decreased intestinal absorption of cholesterol, and at the dose tested, tigogenin cellobioside was the most active compound. On a weight

TABLE 1. Effects of Glycosides and Sapogenins on Cholesterol Absorption in Rats[a]

Series	Substance Administered	Number of Rats	Weight (g)	Dose (mg/rat)	Intestinal Absorption of Cholesterol (% I.D.)	Student's *t* test, Versus Control (*P*)	Relative Absorption
I	none	6	242 ± 3	0	74.6 ± 2.3		100
	tigogenin glucoside	6	246 ± 7	14	46.2 ± 1.8	<0.001	62
	diosgenin glucoside	6	245 ± 5	14	52.6 ± 3.7	<0.001	71
	alfalfa saponins	6	249 ± 9	14	60.2 ± 3.7	<0.01	81
II	none	6	290 ± 7	0	74.8 ± 1.6		100
	tigogenin cellobioside	6	291 ± 12	14	39.6 ± 1.8	<0.001	53
	diosgenin cellobioside	6	287 ± 4	14	53.7 ± 1.3	<0.001	72
	alfalfa saponins	6	275 ± 8	14	66.3 ± 1.4	<0.01	89
III	none	6	268 ± 5	0	78.0 ± 2.1		100
	tigogenin	6	259 ± 5	15	80.4 ± 1.4	N.S.	103
IV	none	6	328 ± 4	0	73.5 ± 2.0		100
	diosgenin	6	330 ± 4	15	76.4 ± 2.6	N.S.	104

[a]Values are means ± SE. Abbreviations: I.D. = injected dose; N.S. = not significant. The excretion of ^{3}H-neutral steroids was determined in feces collected for 72 h after intragastric administration of glycosides or sapogenins and 2 mg of [^{3}H]cholesterol (see text).

basis, the synthetic glycosides, especially the tigogenin glycosides, were more effective than the alfalfa saponins. The table also demonstrates that tigogenin and diosgenin at comparable doses were ineffective.

These results indicate that certain glycosides of spirostane derivatives decrease intestinal absorption of cholesterol in rats and that they are even more effective than the triterpenoid saponins of alfalfa.[1] Moreover, the aglycones of the synthetic glycosides were devoid of activity, although Cayen and Dvorik[15] did observe inhibition of cholesterol absorption when they gave single doses of diosgenin to rats in amounts several orders of magnitude larger than the ones I used. The effects of the synthetic glycosides are consistent with the prevention of hypercholesterolemia observed in monkeys fed digitonin,[9] a mixture of saponins whose main aglycones are tigogenin or closely related compounds.[8] If the synthetic glycosides have effects on cholesterolemia and atherogenesis similar to those of glycosides present in alfalfa,[4,5] and if they exhibit the same lack of toxicity,[14,16] they might be of use in the treatment of human hypercholesterolemia and atherosclerosis.

REFERENCES

1. MALINOW, M. R. 1984. Triterpenoid saponins in mammals: Effects of cholesterol metabolism and atherosclerosis. *In* Biochemistry and Function of Isopentenoids in Plants. W. D. Nes, G. Fuller & L. S. Tsai, Eds.: 229–246. Marcel Dekker. New York.
2. MALINOW, M. R., P. MCLAUGHLIN, G. O. KOHLER & A. L. LIVINGSTON. 1977. Prevention of elevated cholesterolemia in monkeys by alfalfa saponins. Steroids **29:** 105–109.
3. MALINOW, M R., W. E. CONNOR, P. MCLAUGHLIN, C. STAFFORD, D. S. LIN, A. L. LIVINGSTON, G. O. KOHLER & W. P. MCNULTY. 1981. Cholesterol and bile acid balance in *Macaca fascicularis:* Effects of alfalfa saponins. J. Clin. Invest. **67:** 156–162.
4. MALINOW, M. R., P. MCLAUGHLIN, C. STAFFORD, A. L. LIVINGSTON & J. W. SENNER. 1983. Effects of alfalfa saponins on regression of atherosclerosis in monkeys. *In* Rheinisch-Westfalische Akademie der Wissenschaften, Abhandlung Band 70. Second Munster International Arteriosclerosis Symposium: Clinical Implications of Recent Research Results in Arteriosclerosis. W. H. Hauss and R. W. Wissler, Eds.: 241–254. Westdeutscher Verlag. Opladen, West Germany.
5. MALINOW, M. R., P. MCLAUGHLIN, C. STAFFORD, A. L. LIVINGSTON & G. O. KOHLER. 1980. Alfalfa saponins and alfalfa seeds—dietary effects in cholesterol-fed rabbits. Atherosclerosis **37**(3): 433–438.
6. MALINOW, M. R., P. MCLAUGHLIN, L. PAPWORTH, C. STAFFORD, G. O. KOHLER, A. L. LIVINGSTON & P. R. CHEEKE. 1977. Effect of alfalfa saponins on intestinal cholesterol absorption in rats. Am. J. Clin. Nutr. **30:** 2061–2067.
7. MALINOW, M. R., P. MCLAUGHLIN, C. STAFFORD, A. L. LIVINGSTON, G. O. KOHLER & P. R. CHEEKE. 1979. Comparative effects of alfalfa saponins and alfalfa fiber on cholesterol absorption in rats. Am. J. Clin. Nutr. **32**(9): 1810–1812.
8. TSCHESCHE, R. & G. WULFF. 1963. Uber Saponine der Spirostanolreihe—IX Die Konstitution des Digitonins. Tetrahedron **19:** 621–634.
9. MALINOW, M. R., P. MCLAUGHLIN & C. STAFFORD. 1978. Prevention of hypercholesterolemia in monkeys (*Macaca fascicularis*) by digitonin. Am. J. Clin. Nutr. **31:** 814–818.
10. CHIANG, C. 1979. 6-aminohexyl glycopyranosides as ligands for the preparation of affinity adsorbents for the purification of carbohydrate binding proteins. Carbohydrate Research **70:** 93–102.
11. ROSEVEAR, P., T. VAN AKEN, J. BAXTER & S. FERGUSON-MILLER. 1980. Alkyl glycoside detergents: A simpler synthesis and their effects on kinetic and physical properties of cytochrome C oxidase. Biochemistry **19:** 4108–4115.
12. HANESSIAN, S. & J. BANOUB. 1980. Preparation of 1,2-trans-glycosides in the presence of stannic chloride. *In* Methods in Carbohydrate Chemistry. R. L. Whistler and J.N. BeMiller, Eds.: 243–245. Academic Press. New York. London. 1980.

13. MALINOW, M. R., P. MCLAUGHLIN, G. O. KOHLER & A. L. LIVINGSTON. December 30, 1980. Enhancement of cholesterol combining properties of saponins. U.S. Patent no. 4,242,502.
14. MALINOW, M. R., W. P. MCNULTY, P. MCLAUGHLIN, C. STAFFORD, A. K. BURNS, A. L. LIVINGSTON & G. O. KOHLER. 1981. The toxicity of alfalfa saponins in rats. Food Cosmet. Toxicol. **19:** 443–445.
15. CAYEN, M. N. & D. DVORNIK. 1979. Effect of diosgenin on lipid metabolism in rats. J. Lipid Res. **20:** 162–174.
16. MALINOW, M. R., P. MCLAUGHLIN, W. P. MCNULTY, D. C. HOUGHTON, S. KESSLER, P. STENZEL, S. H. GOODNIGHT, JR., E. J. BARDANA, JR. & J. L. PALOTAY. 1982. Lack of toxicity of alfalfa saponins in monkeys. J. Med. Primatol. **11:** 106–118.

The Role of Individual Differences in Lipoprotein, Artery Wall, Gender, and Behavioral Responses in the Development of Atherosclerosis[a]

THOMAS B. CLARKSON, JAY R. KAPLAN, AND MICHAEL R. ADAMS

Arteriosclerosis Research Center
Bowman Gray School of Medicine
of Wake Forest University
Winston-Salem, North Carolina 27103

INTRODUCTION

It has become apparent that within both human and experimental animal populations, striking individual differences exist in responses to virtually every stimulus. We would suggest that such individual differences are highly relevant to our understanding of atherosclerosis and its sequelae. For example, it has been recognized for many years that there is considerable interindividual variability among both human beings and animals in the extent to which plasma lipid and lipoprotein concentrations change in response to increases in dietary cholesterol. These individual differences in responses to dietary cholesterol are perplexing, but at the same time offer research opportunities to better understand pathophysiologic mechanisms. Over the past twenty years, this phenomenon has been referred to as hyper- and hyporesponsiveness to dietary cholesterol, and much research has been done to understand better the strength of genetic influences on this trait, as well as metabolic explanations for such individual differences.

Another aspect of individual differences relates to a puzzling observation in the natural history of human atherosclerosis: some individuals with heavy burdens of the commonly recognized risk factors may have minimal atherosclerosis, while other individuals with minimal burdens of the common risk factors will have extensive atherosclerosis. The phenomenon of discordance between atherosclerosis extensiveness and risk factor exposure is often referred to as "mesenchymal susceptibility."

Yet another poorly understood aspect of the natural history of human atherosclerosis is the mechanism by which premenopausal women of some races and some societies are protected from coronary artery atherosclerosis. Research in this area has been hampered by lack of a suitable animal model. The recent characterization of cynomolgus macaque females for studies of male-female differences in coronary artery atherosclerosis has begun to provide some better understanding of mechanisms of gender differences in susceptibility to coronary artery atherosclerosis.

Although the effect of Type A ("coronary prone") personality on coronary heart disease (CHD) risk has been long recognized, personality type and its interaction with

[a]This work was supported in part by NHLBI SCOR grant no. HL–14164, and NHLBI contract nos. HV–53029 and HV–72978.

social environment generally have not been accepted as contributing significantly to variation in the development of experimental atherosclerosis. However, over the past three years, much evidence has accumulated suggesting that certain psychosocial traits affect plasma lipid and lipoprotein concentrations and the extent of coronary artery atherosclerosis in appropriate animal models.

In this brief review, we shall summarize individual differences in response to dietary cholesterol, approaches being taken to studies of "mesenchymal susceptibility," gender differences in lipoprotein concentrations, gender differences in coronary artery atherosclerosis, and finally, the effect of personality type and social situation on atherogenesis. Understanding in these areas is based largely on experiments on nonhuman primates, and for that reason, we have limited our review to studies of nonhuman primates. By and large, users of nonhuman primates in cardiovascular research represent a minority of scientists. Since our center has always had a heavy emphasis on monkey studies, it is perhaps not surprising that many of the studies cited are from our own laboratories.

Individual Differences in Response to Dietary Cholesterol

Hyper- and hyporesponsiveness to dietary cholesterol have been most studied in squirrel monkeys (*Saimiri sciureus*), rhesus monkeys (*Macaca mulatta*), cynomolgus macaques (*Macaca fascicularis*), and baboons (*Papio species*). The results from studies of squirrel monkeys have been particularly intriguing. Individual differences in the response of squirrel monkeys to dietary cholesterol have been studied extensively. Although marked differences in plasma cholesterol concentrations are not apparent among monkeys fed cholesterol-free diets, some monkeys (hyperresponders) fed cholesterol-containing diets (1 mg/Cal) develop considerable hypercholesterolemia with total serum cholesterol levels in the range of 700 to 1,000 mg/dl; other monkeys (hyporesponders) fed the same diet maintain plasma cholesterol concentrations around 200 to 300 mg/dl (FIGURE 1). Still other individuals are intermediate in their responsiveness.[1,2]

In studies from our laboratory, we showed that squirrel monkey hyporesponders fed cholesterol-containing diets for long periods of time had minimal arterial lesions, while hyperresponders fed the same diet had markedly exacerbated atherosclerosis.[2,3] Approximately 65% of the variability in the level of plasma cholesterol concentrations of cholesterol-fed squirrel monkeys is attributable to genetic factors, a figure similar to that describing the human situation. This strong genetic influence on variation in response to dietary cholesterol has made possible the development of colonies of hyper- and hyporesponsive squirrel monkeys through selective breeding programs.[2] By studying such colonies, Lofland *et al.*[4] demonstrated that hyporesponders fed a cholesterol-containing diet have a greater and more rapid increase in fecal excretion of bile salts than do hyperresponders. The investigators speculated that the mechanism of control of the level of plasma cholesterol is related to the rate of conversion of cholesterol to bile salts.

Jones *et al.*[5] analyzed further the mechanisms for control of plasma cholesterol concentrations and the excretion of bile acids and cholesterol in hyper- and hyporesponders fed safflower oil or butter as 40% of calories. In hyporesponders fed safflower oil, almost no increase in total plasma cholesterol concentrations occurred; however, when the monkeys were fed butter, an early and large increase in plasma cholesterol concentration developed and was found to be due to increased absorption of ingested cholesterol. This early rise in plasma cholesterol concentration was followed by a decrease and plateauing to concentrations near baseline due to an increase in bile acid excretion. It was noted that the excretion of cholesterol via enhanced catabolism to bile acids occurred too late to prevent the initial rise seen in hyporesponders. Hyperresponders fed safflower oil developed increases in plasma cholesterol concentrations due to increased absorption of ingested cholesterol and decreased bile acid excretion, and when they were fed butter, their levels climbed even higher. In both cases of dietary manipulation, hyperresponders had increased amounts of bile acid excretion, eventually allowing for a plateauing of plasma cholesterol; unlike the situation for hyporesponders, the concentrations in hyperresponders plateaued at a much higher level. Hyperresponders absorbed a higher mean percentage of ingested cholesterol than did hyporesponders, and hyperresponders were more sensitive to a given amount of absorbed cholesterol than were hyporesponders.

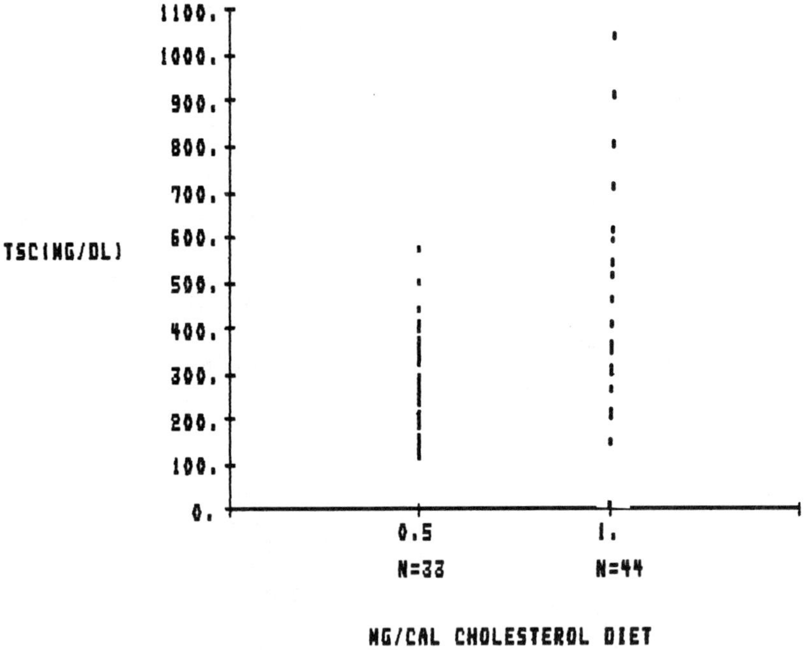

FIGURE 1. Individual differences in the plasma cholesterol response of squirrel monkeys to two levels of dietary cholesterol (0.5 mg/Cal. and 1 mg/Cal.).

Rhesus monkeys, like other nonhuman primates, are variable in the extent to which plasma cholesterol concentrations increase when fed cholesterol-containing diets. Shown in FIGURE 2 is a typical example of the variability seen when young adult rhesus monkey males are fed diets containing 1.0 mg/Cal of cholesterol. As was the case with squirrel monkeys, those animals making a large response have arbitrarily been called hyperresponders, while those making a small response have been called hyporesponders.

Rhesus monkeys have been the subjects of extensive studies to understand better the mechanisms of hyper- and hyporesponsiveness to dietary cholesterol. Unlike some of the other species, hyper- and hyporesponsive rhesus monkeys are significantly

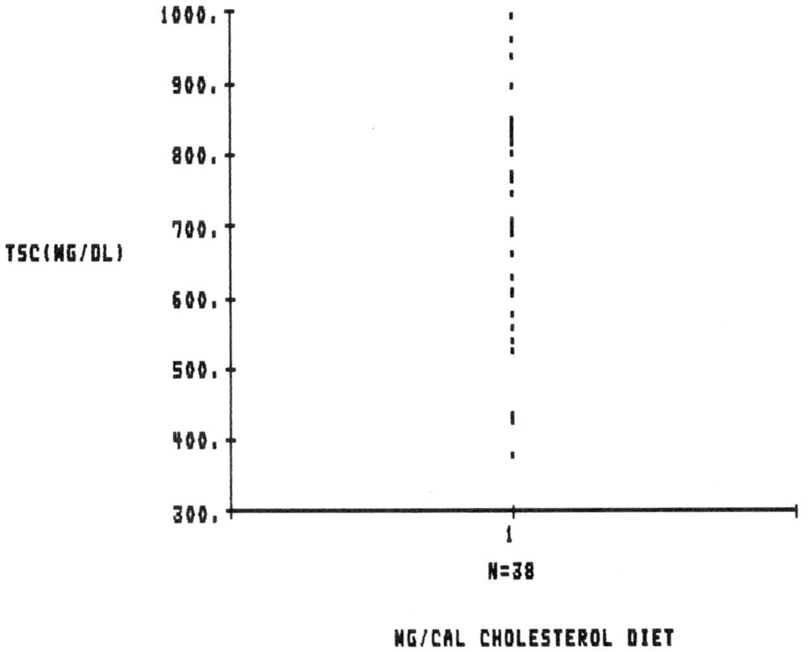

FIGURE 2. Variability in plasma cholesterol concentrations of rhesus monkeys fed a cholesterol-containing diet (1 mg/Cal.).

different in total plasma cholesterol concentrations while cholesterol-free diets are being fed, but like other species, the trait is accentuated by consumption of a high cholesterol diet.[6]

Differences in cholesterol absorption appear to be of major importance in hyper- and hyporesponsiveness of rhesus monkeys.[7–9] In TABLE 1, we have summarized some of the data illustrating differences in cholesterol absorption between hyper- and hyporesponsive rhesus monkeys. The differences in cholesterol absorption were highly significant statistically. It has also been reported that cholesterol synthesis is less inhibited by dietary cholesterol among hyporesponders than in hyperresponders.[10] However, these authors conclude that the cholesterol synthesis rate is probably being

TABLE 1. Plasma Cholesterol Concentration and Intestinal Cholesterol Absorption of Rhesus Monkeys Hyper- and Hyporesponsive to Dietary Cholesterol[a]

Group	No.	Plasma Cholesterol[b] (mg/dl)	Cholesterol Absorption (%)
Hyperresponders	5	697 ± 36	52.9
Hyporesponders	5	256 ± 32	45.4

[a]Adapted from BHATTACHARYYA, A.K. & D.A. EGGEN. 1977. Cholesterol metabolism in high- and low-responding rhesus monkeys. *In* Atherosclerosis, vol. IV., Proceedings of the Fourth International Symposium. G. Schettler, Y. Goto, Y. Hata & G. Klose, Eds.: 293–298. Springer-Verlag. New York.

[b]Variance is standard error of the mean.

modulated by differences in the intestinal absorption of cholesterol. Baker and co-workers have studied the lipoprotein profiles of rhesus monkeys hyper- or hyporesponsive to dietary cholesterol.[11] From a group of 53 young adult rhesus monkey males they selected six hyperresponsive and six hyporesponsive monkeys for lipoprotein studies. In TABLE 2, we have summarized their observations on the total plasma cholesterol concentrations of the colony as a whole and of the six hyper- and six hyporesponsive animals. Also summarized in that table is their observation of the differences in plasma apo B concentrations. In addition to the differences in plasma apo B concentrations, the hyperresponder animals had much higher plasma apo E concentrations and much lower plasma apo A1 concentrations than did the hyporesponders.

Except for breeding studies, cynomolgus macaques have not been used extensively for studies of hyper- and hyporesponsiveness to dietary cholesterol. In FIGURE 3, we have depicted the usual amount of variability seen in a group of 32 young adult male animals fed a diet containing 0.3 mg/Cal.

In 1977, we initiated a program of selective breeding of hyper- and hyporesponsive cynomolgus macaques and have also maintained control groups of animals fed monkey chow. The animals were selected from a large group of cynomolgus macaques fed the

TABLE 2. Plasma Cholesterol and Apo B Concentrations of Rhesus Monkeys Hyper- and Hyporesponsive to Dietary Cholesterol[a]

Group	No.	Plasma Cholesterol[b] (mg/dl)	Plasma Apo B[b] (mg/dl)
Hyperresponders	6	632 ± 103	200 ± 33
Total Colony	53	394 ± 127	122 ± 45
Hyporesponders	6	216 ± 35	56 ± 6

[a]Adapted from BAKER, H.N., D.A. EGGEN, G.W. MELCHIOR, P.S. ROHEIM, G.T. MALCOM & J.P. STRONG. 1983. Lipoprotein profiles in rhesus monkeys with divergent responses to dietary cholesterol. Arteriosclerosis **3:** 223–232.

[b]Variance is expressed as standard deviation.

cholesterol-containing diet in 1977. They were then established as breeding groups and have, in general, retained that metabolic trait since that time. Summarized in TABLE 3 are the plasma cholesterol concentrations and high density lipoprotein cholesterol (HDLC) concentrations of those animals in 1984.

One of our major objectives was to determine if we could produce progeny from that group that would resemble their parents in terms of responsiveness to dietary cholesterol. In FIGURES 4 and 5 we have plotted the total plasma cholesterol concentrations of all of the male and female progeny produced over the first five years of that activity. The data are based on approximately 60 progeny. The data that are presented are cross-sectional in nature, in that they represent all of the male or female progeny in the colony at the times indicated, regardless of the age of the progeny at that time point. It is apparent from the data that the animals produced by hyper- and hyporesponder parents are distinctly different.

Baboons comprise another nonhuman primate taxon in which hyper- and hyporesponsiveness to dietary cholesterol have been studied extensively.[12] In one important study, six male and 134 female adult baboons were assigned to breeding groups on the basis of their hyper- or hyporesponsiveness to dietary cholesterol. Progeny produced from those matings were used to estimate the heritability of the trait. Estimates of

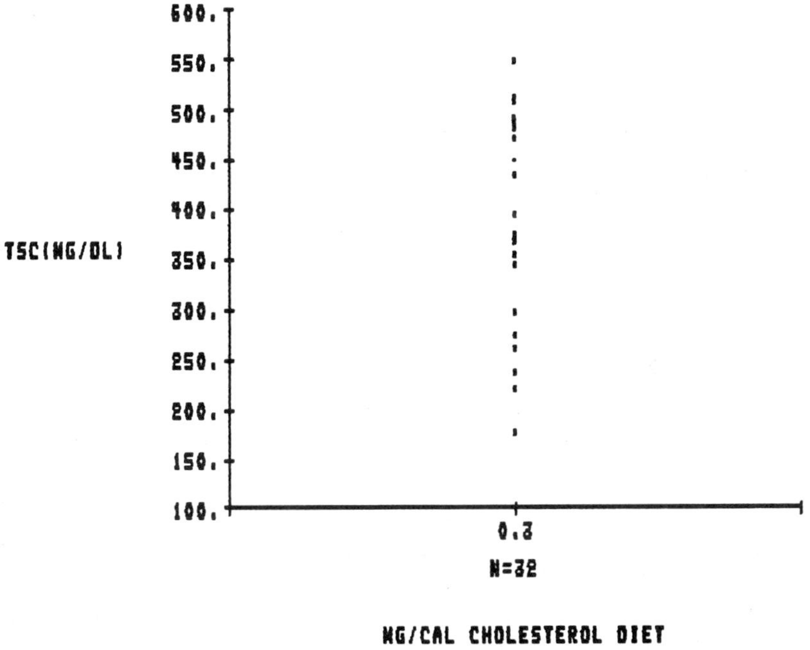

FIGURE 3. Individual differences in plasma cholesterol concentrations among young adult male cynomolgus macaques fed a cholesterol-containing diet (0.3 mg/Cal.).

heritability of serum cholesterol concentration at birth were low, but from three weeks to one year of age they range from 0.25 to 0.80 and averaged about 0.45.

The strength of genetic influence on various aspects of cholesterol metabolism has also been studied in baboons.[13] Here, the heritability estimate for cholesterol production rate was found to be 0.56, while that for the cholesterol turnover rate was estimated to be 0.71.

Flow and his co-workers studied genetic effects on serum lipoprotein and apoprotein concentrations using a paternal half-sib design with 79 progeny of six sires. Some of their observations are summarized in TABLE 4. It appears that the major genetic

TABLE 3. Total Plasma Cholesterol and High Density Lipoprotein Cholesterol Concentrations of Breeding Groups of Cynomolgus Macaques Selected to Be Hyper- or Hyporesponsive to Dietary Cholesterol

Dietary Cholesterol (mg/Cal)	Group	Sex	No.	Plasma Cholesterol (mg/dl)	High Density Lipoprotein Cholesterol (mg/dl)
0.39	Hyperresponder	Male	22	544 ± 24	31 ± 4
0.39	Hyperresponder	Female	32	480 ± 30	31 ± 5
0.39	Hyporesponder	Male	6	219 ± 56	51 ± 9
0.39	Hyporesponder	Female	14	228 ± 28	34 ± 4
None	Control	Male	7	143 ± 23	50 ± 3
None	Control	Female	25	123 ± 8	47 ± 4

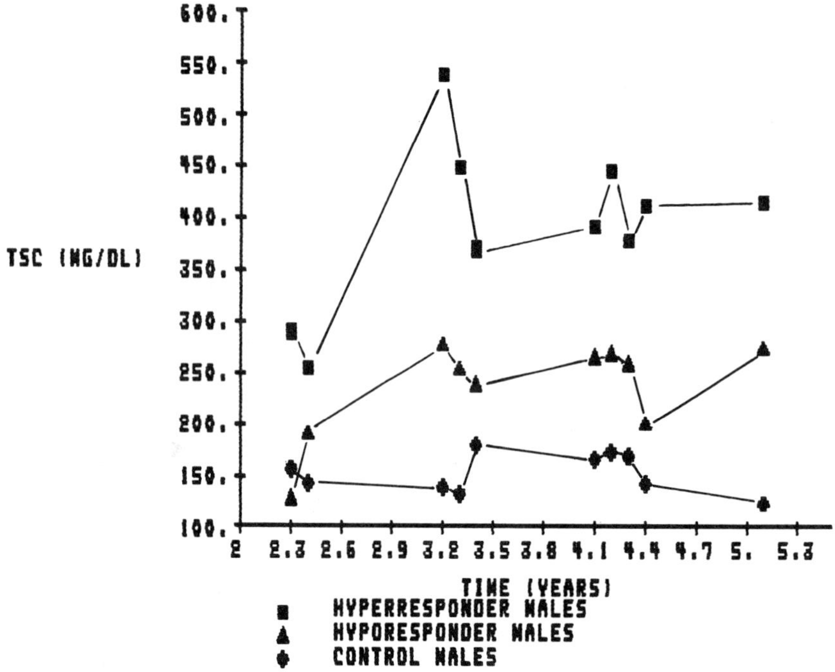

FIGURE 4. Total serum cholesterol concentrations of cross-sectional samples over time of male cynomolgus macaque progeny produced by hyper- or hyporesponsive parents.

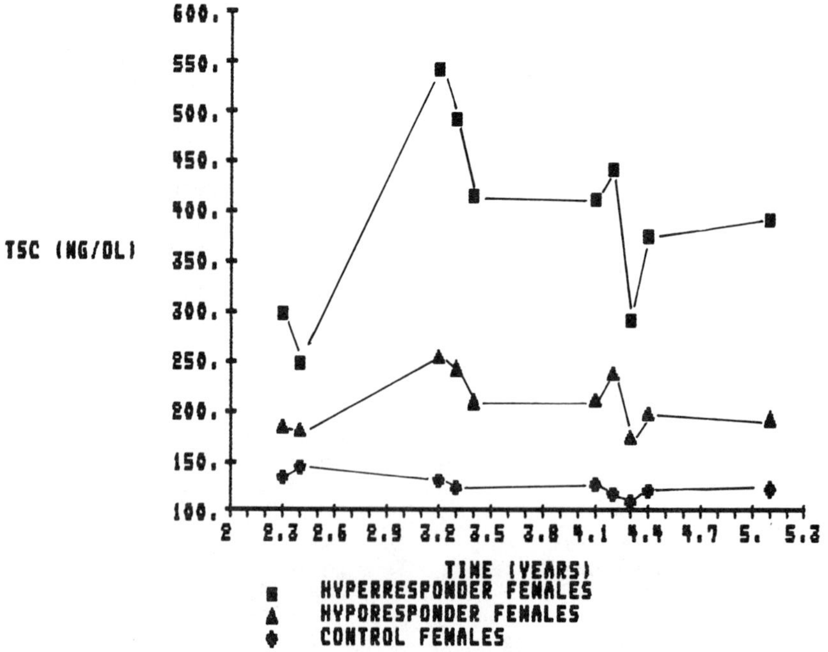

FIGURE 5. Total serum cholesterol concentrations of cross-sectional samples over time of female cynomolgus macaque progeny produced by hyper- or hyporesponsive parents.

influence on total plasma cholesterol concentration is mediated through the HDLC concentration.

Because of the high heritability estimates for both cholesterol metabolism and HDLC concentration, Flow and Mott investigated the relationships between these two metabolic parameters.[14] The results of that study provided strong evidence that the size of the rapidly miscible pool of body cholesterol and the movement of cholesterol in and out of that pool is influenced to a large degree by the same genes that regulate the plasma concentrations of HDLs.

Individual Differences in Susceptibility to Coronary Artery Atherosclerosis ("Mesenchymal Susceptibility")

Both human and nonhuman primates vary considerably in the extensiveness of coronary artery atherosclerosis at each level of plasma cholesterol concentration. In FIGURE 6, we have adapted some findings from the Oslo Study to illustrate the considerable variation that is seen in the percent of coronary artery intimal surface involved with raised atherosclerotic lesions at moderate levels of hypercholesterolemia.

TABLE 4. Strength of Genetic Influence on Hyper- and Hyporesponsiveness of Baboons[a]

Plasma Lipid Component	Estimate of Heritability (h^2)
Total Serum Cholesterol Concentration	0.54
"Low Density" Lipoprotein Cholesterol Concentration[b]	0.32
High Density Lipoprotein Cholesterol Concentration	0.78
ApoB Concentration	0.20
ApoA-I Concentration	0.56

[a]Adapted from FLOW, B.L., G.E. MOTT & J.L. KELLEY. 1982. Genetic mediation of lipoprotein cholesterol and apoprotein concentrations in the baboon (*Papio sp.*). Atherosclerosis **43:** 83–94.

[b]"Low Density" is VLDL + LDL Cholesterol.

As can be seen in FIGURE 6, individuals with total plasma cholesterol concentrations between 280 and 320 mg/dl vary from having minimal to extensive coronary artery atherosclerosis. Some of the differences in atherosclerosis extent with moderate hypercholesterolemia can be attributed to differences in plasma lipoprotein concentrations. It is agreed generally, however, that taking into account all of the characteristics of the plasma lipoproteins one can explain only about half of the variability in the extent and severity of coronary artery atherosclerosis. It seems likely that research to explain the other half of the variability in coronary artery atherosclerosis will be an important research area over the next ten to fifteen years. In order to study this individuality in susceptibility, it will be necessary to have nonhuman primate models that mimic man in this trait.

The macaques appear to be potentially useful for studies of individuality in susceptibility to diet-induced coronary artery atherosclerosis. Malinow and his co-workers[15] were among the first to focus attention on individual differences among cynomolgus macaques in the development of coronary artery atherosclerosis. They refer to the occurrence of hyperreactivity and hyporeactivity in coronary artery lesion extent independent of plasma cholesterol concentrations.[15] We have observed similar variations in the extensiveness of coronary artery atherosclerosis among cynomolgus macaques fed moderately atherogenic diets. We have summarized some of those observations in FIGURE 7. To illustrate that variability, we determined the mean plaque or intimal area for each of the three major coronary arteries of each animal, and then rank ordered the group by their average total plasma cholesterol concentration. We then plotted, separately, each third of the distribution of plasma cholesterol concentrations, indicating the mean plaque size or intimal area for each animal. As can be seen, there is considerable variation in the middle third of the distribution of plasma

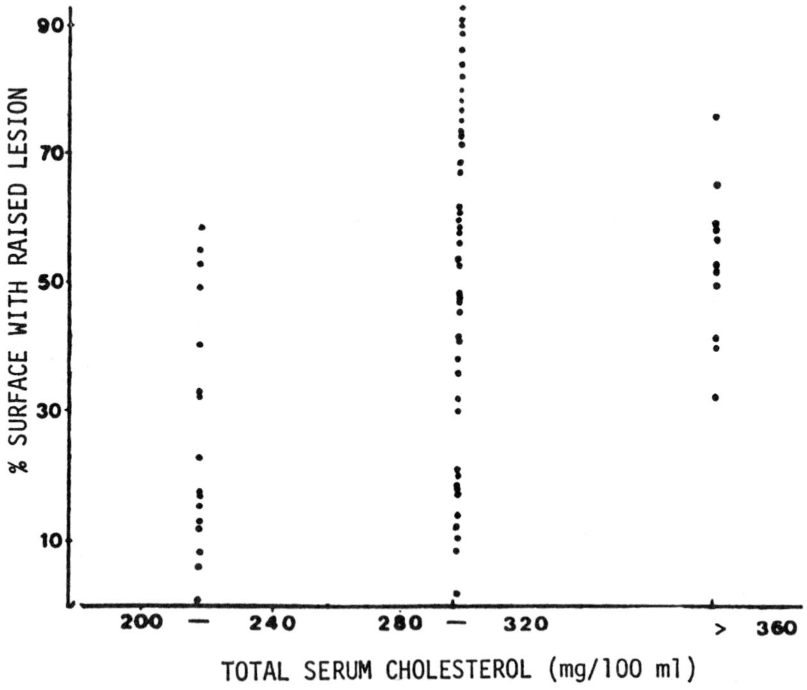

FIGURE 6. Raised atherosclerotic lesion extent of human coronary arteries of individual cases by three intervals of total serum cholesterol showing minimal to extensive coronary artery atherosclerosis at each interval. Adapted from SOLBERG, L. A., S. C. ENGER, I. HJERMANN, A. HELGELAND, I. HOLME, P. LEREN & J. P. STRONG. 1980. Risk factors for coronary and cerebral atherosclerosis in the Oslo study. *In* Atherosclerosis, Vol. V. Proceedings of the Fifth Symposium. A. M. Gotto, Jr., L. C. Smith & B. Allen, Eds.: p. 60. Springer-Verlag. New York, Heidelberg, Berlin.

cholesterol concentrations, and that variation increases in the highest third of the plasma cholesterol concentration.

Rhesus monkeys are the species that have been studied the most in an attempt to develop colonies of animals susceptible or resistant to diet-induced atherosclerosis independent of the traditional risk factors. Considerable variation exists in the response of male rhesus monkeys to an atherogenic diet containing 1.0 mg/Cal of cholesterol. In FIGURE 8, we have summarized the differences in coronary artery atherosclerosis among a group of rhesus monkeys fed such an atherogenic diet for 38

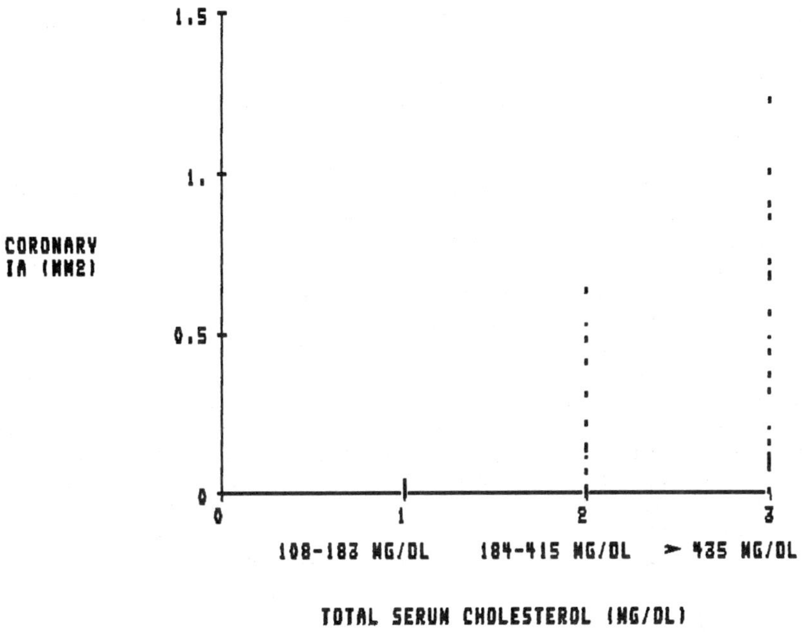

FIGURE 7. Individual differences in extensiveness of coronary atherosclerosis of male cynomolgus macaque monkeys shown by three intervals of increasing total serum cholesterol concentration. (Over 24 months.)

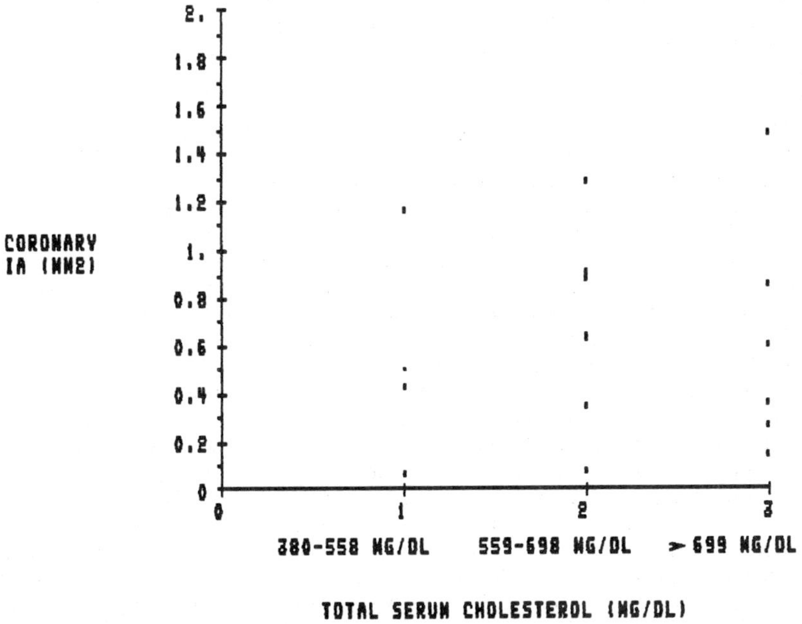

FIGURE 8. Individual differences in extensiveness of coronary atherosclerosis of rhesus monkeys shown by three intervals of increasing total serum cholesterol concentration. (Over 38 months.)

months. Again, coronary artery atherosclerosis is expressed as the mean plaque area or intimal area (in mm^2) derived from evaluation of five sections of each of the three major coronary arteries. We then determined the extent of coronary artery atherosclerosis for each third of the distribution of total plasma cholesterol concentrations that were observed in that experiment. As can be seen from FIGURE 8, at each third of total plasma cholesterol concentrations, some animals have negligible coronary artery atherosclerosis, while others have considerable lesion development.

Since 1975, we have been engaged in an effort to determine the feasibility of developing colonies of rhesus monkeys that are either responsive or non-responsive to diet-induced coronary artery atherosclerosis. Our approach has been to select sires with comparable traditional risk factors on the basis of the amount of coronary artery atherosclerosis seen at thoracotomy. These "susceptible" or "resistant" sires are then bred to randomly selected females, and the progeny are then evaluated at three years of age, having consumed a moderately atherogenic diet until that time. The results are preliminary at this time, but would tend to suggest that resistant males tend to produce resistant offspring, while susceptible males produce some animals that are susceptible and others that are not. These differences in progeny from susceptible sires may relate to the genetic contribution of the dams. Hopefully, in another few years, these colonies will supply a consistent source of animals for research on this trait.

Factors Influencing Plasma Lipids and Atherosclerosis among Female Macaques

The results of two studies have shown that female cynomolgus macaques share with premenopausal white women a relative protection against coronary artery atherosclerosis. Hamm *et al.*[16] studied sixteen male and sixteen female cynomolgus macaques fed an atherogenic diet containing 0.56 mg cholesterol/Cal for sixteen months. TSC did not differ between males and females and averaged about 430 mg/dl. HDLC was 31 mg/dl in males and 38 mg/dl in females, but this difference was not significant statistically. The ratio of TSC to HDLC was significantly greater in males, averaging 17.5 as compared to 13.3 in the females. Coronary artery lumen stenosis was significantly greater among the males averaging 33.8% as compared to 15.5% in the females. Importantly, an analysis of covariance indicated that the male-female differences in coronary artery atherosclerosis were statistically independent of differences in TSC:HDLC. A further finding was that among the females, those judged to be most dominant (in repeated competition for preferred food bits) had significantly less coronary artery atherosclerosis than their subordinate counterparts. Again, an analysis of covariance showed this effect to be independent of plasma lipid differences.

The findings of Kaplan *et al.*[17] generally confirmed and extended those of Hamm *et al.* In this study, 23 female and 15 male cynomolgus monkeys were fed a moderately atherogenic diet containing 0.4 mg cholesterol/Cal for 30 months. This diet resulted in relatively modest hyperlipoproteinemia (median TSC approximately 275 mg/dl), and for this reason, perhaps, male-female differences were less striking. Males and females had similar TSC concentrations (approximately 275 mg/dl), but males had significantly lower HDLC concentrations (33 versus 39 mg/dl). The ratio of TSC to HDLC was not different (males = 8.5, females = 8.1). Due to the mild hypercholesterolemic stimulus, coronary artery atherosclerosis was only extensive in 25% of the animals. Also for this reason, perhaps, differences between males and females in mean intimal area were not significant statistically. However, 40% of the males were affected with more advanced lesions (i.e., plaques), while only 13% of females were affected. Although this difference was of only borderline statistical significance ($p = 0.06$, Fisher's Exact Test), a related finding was that socially "stressed" (subordinate) females were markedly affected with coronary artery atherosclerosis, while their "unstressed" (dominant) counterparts were relatively spared.

A particularly interesting finding from this study was that among males and females with similar plasma lipids, males had significantly more extensive atherosclerosis at the carotid bifurcation than did females (intimal plaque area = 0.912 mm^2 versus 0.324 mm^2, $p < 0.02$). While plasma lipids may be ruled out as a contributor to this gender difference in atherosclerosis, it was observed that males had significantly higher systolic blood pressures than females (107 mm Hg versus 97 mm Hg); this difference may have, in part, accounted for the male-female differences in carotid bifurcation atherosclerosis.

The two studies described above indicate that female cynomolgus macaques share with premenopausal white women a relative protection against atherosclerosis compared to white males of the same age. Much of this relative protection remains unexplained by differences in "traditional" risk factors, suggesting that male-female differences in susceptibility may be mediated, ultimately, at the level of the artery wall, and that intervening characteristics, such as psychosocial phenomena, may be important. In both experiments on females the mechanism for the psychosocial effect, i.e., the less extensive atherosclerosis in the dominant animals, remains unclear. However, the hormonal characteristics of dominant and subordinate females provided important clues regarding mechanisms of pathogenesis. For example, subordinate females differed from dominant females not only in fighting behavior, but also in having impaired ovarian function and relatively enlarged adrenal glands. These findings led to our suggestion that subordinate females were experiencing social "stress." The evidence of impaired ovarian function was deduced from the findings that subordinate females, in comparison to dominants, had a higher percentage of anovulatory cycles, a higher percentage of progesterone-deficient cycles, and overall, lower peak luteal phase plasma progesterone concentrations. Further, various measures of ovarian function (such as peak luteal phase plasma progesterone concentration) were themselves significantly associated with atherosclerosis extent and severity. Significantly, dominant and subordinate females, though differing in coronary artery atherosclerosis extent and severity, did not differ in any of the plasma lipid variables.

Effects of Ovariectomy on Plasma Lipids and Atherosclerosis

An additional approach to the study of gender differences in atherosclerosis (i.e., female "protection") is to examine the effect of alterations in female hormonal status (such as occur at menopause) on atherosclerosis pathogenesis. The evidence regarding the effects of natural or surgical menopause on female protection against coronary artery atherosclerosis is somewhat contradictory, though most human population studies have found evidence for increased severity of coronary artery atherosclerosis[18,19] and increased risk of ischemic heart disease[20–27] in women experiencing natural or surgical menopause. Other studies have found no relationship.[28–31]

A recent study by our group[32] addressed the influence of surgical menopause (ovariectomy) on plasma lipids and extent of atherosclerosis in the cynomolgus macaque. This study also compared the effects of ovariectomy to the effects of stress-induced chronic ovarian dysfunction. Ovariectomy resulted in 15% increases in TSC and low density lipoprotein cholesterol (LDLC), a twofold increase in extent of coronary artery atherosclerosis, and two to tenfold increases in the extent of carotid and iliac-femoral artery atherosclerosis.

Among the intact (i.e., control) females of this study, seven of twelve subordinates and zero of eleven dominants had high rates of ovarian endocrine dysfunction.

Importantly, the seven individuals with a high rate of ovarian endocrine dysfunction (mean = 70% of cycles) could not be distinguished from ovariectomized females as regards plasma lipids, i.e., elevated TSC and LDL cholesterol, and increased extent of coronary artery atherosclerosis. Normal ovarian function was associated with significantly lower ratios of TSC to HDLC, significantly higher HDLC concentrations, and protection against advanced coronary artery atherosclerosis. We speculated that in this study, ovarian dysfunction was the result of altered hypothalamo-pituitary or adrenocortical function associated with the stress of social subordination, and, further, that chronic ovarian endocrine dysfunction may approximate the endocrine deficiencies resulting from ovariectomy. The observed alterations in plasma lipids and lipoproteins are in a direction that would be expected to be associated with estrogen deficiency.

Though plasma lipid concentrations correlated with extent of coronary artery atherosclerosis, our analysis of the foregoing data indicated that much of the variability in extent of atherosclerosis associated with ovarian deficiency (ovariectomy, ovarian dysfunction) cannot be explained by the "traditional" risk factors studied in this experiment, i.e., plasma lipids, blood pressure, and carbohydrate tolerance. We speculated further that estrogen deficiency may affect atherogenesis directly at the level of the artery wall. This speculation is based on the above finding and evidence in the literature that arterial endothelial and smooth muscle cells have estrogen[33–38] and progesterone[38] receptors, and that estrogen treatment *in vivo* or *in vitro* is associated with reductions in smooth muscle cell proliferation,[39] decreased collagen and elastin production,[40–43] and increased degradation of collagen and elastin[44] in arterial tissue.

Social Status and Environment in Male Cynomolgus Macaques

In addition to our studies of psychosocial effects on female atherosclerosis, we have recently completed a series of experiments utilizing males. Like their female counterparts, male macaque monkeys are highly aggressive primates which live together successfully by virtue of elaborate social mechanisms and relationships.[45] Within social groups, both males and females establish among themselves hierarchies of aggressive dominance in which some monkeys habitually win fights or contests, while others habitually and predictably lose. Our recent efforts have involved, in adult male cynomolgus macaques, evaluation of the effect of social status distinctions (dominant versus subordinate) and social manipulations (in which social strangers are placed together in groups) on coronary artery atherosclerosis. In general, among the males, high social status has a neutral or protective effect if animals are living in stable social situations. However, under unstable conditions, where new animals are being introduced to each other and new groups are being formed, the highly aggressive dominant individuals are at greatly increased risk for the development of coronary artery atherosclerosis.[46–48] This result has been observed among animals fed a low fat diet as well as among animals fed a high fat, high cholesterol diet.[47]

The clearest expression of the above described interaction between social status (dominant-subordinate) and social situation (stable, unstable groupings) involved a study with 28 adult male cynomolgus monkeys fed a diet relatively high in saturated fat and cholesterol for two years (equivalent to a human consumption of 680 mg cholesterol per day, with 43% of calories from fat, and resulting in a mean total plasma cholesterol concentration of 495 mg/dl for the experiment). The monkeys were all maintained in social groups of five animals each. Half of the animals (three groups) were subjected to an experimental (environmental) stressor involving repeated reorganization of social group composition by movement of animals among the affected groups. The other half were maintained in social groups of unchanging composition for the duration of the experiment. In addition to observing the social behavior of the animals, data relating to plasma lipids, carbohydrate metabolism, and certain other variables were collected throughout the experiment, which lasted 22 months.

Importantly, individual social status (as determined by patterns of fight outcomes) and social behavior patterns were consistent over the course of the study in both the stable and unstable social groupings. This consistency in behavior allowed us to use social status as a descriptor for individual animals and allowed us to analyze the data in terms of a two-by-two design ($\text{Condition}_{\text{stable, unstable}}$-by-$\text{Status}_{\text{dominant, subordinate}}$). There were no main effects for either status or social condition; however, the two factors interacted significantly. Dominant, highly aggressive males had more extensive atherosclerosis, but only under conditions of social instability. Animals exhibiting similar behavioral characteristics but living in the stable or unmanipulated social groupings were least affected with atherosclerosis (See TABLE 5).

Also, it was observed that there was a disruption of behavioral patterns (fighting and affiliation) in the unstable as compared to the stable social groupings. The pattern of the disruption suggested that while social status, *per se,* was relatively constant over time in both experimental conditions, the behavioral demands associated with domi-

TABLE 5. Coronary Artery Atherosclerosis in Dominant and Subordinate Cynomolgus Macaque Adult Males[a,b]

	Social Status	
Social Environment	Dominant	Subordinate
Stable	0.32 ± 0.13 mm[b] n = 7	0.45 ± 0.12 mm[b] n = 6
Reorganized	0.74 ± 0.12 mm[b] n = 6	0.38 ± 0.10 mm[b] n = 9

[a]Adapted from KAPLAN, J.R., S.B. MANUCK, T.B. CLARKSON, F.M. LUSSO & D.M. TAUB. 1982. Social status, environment, and atherosclerosis in cynomolgus monkeys. Arteriosclerosis **2:** 359–368.

[b]Coronary artery intimal areas (± SEM).

nant status were different in the unstable and stable social groups. Apparently, the dominant animals in unstable social groupings experienced recurrent challenges to their status and these recurrent challenges provided a potent atherogenic stimulus different from that experienced by dominant animals housed in stable or unchallenging social environments. In general, subordinate monkeys seem able to find their social "places" very quickly, while dominant individuals appear to actively impose their status on others. It would be under conditions of constantly changing group organization that this active "imposition" of rank appears to be most demanding and pathogenic.

These findings with regard to cynomolgus monkeys appear to be consistent with current understanding of the role of individual behavioral characteristics in the development of CHD in human males.[49–50] Specifically, it has been hypothesized for human beings that characteristics associated with the Type A or "coronary prone" personality (hostility, competitiveness) are most predictive of coronary heart disease when susceptible individuals are placed in challenging situations demanding considerable coping. Finally, it could be noted that the behavioral effects reported here were not accompanied by concomitant differences in serum lipids (total plasma cholesterol, HDLC) or blood pressure.

Individual Differences in Heart Rate Responsivity

Because serum lipids and blood pressure differences could not explain the psychosocial effects observed in our experiments on males, we tried to identify alternative mechanisms. In this context, it has been suggested that repeated stimulation of the sympathetic nervous system (for example, as through individual differences in cardiovascular responsivity to psychosocial stress) could promote the development of atherosclerosis through hemodynamic and/or hormonal disruptions accompanying such heart rate and pressor changes.[51,52] We recently tested the hypothesis that individual differences in cardiovascular responsivity to psychosocial stress could be associated with atherosclerosis.[53] In an initial study involving 26 male cynomolgus monkeys, we found that the animals showed consistent differences in heart rate responses to psychological stress, and, further, that animals which were most responsive to such stress had more extensive coronary artery atherosclerosis (in terms of lesion areas measured in cross section) than the least responsive animals (high reactors: 0.79 mm^2; low reactors: 0.38 mm^2; $p < 0.04$ by t-test).

These heart rate data were collected under both baseline and "challenge" conditions, with the use of EKG telemetry devices. The psychological stressor involved a laboratory challenge in which the animals, in their social groups, were threatened with capture and handling by the investigator. Importantly, the observed differences in heart rate responsivity were stable over time. These heart rate findings provide some initial support for the hypothesis that a psychophysiologic hyperresponsivity under stress may be involved in the atherogenesis of monkeys, and thus, perhaps, also of man.

It is tempting to speculate that, in addition to increased atherosclerosis risk associated with individual differences in cardiovascular responsivity, some individuals might, because of the particular demands placed on them by their environment, undergo periodic autonomic arousal independently of individual differences in "inherent" responsivity. These animals, presumably, would also be at increased atherosclerosis risk. Such could be the case with the dominant males in unstable social groups, responding to the periodic challenge of reimposing their status. Indeed, recent work by Glagov indicated that experimental induction of consistently elevated heart rates resulted in increased coronary artery atherosclerosis in monkeys fed a high-fat, high-cholesterol diet.[54] Current work at our laboratories is proceeding in this potentially important area of autonomic correlates of social status and condition.

SUMMARY

Striking individual differences exist in the response of animals to atherogenic diets. In this communication, we have summarized the accumulated data that relate to a better understanding of this individuality in susceptibility to atherosclerosis. Described herein, are the accumulated data concerning individual differences in the ways in which animals respond to dietary cholesterol. Also contained in this review, are beginning efforts to understand individual differences in susceptibility to coronary artery atherosclerosis at the level of the artery wall ("mesenchymal susceptibility"). We have placed special emphasis on individual differences that exist among cynomolgus macaques in certain psychosocial variables that contribute to individual differences in susceptibility. Among male cynomolgus macaques both status and social condition contribute to these individual differences. Additionally, individual differences in cardiovascular reactivity contribute to varying degrees of atherosclerosis development largely independent of plasma lipid concentrations. Among cynomolgus macaque females, stress-ovarian function relationships have a major influence on the relative degree to which these female animals are protected against diet-induced coronary artery atherosclerosis.

REFERENCES

1. LOFLAND, H. B., JR., T. B. CLARKSON & B. C. BULLOCK. 1970. Whole body sterol metabolism in squirrel monkeys (*Saimiri sciureus*). Exp. Mol. Pathol. **13:** 1–11.
2. CLARKSON, T. B., H. B. LOFLAND, JR., B. C. BULLOCK & H. O. GOODMAN. 1971. Genetic control of plasma cholesterol. Studies on squirrel monkeys. Arch. Pathol. **92:** 37–45.
3. CLARKSON, T. B., N. D. M. LEHNER, B. C. BULLOCK, H. B. LOFLAND & W. D. WAGNER. 1976. Atherosclerosis in New World monkeys. Primates Med. **9:** 90–144.
4. LOFLAND, H. B., JR., T. B. CLARKSON, R. W. ST. CLAIR & N. D. M. LEHNER. 1972. Studies on the regulation of plasma cholesterol levels in squirrel monkeys of two genotypes. J. Lipid Res. **13:** 39–47.
5. JONES, D. C., H. B. LOFLAND, T. B. CLARKSON & R. W. ST. CLAIR. 1975. Plasma cholesterol concentrations in squirrel monkeys as influenced by diet and phenotype. J. Food Sci. **40:** 2–7.
6. EGGEN, D. A. 1976. Cholesterol metabolism in groups of rhesus monkeys with high or low response of serum cholesterol to an atherogenic diet. J. Lipid Res. **17:** 663–673.
7. BHATTACHARYYA, A. K. & D. A. EGGEN. 1980. Cholesterol absorption and turnover in rhesus monkeys as measured by two methods. J. Lipid Res. **21:** 518–524.
8. BHATTACHARYYA, A. K. & D. A. EGGEN. 1977. Cholesterol metabolism in high- and low-responding rhesus monkeys. *In* Atherosclerosis, vol. IV., Proceedings of the Fourth International Symposium. G. Schettler, Y. Goto, Y. Hata, G. Klose, Eds.: Workshop **8:** 293–298.
9. BHATTACHARYYA, A. K. & D. A. EGGEN. 1983. Mechanism of the variability in plasma cholesterol response to cholesterol feeding in rhesus monkeys. Artery **11**(4): 306–326.
10. BHATTACHARYYA, A. K. & D. A. EGGEN. 1981. Feedback regulation of cholesterol biosynthesis in rhesus monkeys with variable hypercholesterolemic response to dietary cholesterol. J. Lipid Res. **22:** 16–23.
11. BAKER, H. N., D. A. EGGEN, G. W. MELCHIOR, P. S. ROHEIM, G. T. MALCOM & J. P. STRONG. 1983. Lipoprotein profiles in rhesus monkeys with divergent responses to dietary cholesterol. Arteriosclerosis **3**(3): 223–232.
12. FLOW, B. L., T. C. CARTWRIGHT, T. J. KUEHL, G. E. MOTT, D. C. KRAEMER, A. W. KRUSKI, J. D. WILLIAMS & H. C. MCGILL, JR. 1981. Genetic effects on serum cholesterol concentrations in baboons. J. Hered. **72:** 97–103.
13. FLOW, B. L. & G. E. MOTT. 1982. Genetic mediation of cholesterol metabolism in the baboon (*Papio cynocephalus*). Atherosclerosis **41:** 403–414.
14. FLOW, B. L. & G. E. MOTT. 1984. Relationship of high density lipoprotein cholesterol to cholesterol metabolism in the baboon (*Papio* sp.). J. Lipid Res. **25:** 469–473.
15. MALINOW, M. R., P. MCLAUGHLIN, L. PAPWORTH, H. K. NAITO, L. LEWIS & W. P. MCNULTY. 1976. A model for therapeutic interventions on established coronary atherosclerosis in a nonhuman primate. Adv. Exp. Med. Biol. **67:** 3–31.
16. HAMM, T. E., JR., J. R. KAPLAN, T. B. CLARKSON & B. C. BULLOCK. 1983. Effects of gender and social behavior on the development of coronary artery atherosclerosis in cynomolgus macaques. Atherosclerosis **48:** 221–233.
17. KAPLAN, J. R., M. R. ADAMS, T. B. CLARKSON & D. R. KORITNIK. 1984. Psychosocial influences on female "protection" among cynomolgus macaques. Atherosclerosis. **53:** 283–295.
18. WUEST, J. H., JR., T. J. DRY & J. E. EDWARD. 1953. The degree of coronary atherosclerosis in bilaterally oophorectomized women. Circulation **7:** 801–809.
19. PARRISH, H. M., C. A. CARR, D. G. HALL & T. M. KING. 1967. Time interval from castration in premenopausal women to development of excessive coronary atherosclerosis. Am. J. Obstet. Gynecol. **99:** 155–162.

20. OLIVER, M. F. & G. S. BOYD. 1959. Effect of bilateral ovariectomy on coronary-artery disease and serum-lipid levels. Lancet **2:** 690–694.
21. ROBINSON, R. W., N. HIGANO & W. D. COHEN. 1959. Increased incidence of coronary heart disease in women castrated prior to the menopause. Arch. Intern. Med. **104:** 908–913.
22. SZNAJDERMAN, M. & M. F. OLIVER. 1963. Spontaneous premature menopause, ischaemic heart-disease, and serum-lipids. Lancet **1:** 962–965.
23. BENGTSSON, C. 1973. Ischaemic heart disease in young women. Acta Med. Scand. **549**(Suppl): 1–128.
24. OLIVER, M. F. 1974. Ischaemic heart disease in young women. Br. Med. J. **4:** 253–259.
25. KANNEL, W. B., M. C. HJORTLAND, P. M. MCNAMARA & T. GORDON. 1976. Menopause and risk of cardiovascular disease. The Framingham Study. Ann. Intern. Med. **85:** 447–452.
26. GORDON, T., W. B. KANNEL, M. C. HJORTLAND & P. M. MCNAMARA. 1978. Menopause and coronary heart disease. Ann. Intern. Med. **89:** 157–161.
27. ROSENBERG, L., C. H. HENNEKENS, B. ROSNER, C. BELANGER, K. J. ROTHMAN & F. E. SPEIZER. 1981. Early menopause and the risk of myocardial infarction. Am. J. Obstet Gynecol. **139:** 47–51.
28. NOVAK, E. R. & T. J. WILLIAMS. 1960. Autopsy comparison of cardiovascular changes in castrated and normal women. Am. J. Obstet. Gynecol. **80:** 863–872.
29. RITTERBAND, A. B., I. A. JAFFE, P. M. DENSEN, J. F. MAGAGNA & E. REED. 1963. Gonadal function and the development of coronary heart disease. Circulation **27:** 237–251.
30. MANCHESTER, J. H., M. V. HERMAN & R. GORLIN. 1971. Premenopausal castration and documented coronary atherosclerosis. Am. J. Cardiol. **28:** 33–37.
31. BLANC, J. J., J. BOSCHAT, J. F. MORIN, J. CLAVIER & P. PENTHER. 1974. Menopause *et infarctus du myocarde.* Nouv. Presse. Med. **3:** 2173–2175.
32. ADAMS, M. R., T. B. CLARKSON, J. R. KAPLAN & D. R. KORITNIK. 1985. Ovariectomy, social status and coronary artery atherosclerosis in cynomolgus monkeys. Arteriosclerosis **5:** 192–200.
33. STUMPF, W. E., M. SAR & G. AUMULLER. 1977. The heart: a target organ for estradiol. Science **196:** 319–321.
34. COLLUM, P. & V. BUONASSISI. 1978. Estrogen-binding sites in endothelial cell cultures. Science **201:** 817–819.
35. HARDER, D. R. & P. B. COULSON. 1979. Estrogen receptors and effects of estrogen on membrane electrical properties of coronary vascular smooth muscle. J. Cell Physiol. **100:** 375–382.
36. MCGILL, H. C., JR. & P. J. SHERIDAN. 1981. Nuclear uptake of sex steroid hormones in the cardiovascular system of the baboon. Circ. Res. **48:** 238–244.
37. NAKAO, J., W-C. CHANG, S-I. MUROTA & H. ORIMO. 1981. Estradiol binding sites in rat aortic smooth muscle cells in culture. Atherosclerosis **38:** 75–80.
38. LIN, A. L., H. L. MCGILL, JR. & S. A. SHAIN. 1982. Hormone receptors of the baboon cardiovascular system. Biochemical characterization of aortic and myocardial cytoplasmic progesterone receptors. Circ. Res. **50:** 610–616.
39. FISCHER-DZOGA, K., R. W. WISSLER & D. VESSELINOVITCH. 1983. The effect of estradiol on the proliferation of rabbit aortic medial tissue culture cells induced by hyperlipemic serum. Exp. Mol. Pathol. **39:** 355–363.
40. FISCHER, G. M. 1972. *In vivo* effects of estradiol on collagen and elastin dynamics in rat aorta. Endocrinology **91:** 1227–1232.
41. WOLINSKY, H. 1972. Effects of estrogen and progestogen treatment on the response of the aorta of male rats to hypertension. Circ. Res. **30:** 341–349.
42. FISCHER, G. M. & M. L. SWAIN. 1977. Effect of sex hormones on blood pressure and vascular connective tissue in castrated and non-castrated male rats. Am. J. Physiol. **232:** H617–H621.
43. BELDEKAS, J. C., B. SMITH, L. C. GERSTENFELD, G. E. SONENSHEIN & C. FRANZBLAU. 1981. Effects of 17-β estradiol on the biosynthesis of collagen in cultured bovine aortic smooth muscle cells. Biochemistry **20:** 2162–2167.
44. FISCHER, G. M. & M. L. SWAIN. 1978. *In vivo* effects of sex hormones on aortic elastin and collagen dynamics in castrated and intact rats. Endocrinology **102:** 92–97.

45. BERNSTEIN, I. S., T. P. GORDON & R. M. ROSE. 1974. Aggression and social controls in rhesus monkey (*Macaca mulatta*) groups revealed in group formation studies. Folia Primatol. **21:** 81–107.
46. KAPLAN, J. R., S. B. MANUCK, T. B. CLARKSON, F. M. LUSSO & D. M. TAUB. 1982. Social status, environment, and atherosclerosis in cynomolgus monkeys. Arteriosclerosis **2:** 359–368.
47. KAPLAN, J. R., S. B. MANUCK, T. B. CLARKSON, F. M. LUSSO, D. M. TAUB & E. W. MILLER. 1983. Social stress and atherosclerosis in normocholesterolemic monkeys. Science **220:** 733–735.
48. KAPLAN, J. R. & T. B. CLARKSON. 1983. Social instability and coronary artery atherosclerosis in cynomolgus monkeys. Neurosci. & Biobehav. Rev. **7:** 485–491.
49. GLASS, D. C. 1977. Behavior patterns, stress, and coronary disease. Lawrence Erlbaum Associates. Hillsdale.
50. THE REVIEW PANEL ON CORONARY-PRONE BEHAVIOR AND CORONARY HEART DISEASE. 1981. Coronary-prone behavior and coronary heart disease: A critical review. Circulation **63:** 1199–1215.
51. WILLIAMS, R. B. 1978. Psychophysiological process, the coronary-prone behavior pattern, and coronary heart disease. In Coronary-Prone Behavior. Dembroski, T. M., S. M. Weiss, H. L. Shields, S. G. Haynes & M. Feinleib, Eds. Springer-Verlag. New York.
52. SCHNEIDERMAN, N. 1983. Behavior, autonomic function, and animal models of cardiovascular pathology. In Biobehavioral basis of coronary heart disease. Dembroski, T. M., T. H. Schmidt & G. Blumchen, eds.: pp. 364–394. Karger. Basel.
53. MANUCK, S. B., J. R. KAPLAN & T. B. CLARKSON. 1983. Behaviorally-induced heart rate reactivity and atherosclerosis in cynomolgus monkeys. Psychosom. Med. **45**(2): 95–108.
54. GLAGOV, S. 1983. Low heart rate retards coronary atherosclerosis. Arteriosclerosis **3:** 466a.

Lipoprotein Responses and Artery Wall Responses as Factors Affecting the Development of Atherosclerosis

FRED A. KUMMEROW

The Burnsides Research Laboratory
University of Illinois
Urbana, Illinois 61801

In his presentation of lipoprotein responses and artery wall responses as factors affecting the development of atherosclerosis in nonhuman primates, Dr. Clarkson pointed to individual differences in response to dietary cholesterol, gender differences, and psychological stress. He also stated that it is generally agreed "that taking into account all of the characteristics of the plasma lipoproteins, one can explain only about half of the variability in the extent and severity of coronary artery atherosclerosis." I believe that the variability in the extent and severity of atherosclerosis is dependent on the characteristics of the arterial wall itself.

Both *in vitro* and *in vivo* studies have shown that the fluidity of membranes is altered by exposure to oxidized lipids, such as estrogen, and possibly other risk factors, causing perturbation of membranes. We have studied such perturbations of membranes in both *in vitro* and *in vivo* systems. The *in vitro* system involved the uptake of $^{45}Ca^{2+}$ by liposomes containing cholesterol or vitamin D_3 and their partially oxidized derivatives, 25-hydroxycholesterol or 25-hydroxyvitamin D_3. The uptake of $^{45}Ca^{2+}$ was more rapid in the presence of the oxidized derivatives.[1] Therefore, perturbation of membranes by the polar 25-hydroxy group plays a role in increasing membrane permeability to Ca^{2+} *in vitro*.

Oxidized sterols have also been shown to cause perturbation of membranes in *in vivo* systems. The influence of chemotactic agents on serum lipid levels, such as those used by Clarkson, is evident in mature female chickens fed estrogen or progesterone.[2] The plasma triglyceride, phospholipid, and cholesterol levels of those fed estrogen increased five to seven times in a two-week period. The estrogen must have had a significant influence either on transcytosis or on the receptor sites of liver cells to stimulate this magnitude of increase in lipid synthesis, while progesterone did not. The aorta obtained from five-day-old chicks which had been fed 7-ketocholesterol for four weeks have been shown to contain a significantly greater number of dead and dying smooth muscle cells than the aorta of chicks fed only the basal diet.[3] A similar observation was made in swine fed an increased amount of cholecalciferol (vitamin D_3). From two to six months of age, one group of swine was fed a corn/soybean basal ration, free of cholesterol or added fat, containing 3.75 μg vitamin D_3/lb of basal ration. Their coronary arteries showed significantly less intimal thickening and less smooth muscle cell accumulation than the coronary arteries from another group of swine fed a basal ration containing 50 μg vitamin D_3/lb. The serum 25-hydroxyvitamin D level averaged 15 ng/ml for the former and 40 ng/ml for the latter group of swine.

The serum calcium, cholesterol, and triglyceride levels were not significantly different between the two groups. A larger frequency of lipid-laden foam cells was noted at the transmission electron microscopic level in the intimal layer of the coronary arteries (FIGURE 1) of those fed the higher level of vitamin D_3.[4] The serum 25-hydroxyvitamin D_3 level of man is approximately 27 ng/ml, although the average circulating levels of 25-hydroxy D_3 were found to be 64 ng/ml in lifeguards with a minimum of four weeks of exposure to sunlight.[5] The serum 25-hydroxyvitamin D_3 level of the swine fed 50 μg vitamin D_3/lb of ration was, therefore, in the range of published serum 25-hydroxyvitamin D_3 levels for man.

We have also noted less intimal thickening and less lipid-laden foam cells in coronary arteries of weanling swine obtained from sows which had been fed 3.75 μg vitamin D_3/lb of ration as compared to those from sows fed 25 μg vitamin D_3/lb of ration. The serum 25-hydroxyvitamin D_3 level of the weanling swine averaged 15

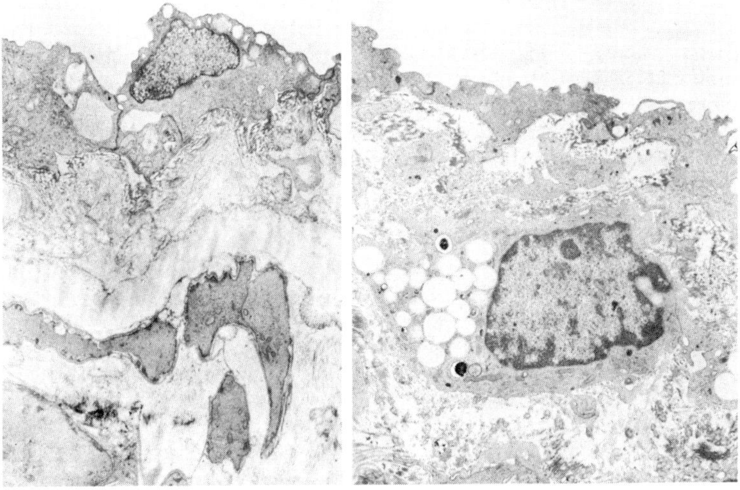

FIGURE 1. (left) e.m. of left anterior descending (l.a.d.) coronary artery from a six-month-old swine fed 2.75 μg vitamin D_3/lb of corn/soybean basal ration from two to six months of age. (right) e.m. of l.a.d. coronary artery from a six-month-old swine fed 50 μg vitamin D_3/lb of ration. Original Magnification: ×6000. Shown here reduced to 45%.

ng/ml and 30 ng/ml, respectively.[6] As weanlings, the two groups of swine, fed 3.75 and 50 μg vitamin D_3/lb of ration, consumed approximately 4 and 60 μg vitamin D_3/day, respectively. A six-month-old human infant of approximately the same weight as these weanling swine has been calculated to consume 35 μg vitamin D_3/day.[7] Thus, the intake levels of vitamin D in the diet of the weanling swine and of human infants are comparable. These data indicate that 25(OH)vitamin D is an oxidized sterol which can perturb the arterial wall sufficiently to initiate intimal thickening in the coronary arteries of swine.

Both *in vitro* and *in vivo* studies have indicated that the fluidity of membranes is also altered by oxidized fatty acids. *In vitro* studies have shown that oxidized preparation of fatty acids facilitated the movement of Ca^{2+} across liposome membranes.[8] Furthermore, unoxidized or oxidized linoleic or linolenic acid treated with stannous chloride did not facilitate the translocation of Ca^{2+}.[9] These data suggested that oxidized di- and trienoic fatty acids which act as calcium ionophores in model bilayers could serve as endogenous ionophores in cells.

In vivo studies that prove oxidized lipids to perturb membranes (so as to alter Ca^{2+} flow through arterial cell membranes) are difficult to devise, as such membranes are protected by antioxidants in the serum.[10] An association between oxidized polyunsaturated fatty acids and atherosclerosis has been suspected for over thirty years.[11] To date, this association has not involved a possible role for intracellular Ca^{2+} in membrane lipid peroxidation. Recently, however, it was shown that calcium treated human erythrocytes exposed to a peroxide generating system showed up to a twofold increase in lipid peroxidation in comparison to untreated cells.[12] This potentiation of membrane lipid peroxidation could be prevented by lipid antioxidants. The presence of oxidized sterols may increase Ca^{2+} flow into the arterial cell, which in turn may stimulate intracellular oxidation of the polyunsaturated fatty acids in the phospholipids of the lipid bilayer in the membrane.

Imai *et al.*[13] have shown that the oxidized derivatives of cholesterol, rather than cholesterol *per se,* caused cell degeneration and induced focal intimal edema in rabbits 24 hr after gavage at 250 mg/dk. Oxidized derivatives of cholesterol are present in the beef tallow which is used to prepare the popular french fries in fast-food chain outlets. Therefore, oxidized sterols are present in food products commonly used, and may contribute to other "risk factors" which perturb membranes. Both the oxidized sterols and fatty acids in the diet could be minimized by eliminating the fortification of milk with Vitamin D, or at least decreasing the level from 400 to 100 I.U./qt, and by limiting the consumption of fried foods and other foods that have been stored long enough to become oxidized.

The mechanism by which oxidized sterols or oxidized fatty acids perturb the membrane, so as to alter Ca^{2+} flow, is not clear. Oxidized sterol molecules may be inserted into the lipid bilayer, or oxidized fatty acids may influence enzyme systems which are involved in the assembly of membranes. The fact that only minute quantities of oxidized sterol are necessary to perturb the membrane was demonstrated in the coronary arteries of swine fed cholecalciferol (vitamin D_3) levels equivalent to those in the average American diet.

Under normal basal conditions, there is a 10,000-fold calcium concentration gradient across the plasma membrane of arterial cells.[14] The concentration of Ca^{2+} is about 0.1 μM in the endothelial cell and 1000 μM in the interstitial fluid. The interstitial fluid is, therefore, rich in calcium, as well as LDL lipoprotein. Although the LDL lipoprotein concentration was only 30% greater in swine interstitial fluid than in swine serum,[15] it was possible to cause intimal thickening of the left anterior descending coronary artery in swine fed levels of vitamin D comparable to the levels in the average American diet. Furthermore, we have shown that calcification of the coronary arteries was more severe in swine fed an excessive dose over a short period of time than the same dosage level fed over a longer period of the life span.[16]

It is possible that intermittent levels of oxidized sterols in the interstitial fluid influence the rate of calcium flux. At times, the flux may be increased enough to cause cell death; at other times, the subendothelial and smooth muscle cells are only damaged to the point of partial interference in protein and lipid metabolism in the cell. Such a hypothesis helps to explain the appearance of the various cell types that have been noted in atherosclerotic arteries.[17]

It seems necessary to study in greater detail the changes in protein and lipid metabolism that may take place in the presence of increasing concentrations of Ca^{2+} ions in the various cell compartments of endothelial and smooth muscle cells. Furthermore, it is still not clear whether lipid oxidation can actually take place *in vivo.*

The autolysis of arterial tissue that takes place so rapidly after death has made it difficult to determine whether auto-oxidation has taken place before or after death. 26-Hydroxycholesterol has been found in the lipid extracted from the plaques that are located in the intimal layer of the aorta.[18] Such observation seems to indicate that auto-oxidation took place *in situ*. If so, such an event adds another dimension to the complex changes that occur in arterial tissue in the process which begins with lipoprotein infiltration into the interstitial fluid and ends with the possible presence of auto-oxidized lipid in the medium.[19]

Recommendations for the treatment of hyperlipidemia are made on the assumption that high serum lipid levels enhance the rate of coronary heart disease (CHD).[20] As oxidized sterols are fat soluble, they may be carried by sterol binding protein or LDL lipoprotein into the interstitial fluid by transcytosis. The level of 25-hydroxyvitamin D increased rapidly in the serum of rabbits fed 200 μg/kilo of body weight for fourteen days.[21] Mitochondrial swelling and dilation of the endoplasmic reticulum of the arterial cells in these rabbits implicated calcium as responsible for membrane perturbation.[14] Therefore, an increased flux of LDL lipoprotein may not enhance CHD

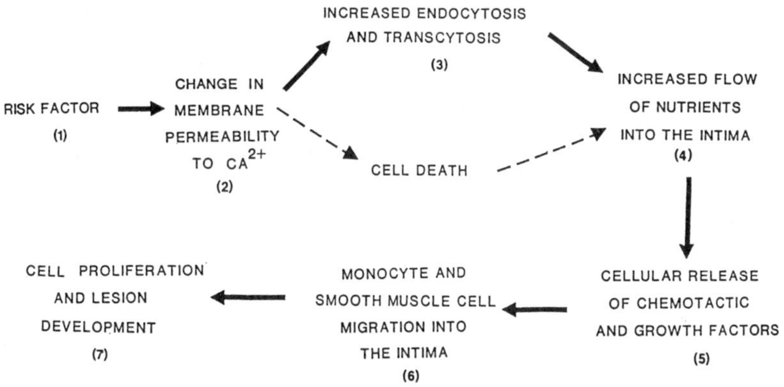

FIGURE 2. A hypothetical scheme outlining the sequence of events associated with the initiation and progression of atherosclerosis.

unless accompanied by oxidized sterols (FIGURE 2). Such an assumption would help to explain why hyperlipidemia does not necessarily result in CHD.[22]

In summary, the rich concentration of nutrients in the interstitial fluid provides a favorable media for subendothelial cell proliferation and for monocyte infiltration into the intima in order to help metabolize LDL lipoprotein that is not needed as a nutrient source by the cells in the internal elastic lamina or by the smooth muscle cells. If the membranes of these cells are perturbed by oxidized sterols or other "risk factors", a change in their fluidity may occur, allowing a change in Ca^{2+} flux, and a change in calcium concentration in the cell large enough to influence the enzyme systems involved in protein and lipid metabolism in the cell. This hypothesis is not dependent on an increased flux of LDL lipoproteins from the blood into the arterial wall as the primary cause for atherosclerosis. Rather, it suggests that the seemingly different risk factors for developing coronary heart disease act through a similar mechanism, all of which accelerate membrane perturbation. The central focus of this hypothesis is that the Ca^{2+} permeability of artial membranes is altered by "risk factors" and sets in motion a sequence of events which results in intimal thickening and lipid accumulation.

ACKNOWLEDGMENTS

I wish to acknowledge Rhonda Gingrich for aid in the preparation, Drs. H. Imai, M. Ito, T. Toda, and R. Tracy for the pathological data, and Drs. S. Cho, R. Holmes, D. Leszczynski, and T. Smith for the biochemical data in this discussion. I also wish to acknowledge the financial support of the Wallace Genetic Foundation and the late Ethel Burnsides.

REFERENCES

1. HOLMES, R. P. & N. L. YOSS. 1984. 25-Hydroxysterols increase the permeability of liposomes to Ca^{2+} and other cations. Biochim. Biophys. Acta **770:** 15–21.
2. HAGEN, R. C., D. E. LESZCZYNSKI & F. A. KUMMEROW. 1984. Comparative plasma lipid response of pullets and laying hens to estradiol and progesterone. Tox. Appl. Pharmacol. **76:** 483–489.
3. TODA, T., D. E. LESZCZYNSKI & F. A. KUMMEROW. 1982. Angiotoxic effects of dietary 7-ketocholesterol in chick aorta. Arterial Wall **7:** 167–176.
4. TAURA, S., M. TAURA, H. IMAI & F. A. KUMMEROW. 1978. Coronary atherosclerosis in normocholesterolemic swine artery. Arterial Wall **4:** 395.
5. HADDAD, J. G. & K. J. CHYU. 1971. Competitive protein-binding radioassay for 25-hydroxycholecalciferol. J. Clin. Endocrinol. **33:** 992–995.
6. HOLMES, R. P. & F. A. KUMMEROW. 1983. The relationship of adequate and excessive intake of vitamin D to health and disease. J. Amer. Coll. Nutr. **2:** 173–199.
7. COMMITTEE ON NUTRITION. AMERICAN ACADEMY OF PEDIATRICS. 1963. The prophylactic requirement and the toxicity of vitamin D. Pediatrics **31:** 512–525.
8. HOLMES, R. P. & N. L. YOSS. 1983. Failure of phosphatidic acid to translocate Ca^{2+} across phosphatidylcholine membranes. Nature **305:** 637–638.
9. SERHAN, C., P. ANDERSON, E. GOODMAN, P. DUNHAM & G. WEISSMANN. 1981. Phosphatidate and oxidized fatty acids are calcium ionophores. J. Biol. Chem. **256:** 2736–2741.
10. VLADIMIROV, Y. A., V. I. OLENEV, T. B. SUSLOVA & Z. P. CHEREMISINA. 1980. Lipid peroxidation in mitochondrial membrane. Adv. Lipid Res. **17:** 173–249.
11. GLAVIND, J., S. HARTMANN, J. CLEMMENSEN, K. E. JESSEN & H. DAM. 1952. Studies on the role of lipoperoxides in human pathology. Acta Pathol. Microbiol. Scand. **30:** 1–6.
12. JAIN, S. K. & S. B. SHOHET. 1981. Calcium potentiates the peroxidation of erythrocyte membrane lipids. Biochim. Biophys. Acta **642:** 46–54.
13. IMAI, H., N. T. WERTHESSEN, C. B. TAYLOR & K. T. LEE. 1965. Angiotoxicity and arteriosclerosis due to contaminants of USP-grade cholesterol. Arch. Pathol. Lab. Med. **100:** 565.
14. RASMUSSEN, H. 1983. Pathways of amplitude and sensitivity modulation in the calcium messenger system. *In* Calcium and Cell Function, vol. IV. W. Y. Cheung, Ed.: pp. 1–61. Academic Press. New York.
15. SMITH, E. B. & E. M. STAPLES. 1982. Plasma protein concentrations in interstitial fluid from human aortas. Proc. R. Soc. London **B217:** 59–75.
16. TAURA, S., M. TAURA, H. IMAI, F. A. KUMMEROW, K. TOKUYASU & S. B. H. CHO. 1979. Ultrastructure of cardiovascular lesions induced by hypervitaminosis D and its withdrawal. Arterial Wall **4:** 245–249.
17. IMAI, H., S. K. LEE, S. J. PASTORI & W. A. THOMAS. 1970. Degeneration of arterial smooth muscle cells: Ultrastructural study of smooth muscle cell death in control and cholesterol–fed animals. Virchows Arch. Pathol. Anat. **350:** 183.
18. VAN LIER, J. E. & L. L. SMITH. 1967. Sterol Metabolism: I. 26-Hydroxycholesterol in the Human Aorta. Biochemistry **6:** 3269–3278.

19. WILSON, R. B. 1976. Lipid peroxidation and atherosclerosis. Critical Reviews in Food Science and Nutrition. **June:** 325–338.
20. GRUNDY, S. M. 1984. Recommendations for the treatment of hyperlipidemia in adults. Arteriosclerosis **4:** 445A–468A.
21. TODA, T., D. E. LESZCZYNSKI & F. A. KUMMEROW. 1983. The role of 25-hydroxyvitamin D_3 in the induction of atherosclerosis in swine and rabbit by hypervitaminosis D. Acta Pathol. Jpn. **33:** 37–44.
22. HOLMES, R. P. & F. A. KUMMEROW. 1985. Membrane perturbations in atherosclerosis. *In* Membrane Fluidity in Biology: Membrane Disease Processes vol. 3. Aloia & Boggs, Eds. Academic Press. NY. In press.

Proteoglycan Structure and Function as Related to Atherosclerosis[a]

WILLIAM D. WAGNER

Department of Comparative Medicine
and
Arteriosclerosis Research Center
Bowman Gray School of Medicine of
Wake Forest University
Winston-Salem, North Carolina 27103

INTRODUCTION

Even though mucosubstances as early as the time of Virchow[1] were recognized to be involved in the atherosclerotic process, it was not until the era of the glycosaminoglycan (or from the 1950's to 1970's) that we began to understand more about the exact nature of these carbohydrates and their role in atherosclerosis. Since the 1970's, we have been able to investigate these arterial carbohydrates as they exist *in situ* as proteoglycans (PG), due in large part to the progress made by those interested in cartilage. Several excellent recent review articles that cover this information are available.[2-9]

Illustrated in FIGURE 1 is a general model of a proteoglycan subunit or monomer. The macromolecule consists of a core protein to which a number of linear and pendant glycosaminoglycan chains are covalently attached. Depending upon the type of tissue and type of proteglycan in that tissue, an average monomer can range from very high molecular weights of 2.5×10^6 for bovine nasal cartilage[10,11] to 59,000 for the chondroitin 4-sulfate PG associated with platelet factor 4.[12] Some proteoglycans have a portion of the core protein termed a hyaluronic acid binding region through which the proteoglycan monomers associate ionically with hyaluronic acid to form supermolecular weight aggregates. The aggregates are stabilized by two link glycoproteins which associate ionically with hyaluronic acid and the hyaluronic acid binding region. For the monomer or aggregate, the anionic glycosaminoglycan chains extend out from the core protein. Thus, in tissues, especially in the intercellular matrix, the proteoglycans occupy a large molecular domain and provide a network for the retention of large amounts of solvent.[3]

Proteoglycan Monomers or Subunits of Artery

Based upon our studies,[13-15] the studies by Oegema *et al.*, and others,[16-21] it is now recognized that there are at least three distinct monomers in arterial tissue—a chondroitin sulfate PG, a dermatan sulfate PG, and a heparan sulfate PG. The glycosaminoglycans of these monomers listed in TABLE 1 have been studied quite extensively (for a review, see reference 5). Each glycosaminoglycan has distinct

[a]This work was supported by grant nos. HL-25161 and HL-14164 from the National Heart, Lung, and Blood Institute.

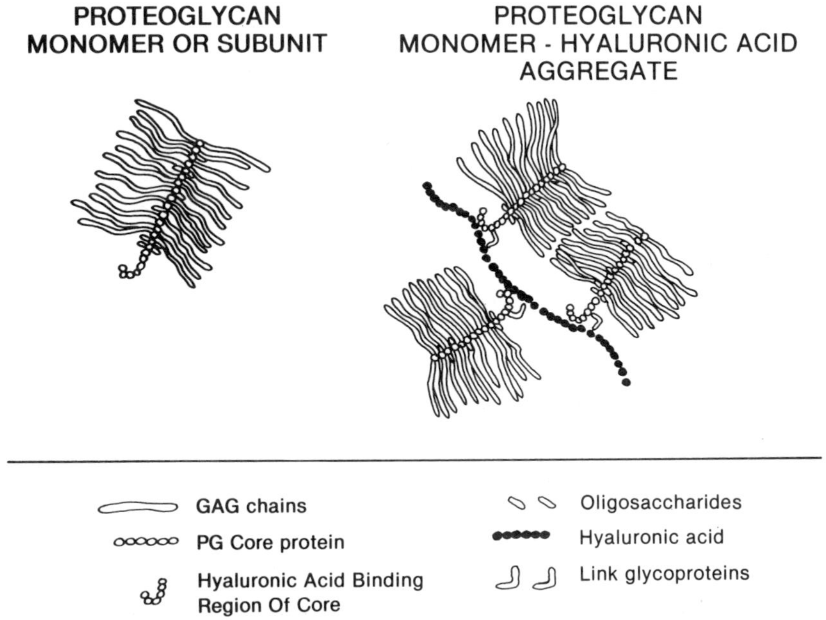

FIGURE 1. General structure of a proteoglycan monomer and a portion of an aggregate.

properties attributed in part to the composition of the repeating disaccharide unit and the positions and degree of sulfation.

Since the advent of an extraction procedure for intact PG by the dissociative conditions proposed by Sajdera and Hascall in 1969,[22,23] our knowledge of the structure of different proteoglycans has expanded vastly. Isolation of tissue proteoglycans as originally proposed included a purification step based upon the *in vitro* reassociation of

TABLE 1. Major Glycosaminoglycans of Artery[a]

	Repeating Disaccharide Unit		
	Hexuronic Acid	Hexosamine	Sulfate
Chondroitin 6-sulfate	D-glucuronic acid	N-acetylgalactosamine	O-sulfate
Chondroitin 4-sulfate	D-glucuronic acid	N-acetylgalactosamine	O-sulfate
Dermatan sulfate	L-iduronic acid or D-glucuronic acid	N-acetylgalactosamine	O-sulfate
Heparan sulfate	D-glucuronic acid or L-iduronic acid	N-acetylglucosamine or D-glucosamine	O-sulfate and N-sulfate
Hyaluronic acid	D-glucuronic acid	N-acetylglucosamine	None

[a]For sulfated GAG—linkage region to core protein via ser-xyl-gal-gal linkage. No protein is known to be associated with hyaluronic acid.

the proteoglycan monomers with hyaluronic acid. Since it later was determined that many tissues, including artery, contained proteoglycan types that did not form high molecular weight aggregates with hyaluronic acid, there have been a number of modifications of the original procedure. However, consistent in all of the procedures is the use of guanidine hydrochloride at concentrations of 4–6 M. This ionic strength is effective in solubilizing the proteoglycans from tissues without the use of homogenization. In fact, studies by Hascall and Sajdera[23] have shown that if tissue is subjected to

Artery Minces

Extract with 4.0 M GdnHCl in 50 mM
sodium acetate pH 4.5
10 mM disodium EDTA
0.1 M 6-aminohexanoic acid
5 mM benzamidine hydrochloride
3 mM phenanthroline
5 mM tryptamine hydrochloride
24 hours, 4°C gentle shaking

↓

Sepharose CL-4B Column

Elute with 4.0 M GdnHCl, 50 mM Sodium Acetate pH 5.8

↓

CsCl Gradients

ρo = 1.40 gm/ml in
4.0 M GdnHCl

↓

Bottom 2/5 ⟶ Expts

↓

DEAE Sephacel Column

Elute with Urea-Tris-NaCl

(NaCl 0 ⟶ 1.0 M) ⟶ Expts

FIGURE 2. An example of a typical isolation procedure for artery proteoglycan designed to separate monomers by size, buoyant density properties, and charge. Where Expts→ is shown, it refers to points at which material can be used for functional or structured studies, depending upon the needed state of purity.

shearing forces during high speed homogenization, the average sedimentation coefficient of the proteoglycans is lowered, indicating a reduction in the molecular weight of the isolated proteoglycans.

One isolation procedure that can be used is outlined in FIGURE 2. Since there is a possibility of degradation of the proteoglycans due to proteolysis, the postmortem interval prior to collection of artery should be short and a variety of protease inhibitors with a broad range of specificities should be added to the extraction solvent. Usually about 10–15 volumes of extraction solution are used per gram of wet weight of tissue. The extraction is done at 4°C with gentle stirring for 24 hours.

The extraction efficiency can be determined by measuring the amount of proteoglycan released into the solvent with time, or by measuring the amount of proteoglycans remaining in the tissue following degradation of that tissue and isolation of the glycosaminoglycan chains. Once the guanidine extract is obtained, then the procedures used in many laboratories are similar but the sequence may be different, depending on the end point of the experiment.

All of the procedures make use of the unique physical and chemical properties of proteoglycans and include size-exclusion chromatography, cesium chloride buoyant density centrifugation, and ion exchange chromatography. For artery proteoglycans, one of the first steps is the separation of monomers on the basis of size on Sepharose CL-4B. The column is eluted with 4.0 M guanidine HCl which maintains the proteoglycans in a dissociated state and facilitates the separation of a chondroitin sulfate-PG that elutes near the column void volume from a dermatan sulfate-PG included with a K_{av} of about 0.4. From the Sepharose CL-4B, appropriate fractions are pooled and then applied to cesium chloride gradients at a loading density of 1.40 g/ml. After centrifugation, the proteoglycans, due to their large size and enrichment in carbohydrate, are localized in the most dense fractions. These are pooled and applied to an ion exchange column.

The size separation of proteoglycans isolated from intima media minces of human aorta is illustrated by FIGURE 3. From the elution profile illustrated by FIGURE 3a, one can see two peaks of hexuronic acid separated from coextracted protein material. Illustrated in FIGURE 3b are the sulfated glycosaminoglycans measured in different fractions, and a separation of the chondroitin sulfate-PG (shown as the white bars) and the dermatan sulfate-PG (shown as the dark bars). The heparan sulfate-PG is polydisperse and has a K_{av} of about 0.11. Hyaluronic acid is not illustrated in the figure but elutes mainly at the column void volume.

The proteoglycan monomers are further purified by density centrifugation and ion exchange chromatography. To separate the smaller dermatan sulfate-PG from the larger chondroitin sulfate-PG, it is essential to use gel permeation chromatography since both of these proteoglycans have similar buoyant density and charge properties. Both chondroitin sulfate-PG and dermatan sulfate-PG elute from DEAE Sephacel at 0.5 M NaCl, while heparan sulfate-PG and hyaluronic acid elute at a lower salt concentration.

Evidence That Chondroitin Sulfate-PG and Dermatan Sulfate-PG Are Distinct Monomers

Prior to the use of procedures to separate individual proteoglycan monomers or subunits, it was unclear from many of the published studies on artery whether or not chondroitin 6-sulfate and dermatan sulfate polysaccharide chains were on the same or different core proteins. Recent evidence, largely structural, functional, and metabolic in nature, has supported the latter. It already has been illustrated in FIGURE 3 that the dermatan sulfate-PG is smaller in hydrodynamic size than the chondroitin sulfate-PG. In studies of the glycosaminoglycan chain composition, we have identified iduronic acid as a component of only the dermatan sulfate-PG. The glycosaminoglycan chains isolated from the chondroitin sulfate-PG migrate on cellulose acetate as authentic chondroitin sulfate and are susceptible to cleavage by both chondroitin ABC and AC II lyase.[24]

The glycosaminoglycan chains of the dermatan sulfate-PG migrate as authentic dermatan sulfate, and are susceptible to chondroitin ABC lyase though resistant to chondroitin AC II lyase. In some preparations of dermatan sulfate-PG, partial cleavage is apparent following treatment with chondroitin AC II lyase, suggesting the presence of blocks of glucuronic acid residues, as has been reported by Fransson and Havsmark,[25] and Kresse *et al.*[26]

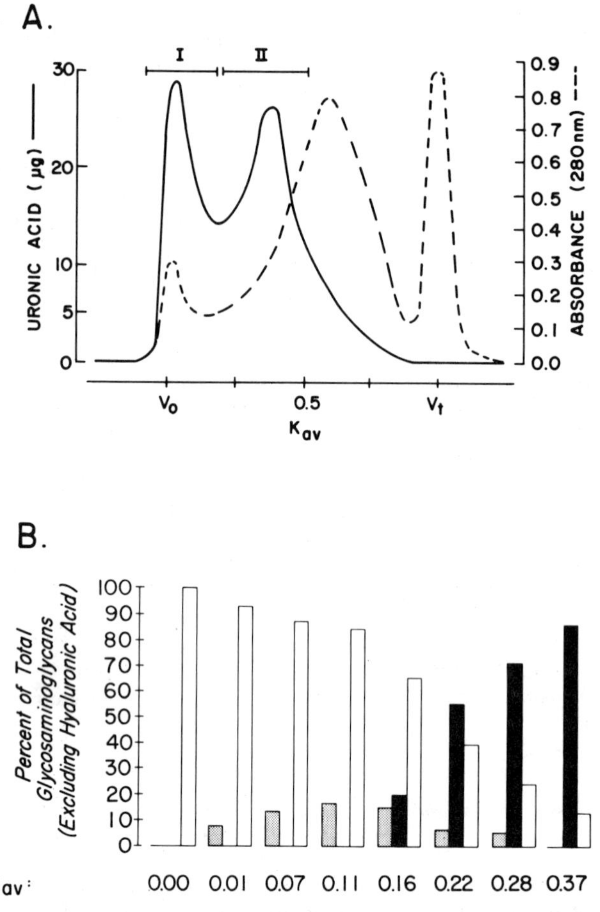

FIGURE 3. (A) Elution profile for the size separation of human aortic proteoglycan extracted with 4.0 M GdnHCl and chromatographed under dissociative conditions (1.4 × 90 cm column of Sepharose CL-4B; 4.0 M GdnHCl, 0.05 M sodium acetate, pH 5.8). Two peaks of hexuronic acid indicated by I and II are resolved. (B) Sulfated glycosaminoglycan composition of Peaks I and II. The numbers below the bars correspond to different K_{av} for fractions of material comprising Peaks I and II. Modified from figures 2 and 5, Salisbury and Wagner,[13] and reproduced with permission.

Core proteins have been prepared following treatments of both proteoglycans with chondroitin ABC lyase. Average molecular weights of 160,000 were determined for the chondroitin sulfate-PG monomer,[27] while the core protein of the dermatan sulfate

TABLE 2. Amino Acid Composition (Residues/1000 Residues) of Artery Core Proteins of Chondroitin Sulfate and Dermatan Sulfate Proteoglycans[a]

	CS-PG	DS-PG
Serine	109	73
Aspartic acid	87	51
Glutamic acid	208	161
Threonine	117	63
Glycine	80	139
Alanine	73	63
Arginine	34	35
Methionine	<10	76
Cysteine	<10	tr
Valine	76	71
Phenylalanine	37	33
Leucine	35	99
Isoleucine	68	57
Lysine	31	62
Tyrosine	29	16
Histidine	16	tr[c]
Proline	n.d.[b]	n.d.[b]

[a]Based on Wagner *et al.*,[24] and Rowe and Wagner.[15]
[b]n.d. = not determined
[c]tr = trace

PG was 50,000.[15] The amino acid compositions of the two core proteins are distinct. Both are rich in acidic amino acids but differ in percent composition (TABLE 2).

A Distinct Functional Property of Chondroitin Sulfate and Dermatan Sulfate Containing Monomers

A functional property of each monomer examined in a number of studies[13,14] is the ability to associate with hyaluronic acid to form high molecular aggregates. FIGURE 4

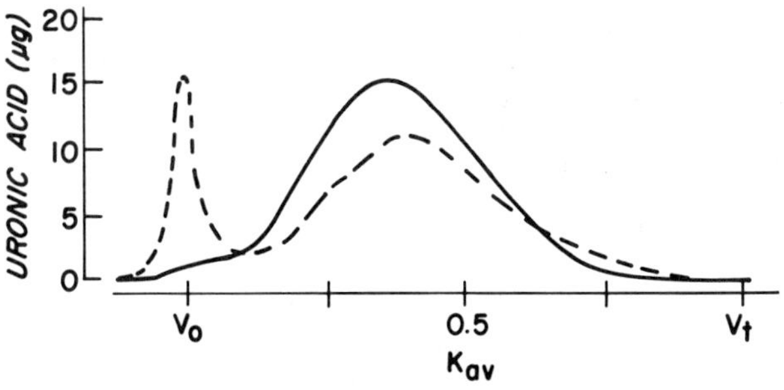

FIGURE 4. Illustration of the formation of proteoglycan-hyaluronic acid aggregate. Chondroitin sulfate-PG containing endogenous hyaluronic acid was divided equally and chromatographed on Sepharose CL-2B. One sample (——) was eluted under dissociative conditions with 4.0 M GdnHCl in 0.05 M sodium acetate, pH 5.8, while the other sample (---) was eluted under associative conditions using 0.5 M sodium acetate, pH 5.8. Reproduced with permission from Salisbury and Wagner,[13] figure 6.

TABLE 3. Characteristics of the Major Proteoglycans Synthesized by Arterial Smooth Muscle Cells and Released into the Medium[a]

	K_{av} on Sepharose CL-2B	GAG Chain Size		
Chondroitin sulfate PG	0.30	43,000	Rich in O- and N-linked oligosaccharides	Associated with hyaluronic acid
Dermatan sulfate PG	0.67	43,000	Poor in O- and N-linked oligosaccharides	No association with hyaluronic acid

[a]Based on data of Chang *et al.*[28] Studies were carried out on third passage, nearly confluent smooth muscle cells derived from the aorta of *M. nemestrina.* After 36 hours, about 80% of PG synthesized were released into the medium and 20% were associated with the cell layer. In addition, the presence of a heparan sulfate-PG was described as a component of the medium.

illustrates that while purified chondroitin sulfate-PG monomers in the presence of hyaluronic acid are included within a large pore Sepharose CL-2B column under dissociative conditions (shown by the solid line), under associative conditions (shown by the broken line), monomers are located in the column void volume, thus suggesting the formation of a high molecular weight species. This association is specific for hyaluronic acid as illustrated in a recent report[14] where removal of endogenous hyaluronic acid and addition of increments of exogenous hyaluronic acid caused a concomitant increase in the amount of aggregate formation. No such association with hyaluronic acid has been seen for the smaller dermatan sulfate-PG. Monomers under dissociative or associative conditions, even with exogenous hyaluronic acid added, elute from Sepharose CL-2B at a similar K_{av}.[13,14]

These findings for differences in chondroitin sulfate-PG and dermatan sulfate-PG are consistent with the recent report by Chang *et al.*[28] on the proteoglycan types synthesized by artery smooth muscle cells in culture. Some pertinent properties of the two major monomers are summarized in TABLE 3. The chondroitin sulfate-PG was larger and was associated with hyaluronic acid in contrast to the dermatan sulfate-PG. An additional difference was seen in the oligosaccharide moiety where the chondroitin sulfate-PG was rich while the dermatan sulfate-PG was poor in content.

The synthetic rate of these two proteoglycans has been reported to differ.[29] Using radioactive sulfate to label the glycosaminoglycan and radioactive serine to label the core protein, proteoglycans synthesized by artery minces *in vitro* were examined. Over 3–9 hours, much more radioactivity was incorporated into the dermatan sulfate-PG suggesting a greater rate of synthesis (TABLE 4). Decreases over time in the ratios of dermatan sulfate-PG to chondroitin sulfate-PG specific activities (FIGURE 5) suggested that the rates of synthesis were distinct for the two PG and that the smaller

TABLE 4. Incorporation of [^{35}S] Sodium Sulfate and [^{3}H] Serine into Chondroitin Sulfate-PG and Dermatan Sulfate-PG of Arteries Incubated *in Vitro*[a]

Incubation Time	% CS-PG of Total PG		% DS-PG of Total PG	
	^{35}S	^{3}H	^{35}S	^{3}H
3 hr	11	7	89	93
6 hr	13	11	87	89
9 hr	25	27	76	73

[a]After Wagner *et al.*[29]

dermatan sulfate-PG was not derived from the degradation of the larger chondroitin sulfate-PG monomer.

Evidence That PG Are Structurally Distinct in Atherosclerotic Plaques

From previous studies,[30-33] it has been demonstrated that the concentration and content of individual glycosaminoglycans change with the progression of atherosclerosis. In contrast, only sparse information is available on qualitative changes in proteoglycan monomers.

In one study,[24] chondroitin sulfate-PG was prepared from intima media minces of normal human aorta and adjacent fatty fibrous atherosclerotic plaques. Both proteoglycans were purified as the 0.5 M NaCl fraction on DEAE Sephacel. The amino acid composition of the core proteins of both PG preparations was similar. Likewise, when core protein molecular weights were determined, both had a similar M_r of about 1.6×10^5.

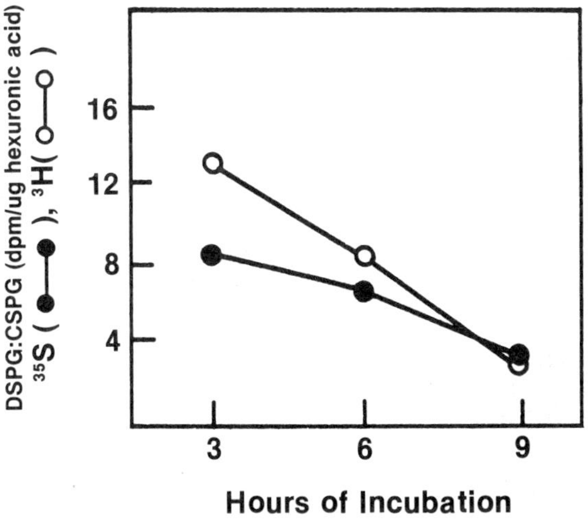

FIGURE 5. Ratio of dermatan sulfate-PG to chondroitin sulfate-PG specific activities over time. Pigeon artery minces were incubated with [^{35}S] sodium sulfate and [^{3}H] serine for the times indicated. Proteoglycan types released into the medium were isolated and specific activities (^{35}S or ^{3}H dpm/μg hexuronic acid) determined. Modified from figure 5, Wagner *et al.*,[29] and reproduced with permission.

Glycosaminoglycan chains were isolated from each monomer and their size properties examined on Ultrogel ACA 54. The chains from normal aorta displayed a normal distribution profile with a K_{av} of 0.48. The peak was polydisperse and had approximately the same upper and lower size limits as the glycosaminoglycans of the atherosclerotic aorta. However, the chains from atherosclerotic aorta displayed a bimodal distribution, showing a major peak with a K_{av} of 0.35 and a smaller peak with a K_{av} of about 0.70. The curve depicting the elution profile was shifted toward the column void volume. The M_r of glycosaminoglycan chains from normal aorta was estimated to be 1.5×10^4. For the atherosclerotic aorta, the majority of chains had an estimated M_r of 2.0×10^4, while the smaller population had a M_r of 1.2×10^4. All three types of glycosaminoglycans migrated as chondroitin sulfate on cellulose acetate. Following digestion with chondroitin ABC lyase, all three chondroitin sulfate preparations were seen to be composed exclusively of disaccharides sulfated at the C-6 position.[24]

Further studies of the monomers were done in an attempt to assess the degree of glycosylation of the core protein. Samples of PG were subjected to β-elimination in the presence of sodium borohydride prior to acid hydrolysis. Chondroitin sulfate-PG from normal aorta had a reduction in serine from 109 to 68 residues/1000 residues following base treatment, with a concomitant increase in alanine from 73 to 114. Threonine decreased from 117 to 55 residues/1000. For the chondroitin sulfate-PG from atherosclerotic plaque, reductions in serine were from 103 to 81 residues/1000, alanine increased from 80 to 110, and threonine decreased from 107 to 77 residues/1000. The results suggest fewer chondroitin sulfate chains and oligosaccharides associated with the core protein in the proteoglycans of atherosclerotic plaque. Compared to normal aorta, substituted serines and threonines in the proteoglycan of atherosclerotic plaque were about half, respectively, 38% vs. 21% serine, 53% vs. 28% threonine. Based upon the serine data, it is estimated that in atherosclerotic plaque there are fewer but longer chondroitin sulfate chains per core protein. This translates to a smaller overall monomer size in atherosclerotic plaque (TABLE 5).

TABLE 5. Characteristics of Human Artery Chondroitin Sulfate-PG Monomer[a]

	Normal Aorta	Adjacent Atherosclerotic Plaque
GAG	Chondroitin Sulfate Δ di 6-SO_4	Chondroitin Sulfate Δ di 6-SO_4
GAG M_r	15,000	20,000 12,000
Core protein M_r	1.6×10^5	1.6×10^5
Substituted serine	38%	21%
Substituted threonines	53%	28%
CS Chains/core (Based upon the number of glycosylated serines)	39	26
Estimated monomer size	7.5×10^5	6.8×10^5

[a]After Wagner *et al.*[24]

Binding Properties of Aortic Proteoglycans to Hyaluronic Acid and Alteration in Atherosclerosis

Although not much is known about the proteoglycan-hyaluronic acid aggregate in artery, in tissues, in general, the aggregate is thought to be responsible for many structural and functional properties of the tissue such as viscoelasticity. It also has been suggested that the aggregate is responsible for an ordered connective tissue structure and, as well, not only serves to retain monomers in the tissue, but also may protect monomers against proteolytic enzymes.[3,34]

In one recent study, we assessed the capacity of artery proteoglycan monomers to form aggregates.[35] The proteoglycan material was prepared from human aorta and adjacent atherosclerotic plaque. It was predominantly chondroitin sulfate-PG and contained 5–7% endogenous hyaluronic acid.

Initially, the ability of the monomers to associate with the endogenous hyaluronic acid to form high molecular weight aggregates was assessed. Preparations were dialyzed to associative conditions and loaded in an analytic ultracentrifuge equipped with Schlieren optics. For both samples, the tracings showed one fast and one slow sedimenting component. The identification of the fast moving component as the aggregate was confirmed by studies showing its disappearance following addition of oligomers of hyaluronic acid (HA_{34}) capable of displacing monomers from hyaluronic acid.

By integrating the area under the peaks, we determined that in normal aorta at least 45% of the monomers were capable of associating with endogenous hyaluronic acid, whereas in atherosclerotic plaque only 28% associated with hyaluronic acid. The sedimentation coefficients for monomer and aggregate were plotted against different concentrations of proteoglycans. The chondroitin sulfate-PG of plaque was distinctly smaller from that in normal aorta; S values were 5.3 vs. 8.7. This difference in monomer size agreed with the estimates of size differences derived from the chemical compositional data. In addition to smaller monomers in the atherosclerotic plaque, the aggregates formed with these monomers were much smaller compared to normal artery. Calculations from a plot of sedimentation coefficients against number of proteoglycan per aggregate published by Hardingham and Muir[36] suggested that the number of monomers per aggregate was 32 for normal aorta but only 12 for atherosclerotic aorta. Additionally, in the study,[35] the potential for the formation of increased amount of aggregate was assessed by adding additional high molecular weight hyaluronic acid in the form of Healon (Pharmacia, Inc., M_r 1.63 × 10^6). For both preparations of chondroitin sulfate-PG, addition of exogenous hyaluronic acid caused additional aggregate formation, suggesting that there were additional monomers in the preparation capable of aggregating to hyaluronic acid. However, the percent aggregate was still much lower for the monomers from atherosclerotic plaque (10% vs. 49%). From the study, it was also deduced that if the reduced monomer size in the atherosclerotic plaque was a significant contributing factor in the formation of smaller aggregates, then the aggregates formed with Healon would have a smaller sedimentation coefficient. However, S_0 values for both monomers were 30. This suggested that monomers in the atherosclerotic plaque that are capable of associating with hyaluronic acid were of a similar average weight as those in normal aorta. Therefore, it appears that the reduced size of the proteoglycan aggregate in the plaque samples was due to a reduced size of endogenous hyaluronic acid in that preparation. The reduced amount of aggregate for the chondroitin sulfate-PG monomer of atherosclerotic plaque was apparently due to some alteration in the hyaluronic acid binding region of the core protein.

Consequences of Reduced Size and Amount of Proteoglycan-Hyaluronic Acid Aggregate

With a reduction in amount and size of the aggregate, one might expect a reduction in the viscoelastic properties of the tissue with a reduction in the ability of the arterial wall to resist compressive force. As a result of the unordered nature of the proteoglycan monomers, the water binding property and maintenance of a hydrated domain might be reduced. All of these conditions could lead to or facilitate an increased transport property of materials through the vessel wall. In addition, monomers not normally bound to hyaluronic acid might be available for association with other vessel wall components and/or plasma components such as low density lipoproteins that enter the intercellular space.[37,38]

Proposed Model for Chondroitin Sulfate-PG

Based upon the chemical studies and the studies on binding of monomers to hyaluronic acid, a proposed model is presented in FIGURE 6. In the atherosclerotic plaques, the monomers are characterized by fewer chondroitin sulfate chains per core protein. Since the charged groups on the linear glycosaminoglycans repel each other and tend to stiffen the molecule, the chains in the monomers from plaques may be less extended as is shown in the monomer to the far right of the illustration. There is a reduced capacity to form aggregates and one can translate this into either an absence or the presence of a conformational change in the hyaluronic acid binding region of the core protein.

Evidence for Distinct Proteoglycan Structure in Animals Predisposed for Atherosclerosis

Arguments can be presented which state that modified proteoglycans in atherosclerotic plaques are a result of the alterations in the metabolism of the atherosclerotic

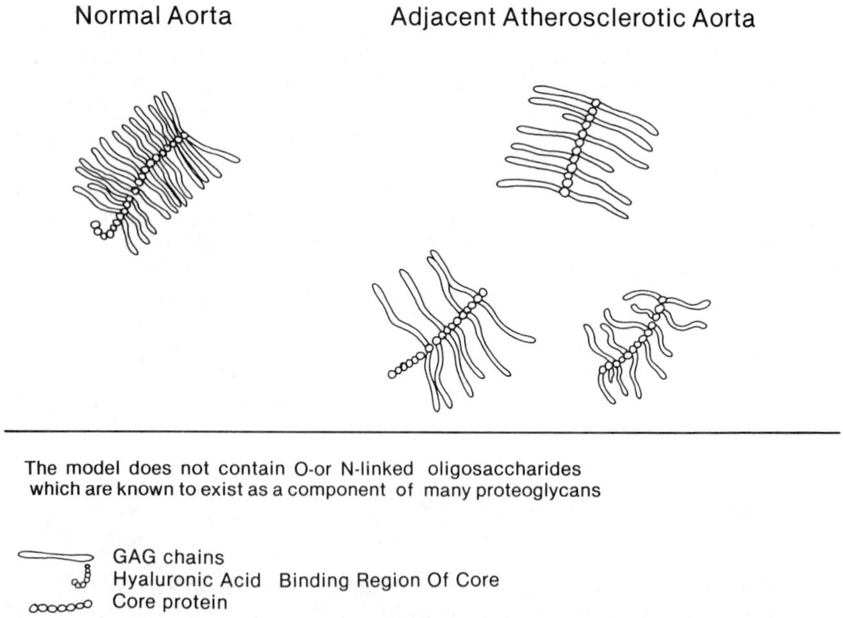

FIGURE 6. A proposed model for chondroitin sulfate-PG isolated from grossly normal aorta (left) or adjacent atherosclerotic plaque (right). One model of a monomer from the atherosclerotic plaque depicts collapsed glycosaminoglycan chains, while the others illustrate the absence or a modification in the hyaluronic acid binding region.

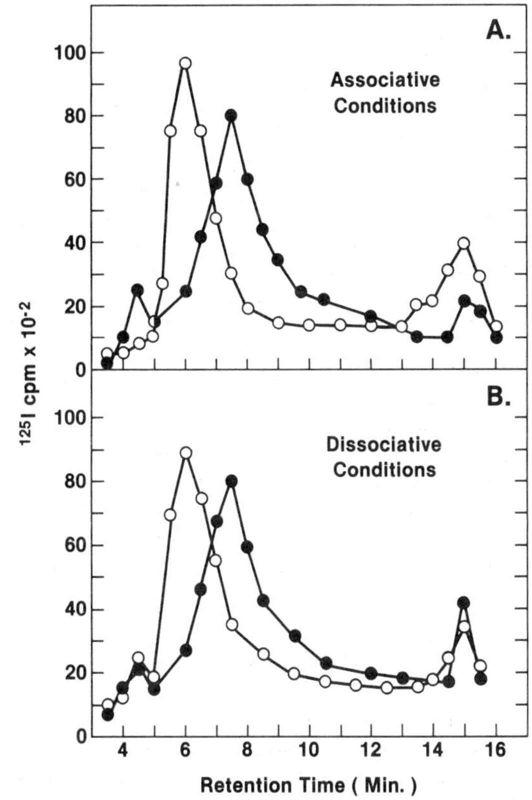

FIGURE 7. Illustration of larger aortic dermatan sulfate-PG monomer size in WC-2 pigeons. Elution profile of ^{125}I-dermatan sulfate-PG monomer isolated from WC-2 (○—○) or randomly-bred White Carneau (RBWC) (●—●) pigeons. A. Associative conditions were 0.25 M Tris-HCl, pH 7.6.; B. Dissociative conditions were 4.0 M GdnHCl, 0.05 M sodium acetate, pH 7.6. TSK G-4000 SW column, V_o = 4.5 min, V_t = 15 min. Reproduced with permission, Rowe and Wagner,[15] figure 5.

tissue, and that this represents a secondary event in atherosclerosis. Therefore, any involvement of proteoglycans in atherogenesis manifested as a chemical compositional alteration or a unique change in the physical property should be evidenced prior to the development of the atherosclerotic lesion. The White Carneau pigeon (WC-2) that has been genetically selected for increased atherosclerosis susceptibility[39] was used to test this hypothesis.

The dermatan sulfate-PG was studied[15] since it has been shown that dermatan sulfate increases with increasing severity of atherosclerosis,[33] and among the arterial glycosaminoglycans, dermatan sulfate has the greatest binding affinity for plasma low density lipoprotein.[40]

The dermatan sulfate-PG was isolated from arteries of 18-day WC-2 or randomly-bred White Carneau pigeon (RBWC) embryos, separated from chondroitin sulfate-PG, purified, and examined. Whether the monomers were examined under associative or dissociative conditions, dermatan sulfate-PG from WC-2 pigeons displayed a greater hydrodynamic size (FIGURE 7). Attempts were made to determine if the carbohydrate or the core protein was different. Core proteins prepared from each had a similar M_r of about 50,000. The amino acid composition of the core proteins were very similar and comparable to the amino acid composition of bovine aorta dermatan sulfate-PG.[17] Average molecular weights of dermatan sulfate chains were smaller for the WC-2 pigeon (about 15,000) compared to 18,000 in RBWC pigeons.

Differences in glycosylation between the two core proteins were apparent. In RBWC, only one or two serine residues appeared to be substituted with carbohydrate, whereas about 30–40% were substituted in WC-2 pigeons. It appeared, therefore, that the monomer from WC-2 pigeons was much more glycosylated. As is summarized in TABLE 6, these data for artery dermatan sulfate-PG are consistent with the proposed structure of a number of dermatan sulfate-PG monomers from a variety of tissues. In all cases, the core protein is about 45,000–50,000 and the difference appears to reside in the carbohydrate moiety, whether it be the glycosaminoglycan chain or the oligosaccharides. This is illustrated by the proteoglycan of ovarian granulosa cells known to contain an unusually high amount of oligosaccharides. Based upon these observations, a proposed model for the dermatan sulfate-PG is illustrated in FIGURE 8. For the WC-2 pigeon, the monomers are larger, probably as a result of more dermatan sulfate chains per core protein. This qualitative difference in the WC-2 pigeon, an animal with a genetic predisposition for atherosclerosis, may be related to the increased atherosclerosis susceptibility through an increased binding affinity to plasma low density lipoproteins. This possibility is likely to exist since the dermatan sulfate is the major active component participating in the ionic association with low density lipoproteins.

CONCLUSION

For the chondroitin sulfate-PG, evidence has been presented that monomers from atherosclerotic plaques are structurally distinct from those in adjacent normal aorta. The fact that the amino acid compositions and molecular weights of the isolated protein cores were similar does not appear to support an argument that these are different basic gene products. Rather, in view of the differences seen in glycosylation, it appears that the monomers were modified through changes in post-translational processing.

An important functional property of the monomer, its binding to hyaluronic acid, was reduced in the atherosclerotic plaque. It was also demonstrated that the size of the aggregate was reduced, perhaps as a result of a reduction in hyaluronic acid molecular weight. This depolymerization of hyaluronic acid may occur as a result of the action of oxygen-derived free reactive species, as has been proposed in synovial fluid in inflammatory arthritis. Should this happen in early stages of atherosclerosis, the artery may then be less able to support compressive loads and be subject to abnormally large deformations under normal blood pressure. In the artery, much of the load then would be supported by collagen fibrils, subjecting them to unphysiological strain. In the same context, the smooth muscle cells, likewise, would be exposed to deformation under the pulsatile force potentially affecting an alteration in the metabolism of these cells.

Studies of the dermatan sulfate-PG in WC-2 pigeon embryos suggested differences in glycosylation of the core protein rather than core protein modifications, again implicating an alteration in post-translational processing. The exact significance of these changes in atherosclerosis is not immediately apparent since we do not know all the functions of the dermatan sulfate-PG. Based upon the work by Scott[50,51] on the specific association of dermatan sulfate-PG with collagen, one possible consequence may be an alteration in this interaction.

TABLE 6. Characteristics of Dermatan Sulfate Proteoglycans Isolated from a Variety of Cells and Tissues

Tissue	Monomer M_r	Core Protein M_r	GAG M_r	Reference
Bovine Aorta	190,000	34,000–73,000[a]	—	Schmidt *et al.*[17]
Skin (Pig)	130,000	—	26,000	Damle *et al.*[41]
Skin (Calf)	—[e]	56,000[b]	17,000	Fuji and Nagai[42]
Human Skin Fibroblasts	—	47,000	—	Carlstedt *et al.*[43]
Human Uterine Cervix	73,000–110,500	47,000	25,000	Uldbjerg *et al.*[44]
Ovarian Granulosa Cells	—	230,000[b,d]	33,000	Yanagishita and Hascall[45]
Bovine Sclera	70,000–130,000	47,000[b]	—	Coster and Fransson[46]
	90,000	42,000[c]	—	Coster *et al.*[47]
Corneal Stroma	100,000–150,000	—	55,000	Hassell *et al.*[48]
Cartilage	500,000	43,000[b]	52,000	Shinomura *et al.*[49]

[a]Calculated from author's data.
[b]Prepared following chondroitin ABC lyase treatment (does not remove oligosaccharides).
[c]Prepared following hydrogen fluoride in pyridine treatment (removes all carbohydrate).
[d]Unusually high oligosaccharide content.
[e]Dash line indicates data not available.

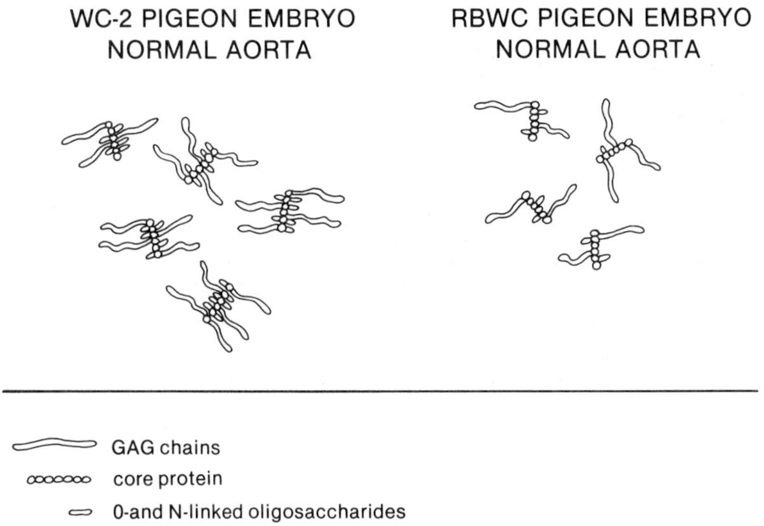

FIGURE 8. A proposed model for the dermatan sulfate-PG isolated from the aorta of pigeons selected genetically for exacerbated atherosclerosis (WC-2) and from the aorta of randomly-bred White Carneau (RBWC) pigeons.

Many more studies, including those on the heparan sulfate-PG, are needed before we can fully understand the function of individual proteoglycans and their role in atherosclerosis. Among areas that deserve attention are: (1) detailed structure and function of the chondroitin sulfate-PG, dermatan sulfate-PG, heparan sulfate-PG, and hyaluronic acid; (2) studies of proteoglycan monomer interaction with other components of the vessel wall such as collagen, elastic fibers, laminin, and fibronectin; (3) studies of the role of proteoglycans in permeability, hemostasis, and thrombosis; (4) studies on the interaction of proteoglycan and plasma derived lipoproteins; and, (5) studies of factors that may influence cell metabolism and thus, the type and amount of proteoglycans synthesized.

REFERENCES

1. VIRCHOW, W. 1971. A more precise account of fatty metamorphosis. *In* Cellular Pathology; as Based upon Physiological and Pathological Histology. 383–408. Dover Publications. New York. (Republication of English translation (of the second German Edition) originally published by J. B. Lippincott and Co. Philadelphia. 1963.)
2. ROSENBERG, L. 1975. Structure of cartilage proteoglycans. *In* Dynamics of Connective Tissue Macromolecules. P. M. C. Burleigh & A. R. Poole, Eds.: 105–124. North-Holland. Amsterdam.
3. HASCALL. V. C. 1977. Interaction of cartilage proteoglycans with hyaluronic acid. J. Supramol. Struct. **7:** 101–120.
4. ROSENBERG, L., H. CHOI, S. PAL & L. TANG. 1979. Carbohydrate-protein interactions in proteoglycans. *In* ACS Symposium Series No. 88. Carbohydrate-Protein Interaction. I. J. Goldstein, Ed.: 186–216. American Chemical Society. Washington, D.C.
5. RODEN, L. 1980. Structure and metabolism of connective tissue proteoglycans. *In* Biochemistry of Glycoproteins and Proteoglycans. W. J. Lennarz, Ed.: 267–371. Plenum. New York.
6. HARDINGHAM, T. 1981. Proteoglycans: Their structure, interactions, and molecular organization in cartilage. Biochem. Soc. Trans. **9:** 489–497.
7. HASCALL, V. C. & J. H. KIMURA. 1982. Proteoglycans: Isolation and characterization. Methods Enzymol. **82:** 769–800.
8. MUIR, H. 1982. Proteoglycans as organizers of the intercellular matrix. Biochem. Soc. Trans. **11:** 613–622.
9. HEINEGARD, D. & M. PAULSSON. 1984. Structure and metabolism of proteoglycans. *In* Extracellular Matrix Biochemistry. K. A. Piez & A. H. Reddi, Eds.: 277–328. Elsevier. New York.
10. HASCALL, V. C. & S. W. SAJDERA. 1970. Physical properties and polydispersity of proteoglycan from bovine nasal cartilage. J. Biol. Chem. **245:** 4920–4930.
11. PASTERNACK, S. G., A. VEIS & M. BREEN. 1974. Solvent-dependent changes in proteoglycan subunit conformation in aqueous guanidine hydrochloride solutions. J. Biol. Chem. **249:** 2206–2211.
12. BARBER, A. J., R. KAISER-GLANZMANN, M. JAKABOVA & E. F. LUSCHER. 1972. Characterization of a chondroitin 4-sulfate proteoglycan carrier for heparin neutralizing activity (platelet factor 4) released from human blood platelets. Biochim. Biophys. Acta **286:** 312–329.
13. SALISBURY, B. G. J. & W. D. WAGNER. 1981. Isolation and preliminary characterization of proteoglycans dissociatively extracted from human aorta. J. Biol. Chem. **256:** 8050–8057.
14. WAGNER, W. D., H. A. ROWE & J. R. CONNOR. 1983. Biochemical characteristics of dissociatively isolated aortic proteoglycans and their binding capacity to hyaluronic acid. J. Biol. Chem. **258:** 11136–11142.
15. ROWE, H. A. & W. D. WAGNER. 1985. Arterial dermatan sulfate proteoglycan structure in atherosclerosis susceptible pigeons. Arteriosclerosis **5:** 101–109.
16. OEGEMA, T. R., Jr., V. C. HASCALL & R. EISENSTEIN. 1979. Characterization of bovine

aorta proteoglycan extracted with guanidine hydrochloride in the presence of protease inhibitors. J. Biol. Chem. **254:**1312–1318.
17. SCHMIDT, A., M. PRAGER, P. SELMKE & E. BUDDECKE. 1982. Isolation and properties of proteoglycans from bovine aorta. Eur. J. Biochem. **125:** 95–101.
18. EISENSTEIN, R., S-E. LARSSON, K. E. KUETTNER, N. SORGENTE & V. C. HASCALL. 1975. The ground substance of the arterial wall. Part 1. Extractability of glycosaminoglycans and the isolation of a proteoglycan from bovine aorta. Atherosclerosis **22:** 1–17.
19. VIJAYAGOPAL, P., B. RADHAKRISHNAMURTHY, S. R. SRINIVASAN & G. S. BERENSON. 1980. Studies of biologic properties of proteoglycans from bovine aorta. Lab. Invest. **42:** 190–196.
20. HORN, M. C., M. BRETON & J. PICARD. 1983. Isolation of arterial wall proteoglycans. Int. J. Biochem. **15:** 309–316.
21. HORN, M. C., M. BRETON, E. DEUDON, E. BERROU & J. PICARD. 1983. The structural characterization of proteoglycans of cultured aortic smooth muscle cells and arterial wall of the pig. Biochim. Biophys. Acta **755:** 95–105.
22. SAJDERA, S. W. & V. C. HASCALL. 1969. Proteinpolysaccharide complex from bovine nasal cartilage. A comparison of low and high shear extraction procedures. J. Biol. Chem. **244:** 77–87.
23. HASCALL, V. C. & S. W. SAJDERA. 1969. Proteinpolysaccharide complex from bovine nasal septum. The function of glycoprotein in the formation of aggregates. J. Biol. Chem. **244:**2384–2396.
24. WAGNER, W. D., B. G. J. SALISBURY & J. R. CONNOR. 1981. Isolation and properties of a chondroitin 6-sulfate proteoglycan from human aorta. Fed. Proc. **40:** 1841.
25. FRANSSON, L-Å & B. HANSMARK. 1970. Structure of dermatan sulfate. VII. The copolymeric structure of dermatan sulfate from horse aorta. J. Biol. Chem. **245:** 4770–4783.
26. KRESSE, H., H. HEIDEL & E. BUDDECKE. 1971. Chemical and metabolic heterogeneity of a bovine aorta chondroitin sulfate-dermatan sulfate proteoglycan. Eur. J. Biochem. **22:** 557–562.
27. WAGNER, W. D. & J. CONNOR. 1981. Aortic proteoglycan modification associated with naturally occurring atherosclerosis in WC-2 pigeons. Fed. Proc. **40:** 342.
28. CHANG, Y., M. YANAGISHITA, V. C. HASCALL & T. N. WIGHT. 1983. Proteoglycans synthesized by smooth muscle cells derived from monkey (*Macaca nemestrina*) aorta. J. Biol. Chem. **258:** 5679–5688.
29. WAGNER, W. D., J. R. CONNOR & E. MULDOON. 1982. High molecular weight proteoglycans biosynthesized in culture by pigeon aorta. Biochim. Biophys. Acta **717:** 132–142.
30. CURWEN, K. D. & S. C. SMITH. 1977. Aortic glycosaminoglycans in atherosclerosis-susceptible and resistant pigeons. Exp. Mol. Pathol. **27:** 121–133.
31. STEVENS, R. L., M. COLOMBO, J. J. GONZALES, W. HOLLANDER & K. SCHMID. 1976. The glycosaminoglycans of the human artery and their changes in atherosclerosis. J. Clin. Invest. **58:** 470–481.
32. TAMMI, M., P. O. SEPPALA, A. LEHTONEN & M. MOTTONEN. 1978. Connective tissue components in normal and atherosclerotic human coronary arteries. Atherosclerosis **29:** 191–194.
33. WAGNER, W. D. & S. R. NOHLGREN. 1981. Aortic glycosaminoglycans in genetically selected WC-2 pigeons with increased atherosclerosis susceptibility. Arteriosclerosis **1:** 192–201.
34. HARDINGHAM, T. E., S. J. PERKINS & H. MUIR. 1983. Molecular conformations in proteoglycan aggregation. Biochem. Soc. Trans. **11:** 128–130.
35. WAGNER, W. D., T. E. HARDINGHAM & I. EDWARDS. 1983. Decreased amount and size of artery chondroitin sulfate proteoglycan-hyaluronic acid aggregate in atherosclerosis. Arteriosclerosis **3:** 471a.
36. HARDINGHAM, T. E. & H. MUIR. 1974. Hyaluronic acid in cartilage and proteoglycan aggregation. Biochem. J. **139:** 565–581.
37. IVERIUS, P-H. 1973. Possible role of the glycosaminoglycans in the genesis of atherosclerosis. *In* Atherogenesis: Initiating Factors. Ciba Foundation Symposium 12. R. Porter & J. Knight, Eds.: 185–196. Associated Scientific Publishers. Amsterdam.

38. CAMEJO, G. 1982. The interaction of lipids and lipoproteins with the intercellular matrix of arterial tissue: Its possible role in atherogenesis. Adv. Lipid Res. **19:** 1–53.
39. WAGNER, W. D. 1978. Risk factors in pigeons genetically selected for increased atherosclerosis susceptibility. Atherosclerosis **31:** 453–463.
40. IVERIUS, P-H. 1972. The interaction between human plasma lipoproteins and connective tissue glycosaminoglycans. J. Biol. Chem. **247:** 2607–2613.
41. DAMLE, S. P., F. J. KIERAS, W-K. TZENG & J. D. GREGORY. 1979. Isolation and characterization of proteochondroitin sulfate from pig skin. J. Biol. Chem. **254:** 1614–1620.
42. FUJII, N. & Y. NAGAI. 1981. Isolation and characterization of a proteodermatan sulfate from calf skin. J. Biochem. **90:** 1249–1258.
43. CARLSTEDT, I., L. COSTER & A. MALMSTROM. 1981. Isolation and characterization of dermatan sulphate and heparan sulphate proteoglycans from fibroblast culture. Biochem. J. **197:** 217–215.
44. ULDBJERG, N., A. MALMSTROM, G. SKMAN, J. SHEEHAN, U. ULMSTEN & L. WINGERUP. 1983. Isolation and characterization of dermatan sulfate proteoglycan from human uterine cervix. Biochem. J. **209:** 497–503.
45. YANAGISHITA, M. & V. C. HASCALL. 1983. Characterization of low buoyant density dermatan sulfate proteoglycans synthesized by rat ovarian granulosa cells in culture. J. Biol. Chem. **258:** 12847–12856.
46. COSTER, L. & L-A. FRANSSON. 1981. Isolation and characterization of dermatan sulphate proteoglycans from bovine sclera. Biochem. J. **193:** 143–153.
47. COSTER, L., D. HEINEGARD & A. MALSTROM. 1983. Dermatan sulfate proteoglycans from bovine sclera. Connect. Tissue Res. **11:** 244.
48. HASSELL, J. R., D. A. NEWSOME & V. C. HASCALL. 1979. Characterization and biosynthesis of proteoglycans of corneal stroma from rhesus monkey. J. Biol. Chem. **254:** 12346–12354.
49. SHINOMURA, T., K. KIMATA, Y. OIKE, A. NORO, N. HIROSE, K. TANABE & S. SUZUKI. 1983. The occurrence of three different proteoglycan species in chick embryo cartilage. J. Biol. Chem. **258:** 9314–9322.
50. SCOTT, J. E., C. R. ORFORD & E. W. HUGHES. 1981. Proteoglycan-collagen arrangements in developing rat tail tendon. An electron-microscopical and biochemical investigation. Biochem. J. **195:** 573–581.
51. SCOTT, J. E. 1984. The periphery of the developing collagen fibril. Biochem. J. **218:** 229–233.

Proteoglycans and Potential Mechanisms Related to Atherosclerosis[a]

GERALD S. BERENSON,[b] BHANDARU RADHAKRISHNAMURTHY,[b,c] SATHANUR R. SRINIVASAN,[b,c] PARAKAT VIJAYAGOPAL,[b] AND EDWARD R. DALFERES[b]

Departments of [b]Medicine and [c]Biochemistry
Louisiana State University Medical Center
New Orleans, Louisiana 70112

INTRODUCTION

Cardiovascular connective tissue plays an important role in the pathogenesis of atherosclerosis. The arterial wall is a well differentiated tissue composed in large part by fibrous materials, collagen and elastin, and ground substance interspersed among organized layers of cells to form lamellar structures. Blood vessels are adapted to be a resilient and flexible conduit for circulating blood components. As products of the vascular cells, components of the interstitial matrix of the arterial wall play fundamental roles in maintaining the integrity of the vessels. Of the interstitial matrix carbohydrate-protein macromolecules, proteoglycans are of particular interest. These materials undergo changes in response to various stimuli, such as stress, inflammation, and hormonal influences, and the changes are generally governed by local cellular activity.

This discussion will focus on the nature of proteoglycans in the arterial wall and potential mechanisms that relate to proteoglycans in atherosclerosis.

NATURE OF ARTERIAL WALL PROTEOGLYCANS

Proteoglycans consist of a core protein covalently linked to many chains of one or more types of glycosaminoglycans (GAG). With the exception of hyaluronic acid, the connective tissue GAG occur in the native state as proteoglycans. Most of our current knowledge of proteoglycan structure is derived from the studies of cartilage, which has a vastly different connective tissue composition than in cardiovascular tissues.

Recently, attention has focused on proteoglycans from the arterial wall because of the involvement in the development of atherosclerotic lesions. From the studies conducted over the past ten years, there is now general agreement that there are at least two types of proteoglycans in the aorta: (1) chondroitin sulfate-dermatan sulfate proteoglycan, and (2) heparan sulfate proteoglycan. The former is present in aorta in greater amounts and can be extracted from the tissue by dissociative solvents like 4 *M*

[a]This work was supported by funds from the National Heart, Lung, and Blood Institute of the United States Public Health Service (HL–02942 and HL–21649) and the National Research and Demonstration Center—Arteriosclerosis (HL–15103).

guanidine hydrochloride or $MgCl_2$.[1] This major proteoglycan isolated from bovine aorta has 12% protein and 21% uronate.

Although little is known about the protein core, the proteoglycan material has chondroitin 4- and 6-sulfates and dermatan sulfate in an 8:3:1 proportion. It is not known precisely how different GAG chains are distributed along the length of the protein core. Studies currently in progress in our laboratory on the organization of GAG in a proteoglycan from bovine aorta suggest that two types of GAG chains are present on the protein core of the proteoglycan: one containing exclusively chondroitin 6-sulfate, and the other containing chondroitin 4-sulfate and dermatan sulfate in a proportion of 4:1. These observations suggest further that in the hybrid GAG chain the dermatan sulfate is not directly linked to the core protein but through chondroitin 4-sulfate. The proportions of GAG to protein and to each other are probably heterogeneous in their native state.

Two different chondroitin sulfate type proteoglycans have been isolated from human aorta[2] and from bovine aorta explant culture media extract:[3] one rich in chondroitin 6-sulfate, and the other rich in dermatan sulfate. Whether these are fragments of one species of proteoglycan or two individual species is not known. It is important to recognize that species differences can occur, and that variations being reported on arterial wall proteoglycans due to species differences or laboratory methods have to be resolved.

In our laboratory, we also have isolated a different type of proteoglycan involving heparan sulfate. Unlike the hybrid chondroitin sulfate-dermatan sulfate proteoglycan, heparan sulfate proteoglycan cannot be easily extracted by dissociative solvents.[4] Only about 10% of this proteoglycan can be extracted by these solvents and the remainder is bound firmly to elastic tissue in the aorta. [Interestingly, heparan sulfate proteoglycan is easily extracted from lung tissue[5]]. Elastase digestion of the arterial tissue provides a method for solubilization of this proteoglycan, but elastase has inherent protease activity that can potentially degrade the protein core. Several protease inhibitors are added to the extraction medium to inhibit spurious protease activity of the enzyme, but, even in the presence of inhibitors, it is possible that some degradation of the core protein can occur. At present, therefore, one should exercise caution in interpreting observations regarding the characteristics of arterial heparan sulfate proteoglycan.

The heparan sulfate proteoglycan isolated by a sequential extraction of bovine aorta by NaCl, followed by digestion of tissue with collagenase and then elastase, has a molecular weight of 300,000 and 19% protein and 18% uronate. The material extracted with guanidine HCl yielded similar results. Interestingly, this material may exist in more than one form with biologic properties, like heparin, that are important in the pathogenesis of atherosclerosis.

AGGREGATION OF PROTEOGLYCANS

Hascall and Sajdera[6] showed that cartilage proteoglycans from bovine nasal tissue form large aggregates in the presence of hyaluronic acid and link proteins. Several investigators have subsequently studied the phenomenon of aggregation. Hardingham and Muir[7] observed that proteoglycans form cartilage aggregate with hyaluronic acid even in the absence of link proteins, but they noted that link proteins stabilize the interaction with hyaluronic acid.

Unlike proteoglycans from cartilage, aorta proteoglycans do not form large aggregates. Only 10% of chondroitin sulfate-dermatan sulfate proteoglycan from bovine aorta formed aggregates with exogenous hyaluronic acid. We[1] isolated two proteoglycan-hyaluronate complexes from bovine aorta and studied their composition.

The GAG found in the complexes were hyaluronic acid and chondroitin sulfates (including dermatan sulfate) in a proportion of 13:87 in Complex I and 24:76 in Complex II.

The presence of link proteins in these complexes has not been established until recently. Gardell *et al.*[8] noted the presence of trace amounts of link proteins in their preparation of proteoglycan aggregates from bovine aorta by immunologic techniques. More recently, we isolated a link protein from a proteoglycan aggregate from bovine aorta in sufficient amounts for partial characterization. The isolated link protein was found to be homogeneous with fewer serine and threonine residues than the core protein, and had a molecular weight of 49,000. It also had 3.1% carbohydrate with galactose, mannose, and fucose in a proportion of 1.5:4:1. The chondroitin sulfate-dermatan sulfate proteoglycan aggregated with the link protein in the presence of hyaluronic acid, and as such, the aggregates may be of particular importance in the pathogenesis of atherosclerosis.

POTENTIAL MECHANISMS RELATED TO ATHEROSCLEROSIS

A number of specific physiologic functions and alterations with aging and atherosclerosis have been attributed to GAG. These include providing structural support to the vessel wall and resistance to infection, influencing fibrillogenesis, regulating fluid and electrolyte balance, influencing blood coagulation, platelet aggregation, calcification and lipoprotein binding, and facilitating lipid clearance and transfer of cholesteryl esters across the endothelium. Some of these properties are specifically related to atherosclerosis as discussed below.

Hemostatic Properties

Even though many of the functions of GAG are not understood clearly, it has been known for many years that GAG, particularly heparin, heparan sulfate, and dermatan sulfate, possess anticoagulant activity. Since GAG occur in the native state as proteoglycans in the tissue, a better understanding of their physiologic functions can be obtained by studying intact proteoglycans.

We[4] studied the hemostatic properties of both the chondroitin sulfate-dermatan sulfate proteoglycan and the heparan sulfate proteoglycan from bovine aorta (FIGURE 1). Heparan sulfate proteoglycan exhibited significantly more anticoagulant activity than chondroitin sulfate-dermatan sulfate proteoglycan. Both proteoglycans, however, also inhibited thrombin-induced platelet aggregation. At comparable uronic acid levels, the heparan sulfate proteoglycan was a more potent inhibitor of platelet aggregation than the chondroitin sulfate-dermatan sulfate proteoglycan. We observed that the protein core of the proteoglycan molecules is not essential for hemostatic properties and that the anticoagulant activity of aorta proteoglycans is due to the nature of specific GAG and to the ability of GAG chains to accelerate the inactivation of serine proteases by antithrombin III. Proteoglycans might achieve inactivation by increasing the binding affinity of proteases for antithrombin III.

Lipoprotein-Lipase Binding

Lipoprotein-lipase (LPL) is the key enzyme involved in the hydrolysis of plasma chylomicrons and very low density lipoprotein-triglycerides. Several lines of evidence suggest that LPL activity is localized at or on the luminal endothelial surface of blood vessels. Heparin or heparin-like compounds are believed to affect the release of LPL either by direct interaction with the enzyme or competition for the LPL binding sites on the cell surface.

We noted that the chondroitin sulfate-dermatan sulfate proteoglycan from bovine aorta when injected into rabbits was about 60% as effective as heparin in causing LPL release.[1] Endothelial cell surface proteoglycan-LPL binding may facilitate cholesteryl ester transfer into the arterial wall from chylomicron remnants, a hydrolytic product of chylomicrons.

Proteoglycan-Lipoprotein Interactions

Lipids of atherosclerotic lesions originate from plasma apoB-containing lipoproteins such as low density (LDL), very low density (VLDL), and Lp(a) lipoproteins. In fact,

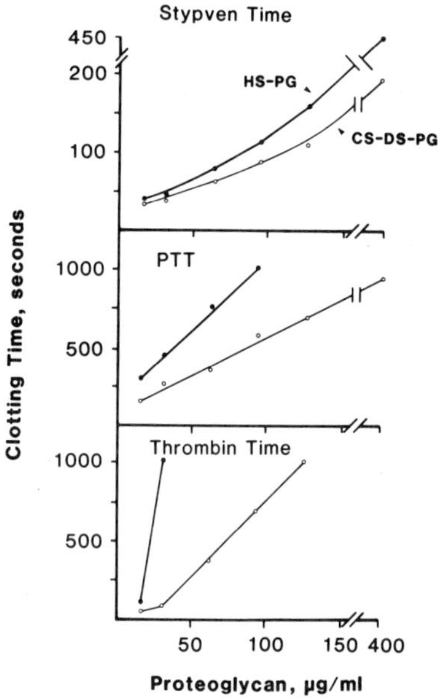

FIGURE 1. Effect of aorta proteoglycan on blood coagulation in Stypven time, partial thromboplastin time (PTT), and thrombin time.

autopsy studies conducted in the Bogalusa Heart Study program showed a high correlation of LDL-cholesterol with atherosclerotic lesions in early life.[9] Modulations in arterial cellular binding and uptake of apoB-containing lipoproteins remain the main focus of attention with respect to lipid accumulation. Histochemical studies have demonstrated a close relationship between arterial GAG, fibrous structures, and lipid deposits of atheromatous lesions in both humans and experimental animals. These observations suggest that connective tissue macromolecules, especially proteoglycans, selectively associate with certain plasma lipoproteins.

Passage of macromolecules across the arterial wall is greatly affected by subendothelial GAG (proteoglycans). The physiochemical properties of proteoglycans and hyaluronic acid allow the formation of a gel-sieve matrix, and the permeability and retention of macromolecules such as lipoproteins that enter the matrix may be modulated by molecular-sieving, steric exclusion, and electrostatic interaction.

Since an increase in lipid content of grossly normal intima with age is greater than the changes of plasma lipids with age, mechanisms other than simple infiltration of plasma lipids into the vessel wall appear to be operative in lipid accumulation. Progressive alterations of connective tissue components likely affect the arterial tissue organization and integrity, which in turn may influence the permeability of macromolecules across the arterial wall. The selective interaction of plasma apoB-containing lipoproteins with proteoglycans and transfer of lipids from LDL to elastin and collagen favor enrichment of normal arterial wall with lipids gradually during life. While all of these changes may be the normal adaptive processes of the arterial wall, focal response to chronic hemodynamic stress and even slightly elevated levels of plasma LDL over time may initiate lesion formation.

In Vitro *Interactions*

The ability of GAG to form both soluble and insoluble complexes with plasma lower density lipoproteins is well known. For selective precipitation of apoB-containing lipoproteins from serum, the nature and concentration of cations appear to be important.[10] The chemical characteristics of isolated GAG seem to influence the complex formation with lipoproteins.

In terms of arterial proteoglycans, we now have demonstrated that the chondroitin sulfate-dermatan sulfate proteoglycan can be as potent and selective as is heparin in producing complex formation.[1] The complex forming abilities of corresponding isolated GAG moieties devoid of protein core were far less, suggesting the importance of net charge density of proteoglycans. It is of interest that the complex forming ability of heparan sulfate proteoglycan is poor when compared to the chondroitin sulfate-dermatan sulfate proteoglycan.[4] These differences may be functionally important because heparan sulfate proteoglycans, which are synthesized predominantly by the endothelial cells, might increase the cell surface negative charge (antithrombogenic) without binding LDL.

The nature of interaction between apoB-containing lipoproteins and GAG at physiologic pH is interesting because both macromolecular species are anionic at this pH. The reaction mechanism between LDL and GAG can be conceived of as an electrostatic binding involving basic amino groups of apoB of LDL and polyanionic groups of GAG. Divalent cations appear to promote aggregates involving anionic groups of GAG and phospholipids of LDL.

In Vivo *Interactions*

Isolation of intact lipoprotein-GAG complexes from human normal intima and atherosclerotic lesions in our laboratory also provided evidence for an *in vivo* interaction.[11] The isolated lipoprotein-GAG complexes fractionate into LDL and VLDL density spectra, with the former being predominant. The presence of Ca^{++} in significant quantities in the complexes[11] and the morphologic evidence that these complexes have a highly aggregated nature[12] indicate an interaction similar to that observed *in vitro*.

Recently, we demonstrated in a rabbit model of atherosclerosis that alterations in GAG metabolism are accompanied by an increase in uptake of LDL by aorta (FIGURE 2).[13] The specific activities of GAG in the complexes obtained by different extraction

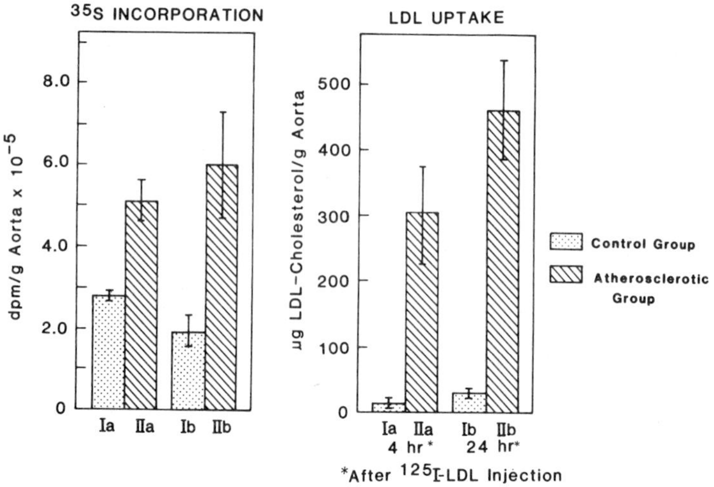

FIGURE 2. ^{35}S-incorporation into GAG and uptake of plasma LDL in aortas of control and atherosclerotic rabbits 4 hours (I_aII_a) and 24 hours (I_bII_b) after ^{125}I-LDL administration.

procedures differed markedly (elastase > collagenase > saline), emphasizing the presence of different pools of complexes.

In vitro and *in vivo* observations now provide evidence that favors a specific role for proteoglycans in selective retention of certain plasma lipoproteins. Further studies are needed to elucidate the dynamic nature and complexity of the physicochemical changes occurring in the extracellular matrix which may affect the lipoprotein flux and retention.

Role of Proteoglycans in Low Density Lipoproteins Uptake by Macrophages

The influence of cellular uptake of lipoproteins is also being considered. The lipid-laden foam cells in the atherosclerotic lesions are derived from both smooth muscle cells and blood monocyte-derived macrophages. The lipids of foam cell predominantly consist of droplets of cholesteryl ester. Attempts to reproduce cholesteryl ester deposition by incubation of macrophages *in vitro* with native LDL have not been successful. However, incubating these cells with LDL that has been made negatively charged by acetylation or malondialdehyde treatment leads to massive accumulation of cholesteryl ester.[14] In addition, the macrophage also takes up β-VLDL, endothelial cell-modified LDL, as well as LDL that has been complexed with dextran sulfate. These studies indicate that modification of LDL either by *in vitro* chemical reaction or by *in vivo* biological process renders the lipoprotein recognizable by macrophages. The property of LDL to form complexes with arterial proteoglycans could be important in promoting the deposition of cholesteryl ester within the scavenger cells.

Recently, Salisbury *et al.*[15] reported that LDL complexed to a proteoglycan from bovine aorta significantly enhanced cholesteryl ester synthesis and accumulation in macrophages. We have observed that the degradation of LDL by mouse peritoneal macrophages is increased sixfold as compared to controls when the cells were incubated with LDL that has been complexed with proteoglycan aggregate rather than proteoglycan monomers. The massive accumulation of intracellular lipids is seen by increase in oil red O-positive droplets, whereas the cells incubated with LDL alone did not show lipid deposition (FIGURE 3). These studies are being pursued further.

GLYCOSAMINOGLYCAN CHANGES IN ATHEROSCLEROSIS

Progression of Atherosclerosis

Histochemical and biochemical studies presented evidence of early and progressive changes in GAG composition in atherosclerotic lesions. The results have been reviewed recently,[1] and fairly extensive studies on arterial GAG changes with atherosclerosis involving both human and experimental animals were performed in our laboratory. Intimal layers have a greater concentration of sulfated GAG than external layers. The initimal concentration of GAG increases as the surface involvement increases from 10 to 30%, and thereafter, the concentration of GAG decreases with further surface involvement and formation of calcified and complicated lesions. Of the individual GAG, hyaluronic acid and heparan sulfate did not change appreciably, while chondroitin 6-sulfate and dermatan sulfate concentrations increased with increasing extensiveness of fatty streaks and fibrous plaques.

Similar GAG changes were also noted in aortas of animals with experimental

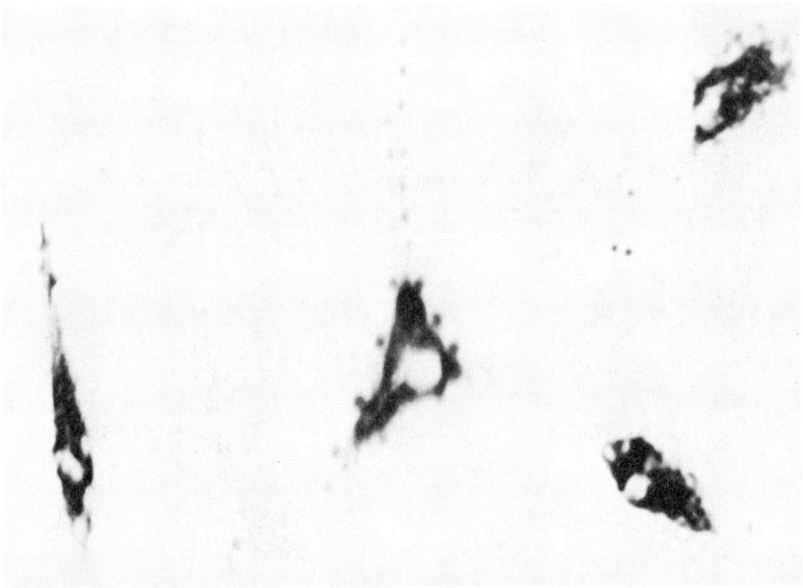

FIGURE 3. Accumulation of lipids in mouse peritoneal macrophages incubated with LDL-proteoglycan complex. Cells were incubated with LDL-proteoglycan complexes for 24 hours and stained for lipids (oil red O). Similar experiment with LDL alone did not show lipid accumulation (data not shown).

atherosclerosis, with some variation in the individual GAG content occurring dependent upon the nature of the lesion.

Regression of Atherosclerosis

Evidence to suggest that atherosclerosis might also be reversible has come from numerous sources. During regression of atherosclerosis, several biochemical and morphologic changes occur in the arterial wall. These include: (a) a decreased rate of proliferation of smooth muscle cells; (b) regeneration of endothelium by endothelial cells; (c) depletion of accumulated lipid; and (d) alterations in the connective tissue components.

Changes in the GAG composition in regressing lesions depend much upon the nature of the lesion and the degree of regression that has occurred. During regression of early lesions of fatty streaks, an increase in hyaluronic acid and a decrease in chondroitin sulfate occur, and additionally, an increase in heparan sulfate occurs during regression of somewhat advanced lesions. Also, when the lesions are induced with peanut oil, marked changes in dermatan sulfate content of aorta occur.

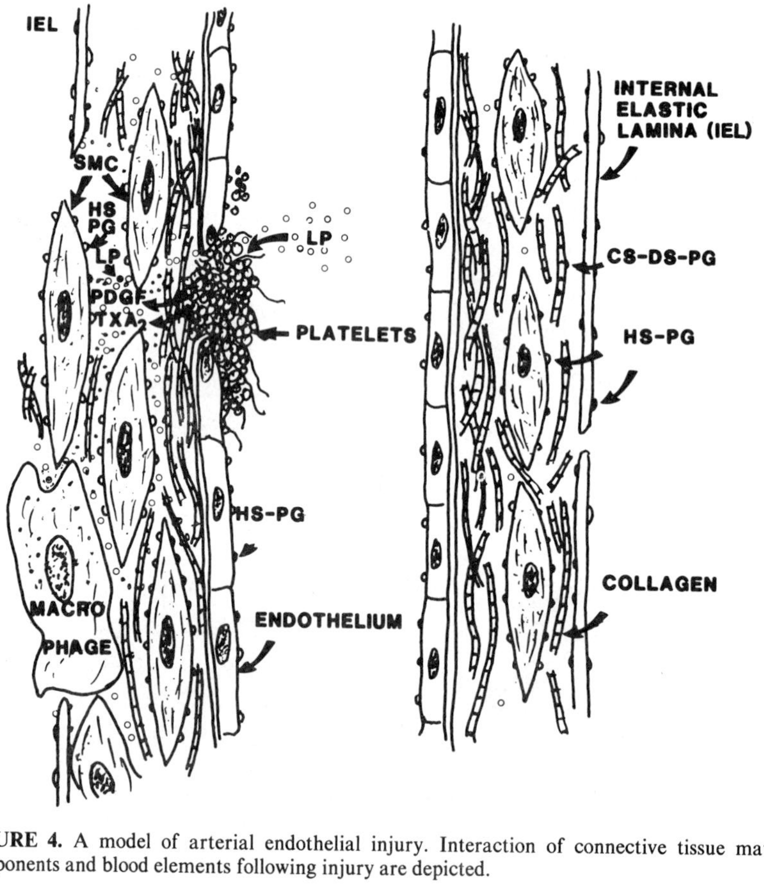

FIGURE 4. A model of arterial endothelial injury. Interaction of connective tissue matrix components and blood elements following injury are depicted.

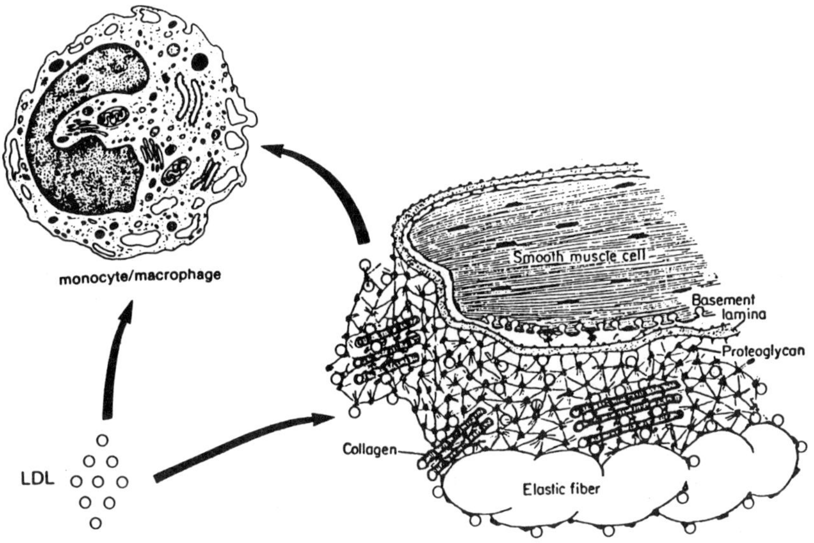

FIGURE 5. Potential role in extracellular and intracellular lipid accumulation in atherogenesis.

These findings are very much the reverse of those noted in development and progression of disease, and are similar to changes in human disease, relating severity of lesions to individual GAG content. The findings further emphasize the importance of GAG in remodelling the arterial wall structure that can occur during regression of atherosclerotic lesions. The observation that the vascular changes parallel GAG changes may be functionally important.

CONCLUSION

The cardiovascular connective tissue proteoglycans play a critical role in maintaining the integrity of the arterial wall and in the pathogenesis of atherosclerosis. Schematically, the various activities and the normal and abnormal functions which take place in injury to the arterial wall and endothelium are depicted in FIGURE 4. The endothelium serves to regulate the influx of plasma macromolecules into the arterial wall. Not only does it act as a molecular sieve, but endothelium alters certain molecules during their passage from blood to subendothelial space. Endothelial cells also secrete extracellular matrix materials that can influence the retention of plasma components within the arterial wall. Endothelial injury leads to proliferation of smooth muscle cells (SMC) and elaboration of connective tissue elements by SMC. In the surrounding connective tissue, a selective interaction of apoB lipoproteins occurs with proteoglycans, particularly chondroitin sulfate-dermatan sulfate proteoglycan (CS-DS-PG), collagen, and elastin. Such interactions make the LDL particles large electronegative aggregates. These altered LDL are taken up by macrophages (and possibly by transformed SMC), and go through a high-affinity process, devoid of feedback control, which results in intracellular lipid accumulation[14] (FIGURE 5). Heparan sulfate proteoglycan (HS-PG) located on the cell surface and in association with internal elastic lamina (IEL) is a potent anticoagulant, inhibits aggregation, and probably binds lipoproteins-lipase to endothelium. Thus, HS-PG may be considered as an antagonist to lesion development. Proteoglycans not only sequester apoB lipoproteins, but become part of the connective tissue responses and fibrous capping of raised plaque lesions. Thus, proteoglycans, as part of the interstitial matrix, enter into a variety of activities important to health and in pathogenesis of disease.

REFERENCES

1. RADHAKRISHNAMURTHY, B., S. R. SRINIVASAN, P. VIJAYAGOPAL, E. R. DALFERES, JR. & G. S. BERENSON. 1982. Mesenchymal injury and proteoglycans of arterial wall in atherosclerosis. *In* Glycosaminoglycans and Proteoglycans in Physiological and Pathological Process of Body systems. R. S. Varma & R. Varma, Eds.: 231–251. Karger. Basel.
2. SALISBURY, B. G. J. & W. D. WAGNER. 1981. Isolation and preliminary characterization of proteoglycans dissociatively extracted from human aorta. J. Biol. Chem. **256:** 8050–8057.
3. SCHMIDT, A., M. PRAGER, P. SELMKE & E. BUDDECKE. 1982. Isolation and properties of proteoglycans from bovine aorta. Eur. J. Biochem. **125:** 95–101.
4. VIJAYAGOPAL, P., S. R. SRINIVASAN, B. RADHAKRISHNAMURTHY & G. S. BERENSON. 1983. Hemostatic properties and serum lipoprotein binding of a heparan sulfate proteoglycan from bovine aorta. Biochim. Biophys. Acta **758:** 70–83.
5. RADHAKRISHNAMURTHY, B., F. SMART, E. R. DALFERES, JR. & G. S. BERENSON. 1980. Isolation and characterization of proteoglycans from bovine lung. J. Biol. Chem. **255:** 7575–7582.
6. HASCALL, V. C. & S. W. SAJDERA. 1969. Protein-polysaccharide complex from bovine nasal cartilage. The function of glycoprotein in the formation of aggregates. J. Biol. Chem. **244:** 2384–2396.
7. HARDINGHAM, T. E. & H. MUIR. 1974. Hyaluronic acid in cartilage and proteoglycan aggregation. Biochem. J. **139:** 565–581.
8. GARDELL, S., J. BAKER, B. CATERSON, D. HEINEGÅRD & L. RODÉN. 1980. Link protein and hyaluronic acid binding region as components of aorta proteoglycans. Biochem. Biophys. Res. Commun. **95:** 1823–1831.
9. BERENSON, G. S., A. W. VOORS, P. GARD, W. P. NEWMAN III & R. E. TRACY. Clinical and anatomic correlates of cardiovascular disease in children from the Bogalusa Heart Study, 1983. In Atherosclerosis VI. Proceedings of the VIth International Symposium on Atherosclerosis F. G. Schettler, A. M. Gotto, Jr., G. Middlehoff, A. G. R. Habenicht and K. R. Jurutke, Eds.: 60–65. Springer-Verlag. New York.
10. SRINIVASAN, S. R., A. LOPEZ-S., B. RADHARISHNAMURTHY & G. S. BERENSON. 1970. Complexing of serum pre-β- and β-lipoproteins and acid mucopolysaccharides. Atherosclerosis **12:** 321–334.
11. SRINIVASAN, S. R., P. DOLAN, B. RADHAKRISHNAMURTHY & G. S. BERENSON. 1975. Lipoprotein-acid mucopolysaccharide complexes of human atherosclerotic lesions. Biochim. Biophys. Acta **388:** 58–70.
12. WOODARD, J. F., S. R. SRINIVASAN, M. L. ZIMNY, B. RADHAKRISHNAMURTHY & G. S. BERENSON. 1976. Electron microscopic features of lipoprotein-glycosaminoglycan complexes from human atherosclerotic plaques. Lab. Invest. **34:** 516–521.
13. SRINIVASAN, S. R., P. VIJAYAGOPAL, E. R. DALFERES, JR., B. ABBATE, B. RADHAKRISHNAMURTHY & G. S. BERENSON. 1984. Dynamics of lipoprotein-glycosaminoglycan interactions in the atherosclerotic rabbit aorta *in vivo*. Biochim. Biophys. Acta **793:** 157–168.
14. BROWN, M. S. & J. L. GOLDSTEIN. 1983. Lipoprotein metabolism in the macrophage: Implications for cholesterol deposition in atherosclerosis. Ann. Rev. Biochem. **52:** 223–261.
15. SALISBURY, B. G. J., D. J. FALCONE & C. R. MINICK. 1984. Arterial proteoglycans enhance lipid accumulation in macrophages (Abstract). Fed. Proc. **43:** 786.

Foam Cells and Atherogenesis[a]

STANLEY D. FOWLER,[b] EUGENE P. MAYER,[c] AND PHILLIP GREENSPAN[b]

[b]*Department of Pathology*
and
[c]*Department of Microbiology and Immunology*
School of Medicine
University of South Carolina
Columbia, South Carolina 29208

Foam cells occur in early atherosclerotic lesions (fatty streaks), as well as in mature grumous plaques. In the latter, they are seen most prominently as clusters of cells surrounding necrotic areas. The foam cells derive their name from the numerous lipid inclusions that swell their cytoplasm (FIGURE 1). Despite their prominence, the origin of arterial foam cells and their significance to atherogenesis have been much debated.[1] Historically, two contrasting views have been held regarding the origin of arterial foam cells. The first of these proposed that foam cells are intimal smooth muscle cells, which gradually transform into foam cells through the intracellular accumulation of lipids that are inadequately metabolized or disposed of by the cells. The second viewpoint maintained that foam cells are wandering blood monocytes that have entered the artery wall and engulfed lipid containing debris. Depending on the viewpoint, foam cells could be considered as passive participants in the disease process or as important contributors to its genesis.

Electron microscopic studies of atherosclerotic lesions reveal the presence of both arterial smooth muscle cells in varying stages of lipid overloading and blood monocytes infiltrating the artery wall.[2-10] However, the origin of most foam cells has remained uncertain in these studies since the numerous lipid inclusions present in the cytoplasm obliterate characteristic ultrastructural features needed to identify the foam cells as being derived from smooth muscle cells or monocyte/macrophages (see FIGURE 1).

CHARACTERIZATION OF LIPID-LADEN CELLS ISOLATED FROM ATHEROSCLEROTIC ARTERIES

Direct evidence for the cell origin of foam cells has come from biological and immunological studies on lipid-laden cells isolated from atherosclerotic arteries. The best preparations are obtained by incubating chunks of diseased arteries with a mixture of purified collagenase and elastase. The cells released by the enzymes are morphologically and biochemically heterogeneous, all exhibiting varying degrees of lipid accumulation. Haley *et al.*[11] showed that these cell mixtures could be separated according to their buoyant density by means of Metrizamide density gradient centrifugation. In studies on cholesterol-fed rabbits, they observed a continuous

[a]These studies were supported by Public Health Service grant no. HL-29940 from the National Heart, Lung, and Blood Institute, grant no. PCM-8212634 from the National Science Foundation, and by grants from the Juvenile Diabetes Foundation and the American Health Assistance Foundation.

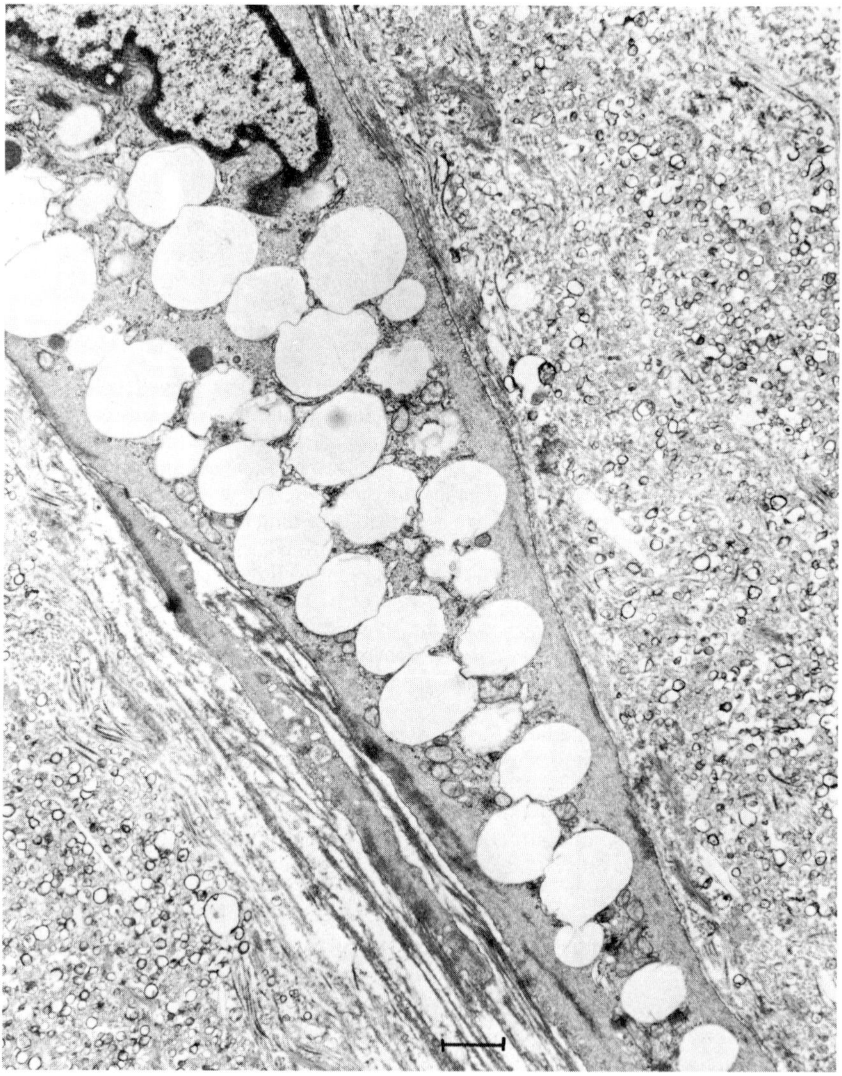

FIGURE 1. Electron micrograph of a foam cell *in situ* in an atheromatous aortic plaque of a cholesterol-fed rabbit. The cell is engorged with lipid inclusions to such a degree that its cell origin is uncertain. Bar = 1 μm. ($\times$8000).

distribution of such cells in the density gradients, although two major populations of cells were evident. The most numerous cells equilibrated at the higher densities in the gradient (d = 1.10–1.14), and were recognizable as smooth muscle cells in varying stages of lipid overloading. A second, smaller population equilibrated at very low densities (d = 1.03–1.07), and consisted of cells excessively laden with lipid inclusions. These cells appeared as typical arterial foam cells, and they possessed great quantities of cholesterol and cholesteryl esters, as well as high levels of catalase and lysosomal enzymes. Compared to aortic smooth muscle cells isolated from normal rabbits, the high-density cell population was also enriched in cholesterol and lysosomal enzymes, although not to the degree shown by the low-density cells. Very similar findings were obtained when cells isolated from atherosclerotic aortas of rhesus monkeys were analyzed by Metrizamide density gradient centrifugation.[12]

Based on sensitive erythrocyte rosetting tests, Fowler *et al.*[13] demonstrated that many of the low-density foam cells isolated from cholesterol-fed rabbits possess Fc and C3 receptors, which indicate their monocyte/macrophage origin. As illustrated in FIGURE 2, the low-density foam cells bound IgG-coated erythrocytes to form richly garnished rosettes. No significant binding was found with uncoated erythrocytes or with erythrocytes coated with $F(ab')_2$, thus demonstrating the presence of authentic Fc receptors. Although 70% or more of the low-density foam cells exhibited Fc receptors, less than 30% showed C3 receptors by rosette testing. The reason for this difference is unclear since both kinds of receptors are present in macrophages. Under appropriate conditions, Fc bearing foam cells could be induced to phagocytize IgG-coated erythrocytes, indicating that these cells can act as phagocytes (see FIGURE 2).

The presence of foam cells bearing typical monocyte/macrophage surface markers has been confirmed by Schaffner *et al.*,[14] using Fc and C3 immunologic tests, and by Pitas *et al.*,[15] who demonstrated receptors on the cells for β-VLDL and chemically modified LDL (acetoacetylated). Also supporting these conclusions, is the report by Spraragen *et al.*[16] that [^{3}H] thymidine-labeled blood monocytes injected into rabbits given an atherogenic diet appeared as foam cells. Furthermore, macrophages can be transformed into "foam cells" in culture by incubation with acetylated low density lipoprotein,[17] β-very low density lipoprotein,[18] altered low density lipoprotein extracted from atherosclerotic arteries,[19] or insoluble complexes of low density lipoprotein, heparin, fibronectin, and denatured collagen.[20]

The above studies have not excluded the possibility that some foam cells are derived instead from smooth muscle cells. Arterial smooth muscle cells do exhibit variable degrees of lipid overloading in atheromatous lesions, as revealed in earlier electron microscopy studies and by their presence as high density cells in enzymically isolated cell preparations.[11] The continued evolution of these cells into foam cells is easily envisioned. Indeed, in the studies cited above, not all foam cells exhibited macrophage markers. Exposure of arterial smooth muscle cells *in vitro* to cationized low density lipoprotein creates lipid-filled cells strikingly similar in appearance to some foam cells seen *in vivo.*[21]

SIGNIFICANCE OF FOAM CELLS IN ATHEROGENESIS

Recognition of the monocyte/macrophage origin of many foam cells has led to renewed interest in the potential role of macrophages in atherogenesis. Very little is really known of the activities of these cells in atherosclerotic lesions, but one can speculate about the consequences of their presence based on current knowledge of the biology of mononuclear phagocytes.[22]

The function of macrophages as scavenger cells is well known, and the appearance of foam cells clustered about the grumous core of atheromas has long been interpreted as macrophages scavenging decaying cells and debriding the area of aggregates of cholesterol, other lipids, and denatured proteins. The membranous whorls and crystals of cholesterol often seen within lysosomes of arterial foam cells[23,24] may well be a reflection of such activity.

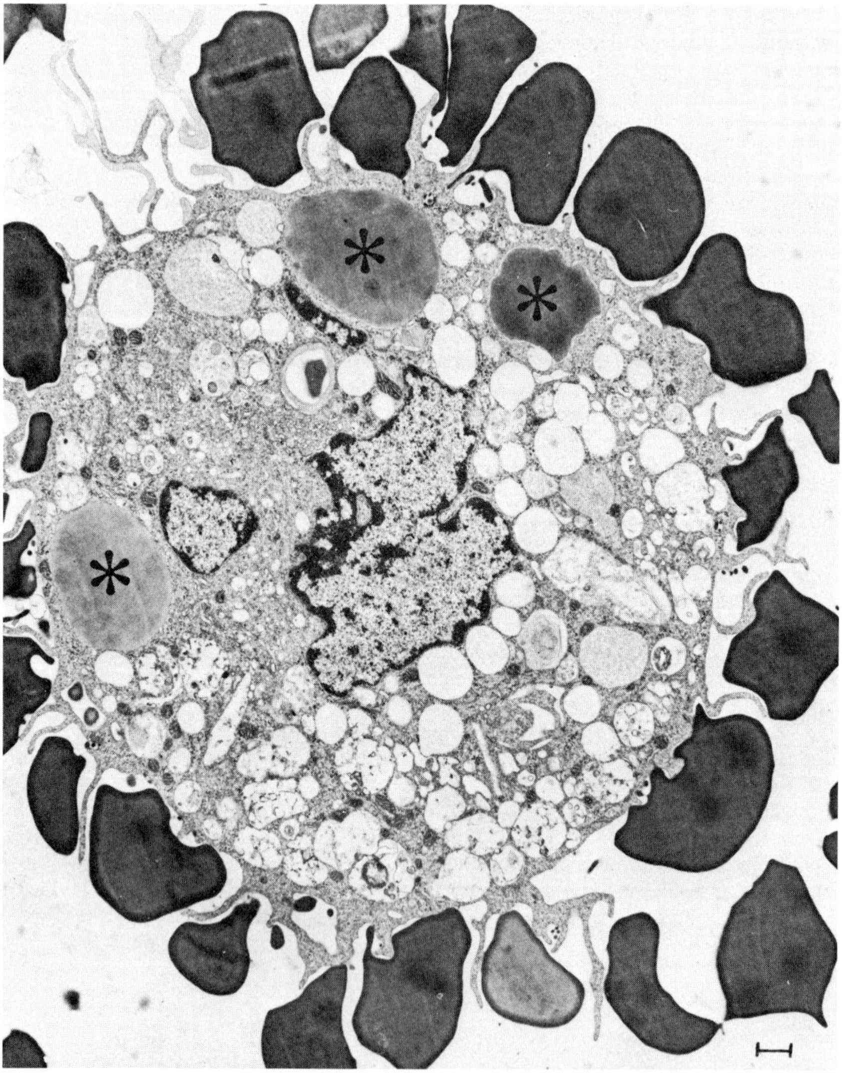

FIGURE 2. Demonstration of a foam cell with Fc receptors on its surface. This electron micrograph shows an enzymically isolated rabbit aortic foam cell rosetted with IgG-coated erythrocytes. Three engulfed erythrocytes (asterisks) are seen in the cytoplasm indicating that the foam cell is phagocytic. Bar = 1 μm. ($\times$5000). (From Fowler *et al.*[13]).

In the past decade, macrophages have become recognized as true secretory cells with a striking repertoire of potent secretory products.[25,26] Through these secretions, macrophages could exercise a profound influence on atherogenesis. TABLES 1 and 2 list macrophage secretion products that could potentially be involved in lesion initiation or evolution. Among these, the most interesting is the macrophage-derived growth factor,

TABLE 1. Macrophage Protein Secretory Products Potentially Influencing Atherogenesis[a]

Neutral Hydrolases	*Complement Components*
Collagenase I	C1
Collagenase II	C2
Collagenase III	C3
Collagenase IV	C4
Collagenase V	C5
Elastase	Factor B
Lipoprotein lipase	Factor D
Plasminogen activator	Factor H
	Factor I
Acid Hydrolases	Properdin
Proteases	
Glycosidases	*Coagulation Factors*
Lipases	Factor V
Nucleases	Factor VII
Phosphatases	Factor IX
Sulfatases	Factor X
Binding Proteins	*Factors Regulating Responses By Other Cells*
Apolipoprotein E	Angiogenesis factor
Fibronectin	Factor stimulating collagen production
α_2-Macroglobulin	Macrophage-derived growth factor
Transferrin	

[a]Sources: Nathan *et al.*[25] and Takemura & Werb.[26]

which can induce the proliferation of both fibroblasts and smooth muscle cells.[27,28] Intimal proliferation of smooth muscle cells, a key feature of atherosclerosis, is likely controlled, or at least moderated, by local growth factors. Because of their position in the artery wall itself, macrophages might well exert a greater influence than platelets on the initiation of localized proliferation of intimal smooth muscle cells.

Macrophages secrete several neutral proteinases, including collagenases,[29,30] elastase,[31] and plasminogen activator.[32] These enzymes have the potential to greatly alter structural components of the arterial wall. For example, among the collagenases produced, one cleaves interstitial collagen, a second cleaves pericellular (type 5) collagen, and a third degrades basement membrane-type collagen. Further, macrophage elastase is a unique metalloproteinase that is especially active against native elastin fibrils. Plasminogen activator, which forms plasmin from plasminogen, is a general protease that can produce lysis of fibrin and can activate components of complement. It may also aid macrophages in their migration through tissue. Most

TABLE 2. Macrophage Non-Protein Products Potentially Influencing Atherogenesis[a]

Reactive Metabolites of Oxygen	*Bioactive Lipids*
Hydrogen peroxide	Prostaglandin E_2
Hydroxyl radical	Prostacyclin
Singlet oxygen	Thromboxane B_2
Superoxide anion	Leukotriene C
	Hydroxyeicosatetraeneoic acids
	Platelet activating factor

[a]Sources: Nathan *et al.*[25] and Takemura & Werb.[26]

significantly, the secretion of all these neutral proteases is induced by macrophage ingestion of particle aggregates, such as scavenging macrophages might find in the extracellular matrix of atheromas.

Under certain conditions, such as during phagocytosis, macrophages also release lysosomal hydrolases into their surroundings.[33] The activity of these enzymes at neutral pH would be limited, but should the pH of the environment surrounding the cells become acidic (for example, by release of lactic acid during anaerobic glycolysis), these enzymes could degrade matrix components of arteries and could even attack arterial cells as well.

In addition to the enzymes just discussed, macrophages can secrete a variety of other proteins that could affect cellular activities in arterial lesions. Among these are the binding proteins fibronectin[34] and apolipoprotein E[35] angiogenesis factor,[36] a factor stimulating collagen production,[37] and lipoprotein lipase.[38] In addition, many of the components of the complement system are produced by macrophages.[39] A number of the degradation products of complement formation are important mediators of inflammation. C5a, notably, is strongly chemotactic to leukocytes. If generated in atheromatous lesions, C5a could further attract macrophages to the affected sites.

Besides the proteins described, macrophages release a variety of potent biological compounds of low molecular weight. These include reactive metabolites of oxygen (superoxide, hydrogen peroxide, hydroxyl radicals, and singlet oxygen[40,41]) which are generated in a metabolic burst triggered by phagocytosis. These products can kill neoplastic cells[42] and could perhaps harm normal arterial cells. Macrophages are especially rich in arachidonic acid, and they can synthesize prostaglandins, thromboxanes, leukotrienes, and hydroxyeicosatetraeneoic acids.[43–45] These compounds could influence arterial lesions in multiple ways, including affecting arterial wall metabolism, histamine production, and platelet reactivity.

Not all of the secretory products are produced by macrophages all the time. Instead, macrophages appear to participate in the inflammatory response and subsequent tissue repair by secreting various products at appropriate stages of the response and repair process.[26] However, it is significant that the influence of excessive lipid overloading of macrophages on their secretion of most of these products is unknown.

Presumably, the smooth muscle cell-derived foam cells take a more passive role in atherogenesis. These cells may be viewed as innocent bystanders attempting to cope with a flood of cholesteryl ester-rich lipoproteins. Following internalization and metabolism of the lipoproteins entering the artery wall, the excess cholesterol is stored in the cytoplasm of the cells as cholesteryl ester droplets.[46,47] In time, the growing cholesterol deposits could block essential cellular activities and cause cell death. The lipid and enzyme contents of the dead cells would then be dumped into the surrounding environment to contribute to the development of a necrotic grumous plaque core.

ANALYSIS OF LIPID-LADEN ARTERIAL CELLS BY FLOW CYTOFLUOROMETRY

An important step to further understand the events in atherogenesis will be to elucidate the biological activities of the various cell types present in arterial lesions. We have recently devised methods to analyze isolated arterial cells by flow cytofluorometry and to purify defined subpopulations by cell sorting. Since lipid overloading is a common feature of the diseased cells, we required the use of a specific fluorescent lipid stain for our investigations. Nile red, 9-diethylamino-5H-benzo[α]phenoxazine-5-one, a trace component of the dye nile blue, was found to be ideally suited for this purpose.

Nile red is intensely fluorescent and, if proper spectral conditions are chosen, it can be used as a sensitive vital stain for the detection of cytoplasmic lipid droplets by fluorescence microscopy and by flow cytofluorometry.[48,49]

When nile red is applied to cell preparations obtained from atherosclerotic aortas, many of the cells are seen to fluoresce intensely. These same cells are readily detected when analyzed with a Coulter EPICS V cell sorter. FIGURE 3 illustrates the differences in fluorescence intensity of the nile red stained cells isolated from an atherosclerotic rabbit aorta compared to the fluorescence intensity of nile red stained smooth muscle cells isolated from a control rabbit aorta. Although some of the cells derived from the atherosclerotic aorta are as dim as the control smooth muscle cells, the majority stain brightly, which indicates that they possess excessive deposits of lipid. The fluorescence distribution of these cells is very broad, showing that a continuous spectrum of cellular

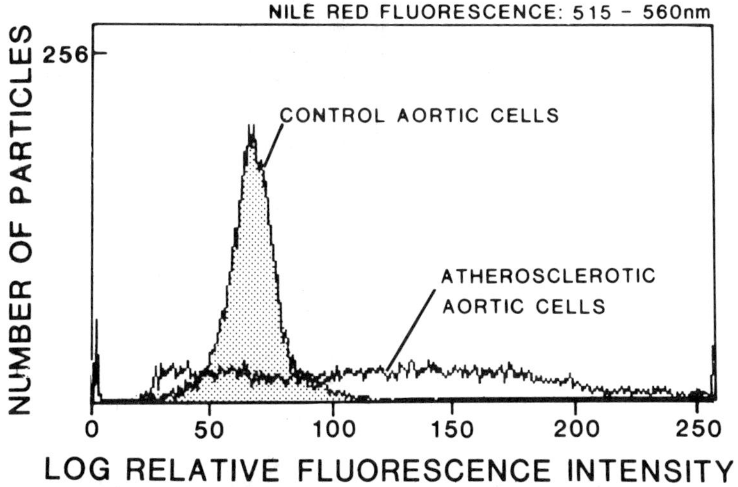

FIGURE 3. Flow cytofluorometric analysis of lipid overloading in diseased arterial cells. Cell preparations obtained by enzymic digestion of atherosclerotic or control rabbit aortas were treated with the fluorescent lipid stain nile red. The relative fluorescence intensities of cells in the two preparations are compared in the form of frequency distribution histograms. The ordinate is given as the log relative fluorescence intensity to indicate that the fluorescence signal was amplified logarithmically before analog to digital conversion.

lipid overloading is present. This observation confirms the results of Haley *et al.*[11] who analyzed similar preparations by density gradient centrifugation. As might be expected, the most lipid-rich cells detected by flow cytofluorometry were also found to be the largest cells of the entire population.

With nile red staining, the lipid-filled cells obtained by enzymic digestion of atherosclerotic arteries can be separated and purified by cell sorting. An example is illustrated in the experiment shown in FIGURE 4. The cell sorter was adjusted to sort and collect two populations: (1) the 33% most fluorescent nile red stained cells, and (2) the 33% least fluorescent nile red stained cells. After sorting, the two cell preparations were clearly distinguishable by their fluorescence profiles. When examined by microscopy, the sorted bright cells consisted only of extensively lipid loaded foam cells, while the sorted dim cells were composed of contracted smooth muscle cells bearing occasional lipid droplets (FIGURE 5). These studies were performed on freshly isolated living cells not exposed to fixatives. Thus, using this cell sorting technique, we can now further study a selected population of living, lipid-laden arterial cells.

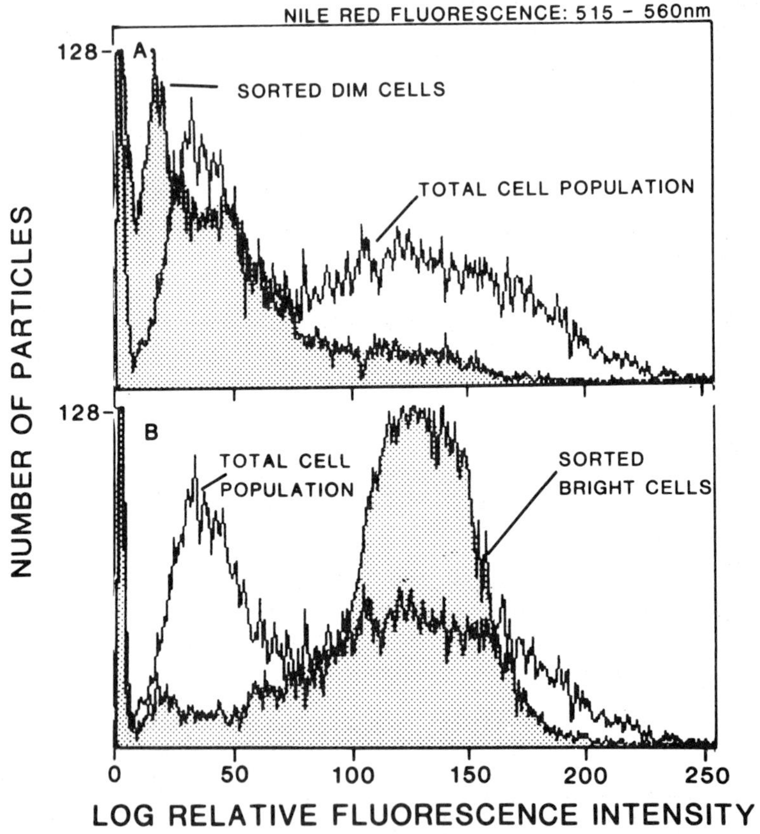

FIGURE 4. Cell sorting of enzymically isolated rabbit diseased aortic cells based on their relative lipid content. Sorting gates on the flow cytofluorometer were set to collect (A) the 33% least fluorescent nile red stained cells and, (B) the 33% most fluorescent nile red stained cells. The histograms, presented as in FIGURE 3, compare the fluorescence distributions of sorted dim and sorted bright cells with the initial unsorted cell preparation. The sorting was performed on freshly isolated, unfixed cells.

We are also employing various immunologic tests to identify cell types in the arterial cell preparations by flow cytofluorometry. In one study, enzymically isolated cells from an atherosclerotic rabbit aorta were incubated with C3 coated fluorescent bacteria and analyzed for C3 receptor-positive cells by flow cytofluorometry. The C3-positive cells (representing 17% of the total cell population in the study) were then separated by cell sorting and assessed for extent of lipid overloading using nile red

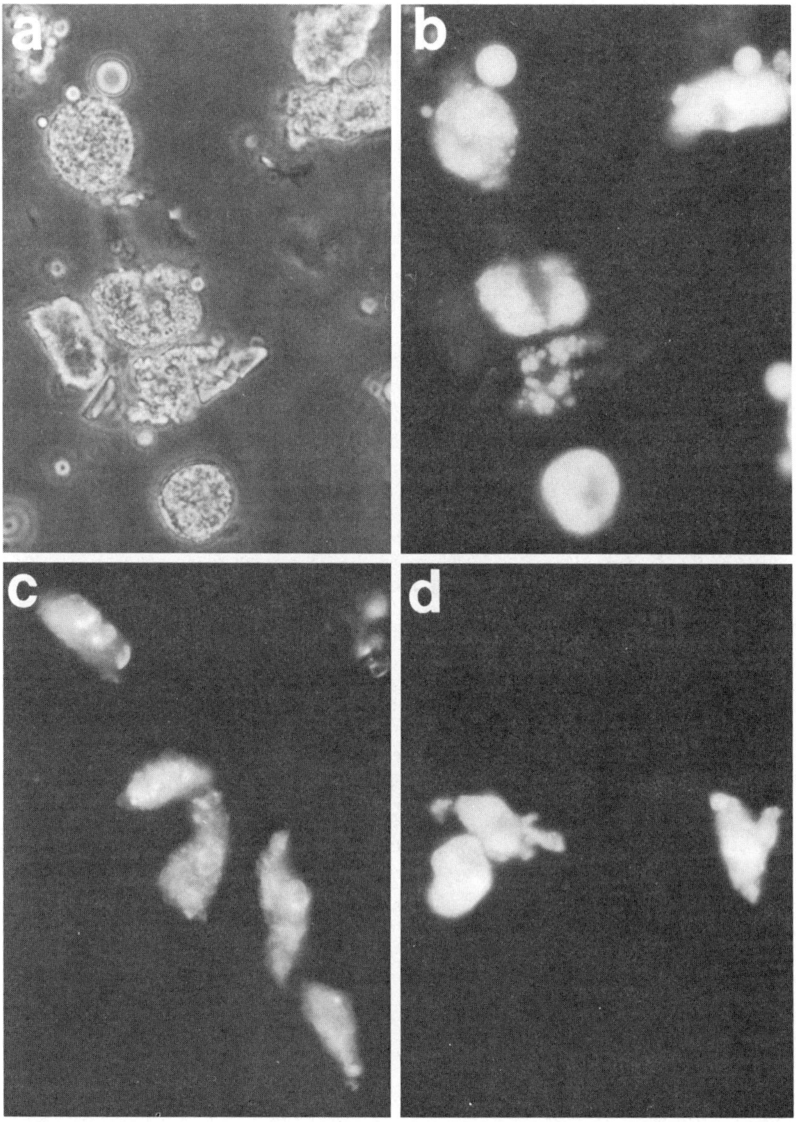

FIGURE 5. Identification of enzymically isolated rabbit diseased aortic cells sorted by flow cytofluorometry based on relative lipid content (FIGURE 4). Shown are the appearance of nile red stained presorted cells seen by (a) phase microscopy and (b) fluorescence microscopy (same field). The sorted dim cells (c) can be identified as contracted smooth muscle cells possessing occasional lipid droplets, while the sorted bright cells (d) are identified as lipid-laden arterial foam cells.

staining. Judged by the flow cytofluorometric analysis, the C3-positive cells represented the most intensely fluorescent cells in the preparation, and they were readily recognized as typical arterial foam cells by fluorescence microscopy. These results demonstrate that flow cytofluorometry is a useful technique for the further investigation of cellular heterogeneity in atherosclerotic arteries.

ACKNOWLEDGMENTS

The authors express their thanks to Ms. Indhira Handy, Susan Maness, and Rebecca Schwiebert for excellent technical assistance, and to Mrs. Dorothea Barwick for typing the manuscript. We are most grateful to Ms. Helen Shio, Rockefeller University, for preparing the electron micrographs shown in FIGURES 1 and 2.

REFERENCES

1. GEER, J. C. & M. D. HAUST. 1972. Smooth muscle cells in atherosclerosis. *In* Monographs on Atherosclerosis, vol. 2. O. J. Pollack, H. S. Simms & J. E. Kirk, Eds.: 1–137. S. Karger. Basel & New York.
2. IMAI, H., K. T. LEE, S. PASTORI, E. PANLILIO, R. FLORENTIN & W. A. THOMAS. 1966. Atherosclerosis in rabbits. Architectural and subcellular alterations of smooth muscle cells of aortas in response to hyperlipemia. Exp. Mol. Pathol. **5:** 273–310.
3. PARKER, F. & G. F. ODLAND. 1966. A correlative histochemical, biochemical, and electron microscopic study of experimental atherosclerosis in the rabbit aorta with special reference to the myo-intimal cell. Am. J. Pathol. **48:** 197–239.
4. GHIDONI, J. J. & R. M. O'NEAL. 1967. Recent advances in molecular pathology: A review. Ultrastructure of human atheroma. Exp. Mol. Pathol. **7:** 378–400.
5. SCOTT, R. F., R. JONES, A. S. DAOUD, O. ZUMBO, F. COULSTON & W. A. THOMAS. 1967. Experimental atherosclerosis in rhesus monkeys. II. Cellular elements of proliferative lesions and possible role of cytoplasmic degeneration in pathogenesis as studied by electron microscopy. Exp. Mol. Pathol. **7:** 34–57.
6. COOKSON, F. B. 1971. The origin of foam cells in atherosclerosis. Br. J. Exp. Pathol. **52:** 62–69.
7. STARY, H. C. 1976. Coronary artery fine structure in rhesus monkeys. The early atherosclerotic lesion and its progression. Prim. Med. **9:** 359–395.
8. GERRITY, R. G. 1981. The role of the monocyte in atherogenesis. I. Transition of blood-borne monocytes into foam cells in fatty lesions. Am. J. Pathol. **103:** 181–190.
9. FAGGIOTTO, A., R. ROSS & L. HARKER. 1984. Studies of hypercholesterolemia in the nonhuman primate. I. Changes that lead to fatty streak formation. Arteriosclerosis **4:** 323–340.
10. ROSS, R., T. N. WIGHT, E. STRANDNESS & B. THIELE. 1984. Human atherosclerosis. I. Cell constitution and characteristics of advanced lesions of the superficial femoral artery. Am. J. Pathol. **114:** 79–93.
11. HALEY, N. J., H. SHIO & S. FOWLER. 1977. Characterization of lipid-laden aortic cells from cholesterol-fed rabbits. I. Resolution of aortic cell populations by metrizamide density gradient centrifugation. Lab. Invest. **37:** 287–296.
12. FOWLER, S., P. A. BERBERIAN, H. SHIO, S. GOLDFISCHER & H. WOLINSKY. 1980. Characterization of cell populations isolated from aortas of rhesus monkeys with experimental atherosclerosis. Circ. Res. **46:** 520–530.
13. FOWLER, S., H. SHIO & N. J. HALEY. 1979. Characterization of lipid-laden aortic cells from cholesterol-fed rabbits. IV. Investigation of macrophage-like properties of aortic cell populations. Lab. Invest. **41:** 372–378.
14. SCHAFFNER, T., K. TAYLOR, E. J. BARTUCCI, K. FISCHER-DZOGA, J. H. BEESON, S. GLAGOV & R. W. WISSLER. 1980. Arterial foam cells with distinctive immunomorphologic and histochemical features of macrophages. Am. J. Pathol. **100:** 57–80.

15. PITAS, R. E., T. L. INNERARITY & R. W. MAHLEY. 1983. Foam cells in explants of atherosclerotic rabbit aortas have receptors for β-very low density lipoproteins and modified low density lipoproteins. Arteriosclerosis **3:** 2–12.
16. SPRARAGEN, S. C., A. R. GIORDANO, T. P. POON & H. HAMEL. 1969. Participation of circulating mononuclear cells in the genesis of atheromata. Circulation **40** (Suppl. III): 24.
17. BROWN, M. S., J. L. GOLDSTEIN, M. KRIEGER, Y. K. HO & R. G. W. ANDERSON. 1979. Reversible accumulation of cholesteryl esters in macrophages incubated with acetylated lipoproteins. J. Cell Biol. **82:** 597–613.
18. GOLDSTEIN, J. L., Y. K. HO, M. S. BROWN, T. L. INNERARITY & R. W. MAHLEY. 1980. Cholesteryl ester accumulation in macrophages resulting from receptor-mediated uptake and degradation of hypercholesterolemic canine β-very low density lipoproteins. J. Biol. Chem. **255:** 1839–1848.
19. GOLDSTEIN, J. L., H. F. HOFF, Y. K. HO, S. K. BASU & M. S. BROWN. 1981. Stimulation of cholesteryl ester synthesis in macrophages by extracts of atherosclerotic human aortas and complexes of albumin/cholesteryl esters. Arteriosclerosis **1:**210–226.
20. FALCONE, D. J., N. MATEO, H. SHIO, C. R. MINICK & S. D. FOWLER. 1984. Lipoprotein-heparin-fibronectin denatured collagen complexes enhance cholesteryl ester accumulation in macrophages. J. Cell. Biol. **99:** 1266–1274.
21. GOLDSTEIN, J. L., R. G. W. ANDERSON, L. M. BUJA, S. K. BASU & M. S. BROWN. 1977. Overloading human aortic smooth muscle cells with low density lipoprotein-cholesteryl esters reproduces features of atherosclerosis *in vitro*. J. Clin. Invest. **59:** 1196–1202.
22. VAN FURTH, R., Ed. 1980. Mononuclear phagocytes: Functional aspects. Martinus Nijhoff BV. The Hague, The Netherlands.
23. SHIO, H., N. J. HALEY & S. FOWLER. 1978. Characterization of lipid-laden aortic cells from cholesterol-fed rabbits. II. Morphometric analysis of lipid-filled lysosomes and lipid droplets in aortic cell populations. Lab. Invest. **39:** 390–397.
24. SHIO, H. N. J. HALEY & S. FOWLER. 1979. Characterization of lipid-laden aortic cells from cholesterol-fed rabbits. III. Intracellular localization of cholesterol and cholesteryl ester. Lab. Invest. **41:** 160–167.
25. NATHAN, C. F., H. W. MURRAY & Z. A. COHN. 1980. The macrophage as an effector cell. N. Engl. J. Med. **303:** 622–626.
26. TAKEMURA, R. & Z. WERB. 1984. Secretory products of macrophages and their physiological functions. Am. J. Physiol. **246:** C1–C9.
27. LEIBOVICH, S. J. & R. ROSS. 1976. A macrophage-dependent factor that stimulates the proliferation of fibroblasts in vitro. Am. J. Pathol. **84:** 501–514.
28. MARTIN, B. M., M. A. GIMBRONE, JR, E. R. UNANUE & R. S. COTRAN. 1981. Stimulation of nonlymphoid mesenchymal cell proliferation by a macrophage derived growth factor. J. Immunol. **126:** 1510–1515.
29. WERB, Z. & S. GORDON, 1975. Secretion of a specific collagenase by stimulated macrophages. J. Exp. Med. **142:** 346–360.
30. MAINARDI, C. L., J. M. SEYER & A. H. KANG. 1980. Type-specific collagenases. A type V collagen-degrading enzyme from macrophages. Biochem. Biophys. Res. Commun. **97:** 1108–1115.
31. WERB, Z. & S. GORDON. 1975. Elastase secretion by stimulated macrophages: characterization and regulation. J. Exp. Med. **142:** 361–377.
32. UNKELESS, J. C., S. GORDON & E. REICH. 1974. Secretion of plasminogen activator by stimulated macrophages. J. Exp. Med. **139:** 834–850.
33. SCHNYDER, J. & M. BAGGIOLINI. 1980. Secretion of lysosomal enzymes by macrophages. *In* Mononuclear Phagocytes: Functional Aspects. R. van Furth, Ed. Nijhoff B.V., The Hague, The Netherlands.
34. ALITALO, K., T. HOVI & A. VAHERI. 1980. Fibronectin is produced by human macrophages. J. Exp. Med. **151:** 602–613.
35. BASU, S. K., M. S. BROWN, Y. K. HO, R. J. HAVEL & J. L. GOLDSTEIN. 1981. Mouse macrophages synthesize and secrete a protein resembling apolipoprotein E. Proc. Natl. Acad. Sci. USA **78:** 7545–7549.
36. POLVERINI, P. J., R. S. COTRAN, M. A. GIMBRONE, JR. & E. R. UNANUE. 1977. Activated macrophages induce vascular proliferation. Nature London **269:** 804–806.

37. AALTO, M., M. POTILA & E. KULONEN. 1976. The effect of silica-treated macrophages on the synthesis of collagen and other proteins in vitro. Exp. Cell. Res. **97:** 193–202.
38. KHOO, J. C., E. M. MAHONEY & J. L. WITZTUM. 1981. Secretion of lipoprotein lipase by macrophages in culture. J. Biol. Chem. **256:** 7105–7108.
39. BENTLEY, C., B. ZIMMER & U. HADDING. 1981. The macrophage as a source of complement components. *In* Lymphokines, Vol. 4. E. Pick, Ed.: 197–230. Academic Press. New York.
40. JOHNSTON, R. B., JR. 1978. Oxygen metabolism and the microbicidal activity of macrophages. Federation Proc. 37: 2759–2764.
41. SOBERMAN, R. J. & M. L. KARNOVSKY. 1981. Biochemical properties of activated macrophages. *In* Lymphokines, Vol. 3. E. Pick, Ed.: 11–31. Academic Press. New York.
42. NATHAN, C. & Z. COHN. 1980. Role of oxygen-dependent mechanisms in antibody-induced lysis of tumor cells by activated macrophages. J. Exp. Med. **152:** 198–208.
43. GEMSA, D., M. SEITZ, W. KRAMER, G. TILL & K. RESCH. 1978. The effects of phagocytosis, dextran sulfate, and cell damage on PGE_1 sensitivity and PGE_1 production of macrophages. J. Immunol. **120:** 1187–1194.
44. ROUZER, C. A., W. A. SCOTT, Z. A. COHN, P. BLACKBURN & J. M. MANNING. 1980. Mouse peritoneal macrophages release leukotriene C in response to a phagocytic stimulus. Proc. Natl. Acad. Sci. USA. **77:** 4928–4932.
45. STENSON, W. F. & C. W. PARKER. 1980. Prostaglandins, macrophages, and immunity. J. Immunol. **125:** 1–5.
46. GOLDSTEIN, J. L. & M. S. BROWN. 1977. The low-density lipoprotein pathway and its relation to atherosclerosis. Ann. Rev. Biochem. **46:** 897–930.
47. BROWN, M. S. & J. L. GOLDSTEIN. 1983. Lipoprotein metabolism in the macrophage: Implications for cholesterol deposition in atherosclerosis. Ann. Rev. Biochem. **52:** 223–261.
48. GREENSPAN, P. & S. D. FOWLER. 1985. Spectrofluorometric studies of the lipid probe, nile red. J. Lipid Res. **26:** 781–789.
49. GREENSPAN, P. E. P. MAYER & S. D. FOWLER 1985. Nile red: A selective fluorescent stain for intracellular lipid droplets. J. Cell Biol. **100:** 965–973.

Foam Cell Characteristics in Coronary Arteries and Aortas of White Carneau Pigeons with Moderate Hypercholesterolemia[a]

JON C. LEWIS, RICHARD G. TAYLOR,
AND W. GRAY JEROME

Department of Pathology
Arteriosclerosis Research Center
Wake Forest University Medical Center
The Bowman Gray School of Medicine
Winston-Salem, North Carolina 27103

INTRODUCTION

Mild hypercholesterolemia of short duration has been associated with the formation of foam cell intimal lesions in a variety of animal models including pigs,[1] rabbits,[2] rats,[3] nonhuman primates,[4] and pigeons.[5–7] Concurrent with the initiation of foam cell lesions in many of these models is the adherence and apparent migration of blood monocytes into the involved intima.[1,3,5–7] These observations have led many investigators to suggest a blood monocyte origin for foam cells in early lesions, a suggestion which is consistent with the often reported mononuclear-macrophage ultrastucture.[1–4] Although mononuclear-macrophages may comprise a significant proportion of the cells in lesions with mild hypercholesterolemia, numerous investigators have also documented the contribution of smooth muscle cells to the foam cell population,[8–10] and recent evidence following cell isolation from the intima of hypercholesterolemic rabbits documents a multicellular character to lesion homogenates.[11,12] These observations raise questions about the kinetics of foam cell character and origin during lesion progression. Conceivably, as lesions progress, there occurs a shift in foam cells with mononuclear cells predominating during the early stages and smooth muscle cells becoming more prevalent as lesions age and become more biochemically and structurally complex.

Reported is a study of foam cell characteristics in aortic and coronary artery lesions of the hypercholesterolemic White Carneau pigeon. Through the correlative use of cytochemistry and morphometric analysis, we document both a shift in foam cell nature and structural complexity as lesions progress.

MATERIALS AND METHODS

White Carneau pigeons used in this study were obtained from a closed breeding colony at the Animal Resource Unit of Bowman Gray School of Medicine. Complete

[a]This work was supported by Specialized Center of Research in Arteriosclerosis (SCOR) Grant HL-14164 from the National Heart, Lung, and Blood Institute, and by National Research Service Award Institutional Grant HL-07115.

details of animal handling, diets, and processing tissues for microscopic analysis have been published,[5–7] but a brief description is given below for clarity.

All animals were entered into the study at the age of eight weeks when they began to receive a pigeon pellet diet supplemented with cholesterol. The levels of cholesterol in the diet ranged from 0.2 to 0.5% and resulted, over a twelve week course, in serum cholesterol levels above 450 mg/dl (normal cholesterol levels in the pigeon are in the range 200–250 mg/dl). The animals, following anesthesia, were necropsied by intraventricular perfusion with 2.5% glutaraldehyde buffered to pH 7.2 with 0.1 M sodium cacodylate. Tissues for transmission electron microscopy were further fixed in buffered, 1% osmium tetroxide, dehydrated through a series of ethanols and embedded in epoxy resin. Thin sections were double stained with lead citrate and uranyl acetate, and observed in Philips EM-400 microscope. Typically, sections were first obtained at the lesion developing edge. The blocks were then serially sectioned into older (more advanced) portions of the lesion. This approach was possible in the pigeons since both the site of lesion origin and the direction and rate of progression have been well characterized. Scanning electron microscopy samples were dehydrated through the ethanol series, dried from CO_2 by the critical point method, and sputter coated with gold:palladium prior to observation in a Philips SEM-500. Lysosomal enzyme cytochemistry, as an indication of foam cell complexity, was carried out by a modification of the Gomori reaction.[13] Tissues for cytochemistry, subsequent to initial fixation, were washed extensively on ice in cacodylate buffer (0.1 M, pH 7.2) containing sucrose (2–5%). The cytochemical reaction, carried out at 37°C for one hour in Tris buffer containing β-glycerophosphate as a substrate and lead as the capture ion, was followed by staining en bloc with uranyl acetate. Embedding and sectioning were as described above. However, sections for cytochemistry were observed and photographed without on-grid staining.

Foam cell identity during the early stages of hypercholesterolemia was established using autoradiography to identify tritium labeled mononuclear cells in arterial lesions. The experiment was carried out through the use of parentally matched pairs of animals, all of which had been maintained on the cholesterol supplemented diet as described above. In the study, one member of each pair was designated donor and received multiple infusions of tritiated thymidine. Thymidine infusion was followed by stress bleeding to induce blood cell formation. Four such cycles, carried out over a period of ten days, resulted in radiolabeling of approximately 90% of the donor blood cells. Throughout the labeling cycle, leukocytes were harvested from the donor animals using differential centrifugation, washed to remove plasma proteins, and infused into the second member of each matched pair (recipient bird). Each recipient animal received approximately 25×10^6 radiolabeled cells. The half-life for the labeled cells in the recipients was four days, a period sufficient for potential interaction with the artery wall. The animals were necropsied as described above, the tissues were then processed for transmission electron microscopy, and subsequent to lesion sectioning, the grids were coated with Illford L-4 emulsion for autoradiography.[14]

Morphometric analysis of all electron micrographs was accomplished using standard point count techniques.[6,14]

RESULTS

Atherosclerosis in the aorta and coronary arteries of the hypercholesterolemic pigeon occurred at predictable locations where, as observed by scanning electron microscopy, the lesions protruded into the luminal space. Typically, the lesion and nonlesion areas were clearly delineated, resulting in a well-defined interface between the two regions (FIGURE 1). A distinctive feature of the interface region, referred to as the lesion edge, was the concentration of leukocytes. As summarized in TABLE 1, adherent leukocytes were found in all arteries. However, the density of these cells was significantly increased over lesion areas, with dramatically enhanced adhesion at the lesion edge.

Early lesions in the pigeons were primarily foam cell in nature, and were characterized by the lipid-filled cells positioned between an intact endothelium on one side and the internal elastic lamina on the other side (FIGURE 2). Within the expanded intima, foam cells occupied the majority of the volume, with extracellular matrix accounting for less than 10%. Smooth muscle cells were rarely observed in the early lesions of either the aorta or the coronary artery, and several ultrastructural characteristics suggested a macrophage origin for the foam cells. Prominent among these features were the characteristic macrophage-like nucleus, the frequent presence of cytoplasmic granules and numerous residual lysosomes, and the conspicuous absence of a basement membrane (FIGURE 2). In order to determine whether the foam cells were of monocyte/macrophage origin, autoradiography was done on the arteries from birds which had received radiolabeled leukocytes. As exemplified in FIGURE 3, radioisotope in the leukocytes harvested from the donors and infused into the recipients was predominantly in cell nuclei, with 95% of the silver grains specifically located to the nucleus and 100% of the grains within one-half grain radius of the nucleus. On arterial sections from both coronaries and aortas of the recipient birds, silver grains were consistently found within foam cell lesions. Specificity of label location was established through morphometric analysis, and by this approach, 95% of all grains in the autoradiograms have been located over the lesion regions. Adjacent nonlesion regions in the same tissue sections had grain counts at background levels. TABLE 2 summarizes data obtained from three separate labeling experiments, and as noted within the recipient bird arteries, 66% of all label was located in foam cells. This represented approximately eight grains per foam cell, a level which exceeds that found for other cell types.

Although early lesions and the developing edge of large lesions were primarily lipid-filled monocyte/macrophage foam cells, the composition of older lesion regions was more complex, consisting of increased extracellular matrix and the presence of lipid-containing smooth muscle cells (FIGURE 4). When morphometrically analyzed, it was found that foam cells accounted for approximately 60% of mature lesion volume, and smooth muscle cells comprised another 25%. Smooth muscle cells, as already noted, were not identified in small early lesions; and, at the developing edge of mature lesions, these cells accounted for less than 5% of the intimal volume.

This shift in cellularity with lesion maturation was accompanied by an intracellular redistribution of lipid and a change in lysosomal complexity (FIGURE 5). Intracellular lipid in the macrophage foam cells of early lesions accounted for approximately 80% of total cell volume and of this lipid, 88% was cytoplasmic. In these early lesions and at the developing edge of mature lesions, the remaining 12% of the lipid was in acid phosphatase positive lysosomes. There was not a dramatic change in the total percent of cell volume occupied by lipid in foam cells of more mature lesions; however, in marked contrast to the early lesions, the lipid in the mature lesion regions was 66% lysosomal and 34% cytoplasmic. Differences of a consistent nature were not noted in the location of lipid in either non-foam cell macrophages or smooth muscle cells.

DISCUSSION

Blood monocytes have been observed on the luminal surface and in intimal lesions from a variety of species including young humans who have come to autopsy, and it has been suggested that these cells are precursors for foam cells in early atherosclerosis.[1-7]

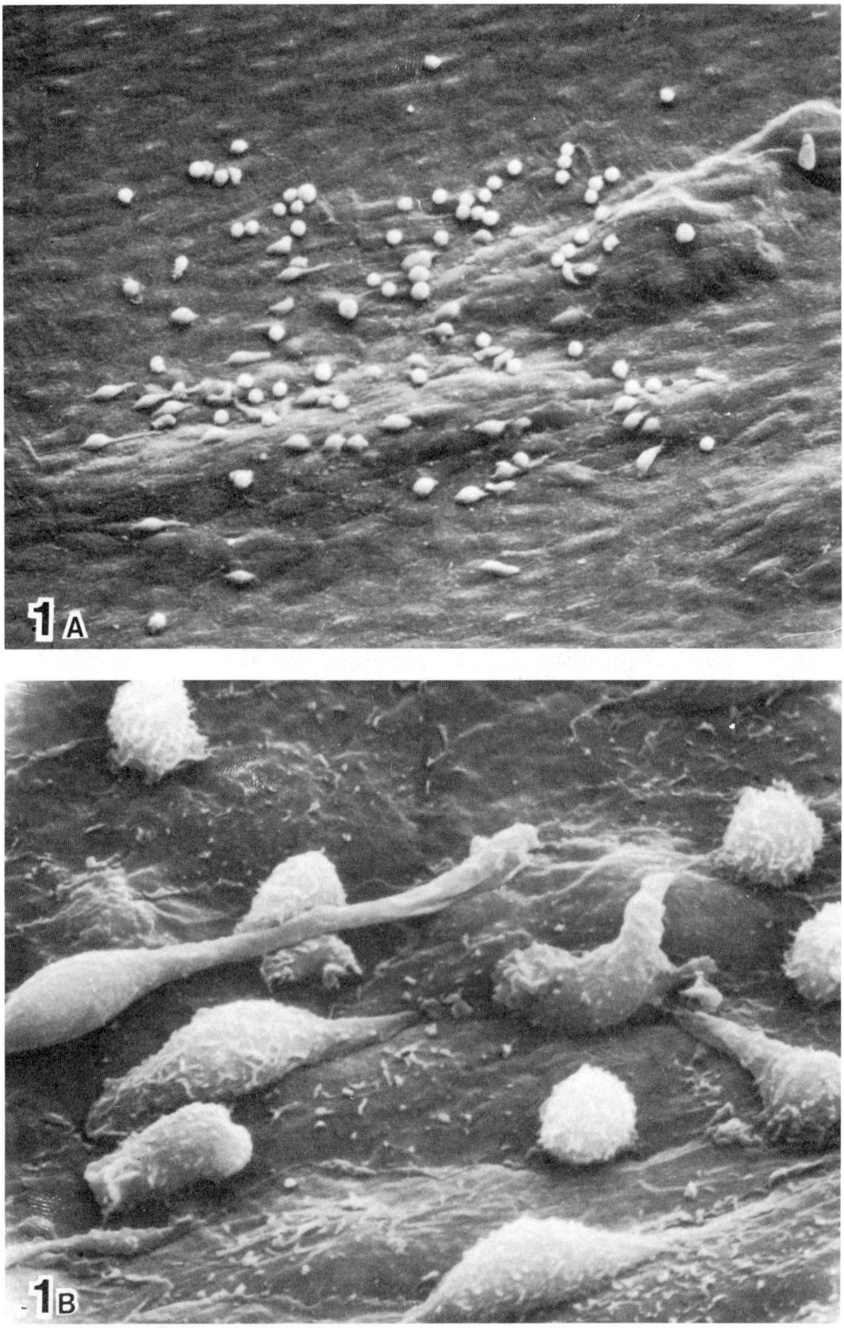

FIGURE 1. Scanning electron micrographs of the luminal surface of the coronary artery in a hypercholesterolemic pigeon. A. Leukocytes are shown focally adherent to small lesions which protrude into the vessel lumen. (×500). B. High magnification micrograph of the adherent leukocytes illustrating the "migratory" morphology of these cells. (×5500).

TABLE 1. Leukocyte Density[a] on Pigeon Arteries

	Region of Artery		
	Nonlesion	Lesion	Lesion Edge
Coronary Artery	35	150	575
Aorta	200	960	2240

[a]Density is shown as cells/mm^2. Data based upon morphometric analysis of coronary arteries from 50 animals and aortas from 80 animals.

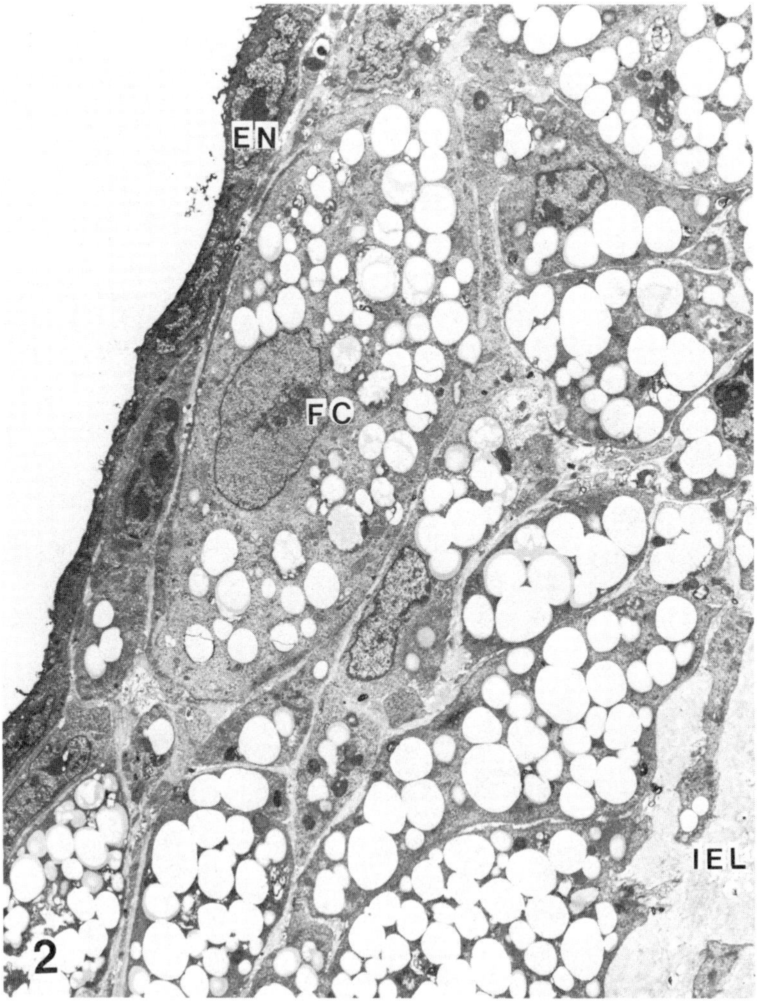

FIGURE 2. Transmission electron micrograph through an early coronary lesion in the hypercholesterolemic pigeon. Numerous macrophage-like foam cells (FC) are shown between the intact endothelium (EN) and the underlying internal elastic lamina (IEL). (×3900).

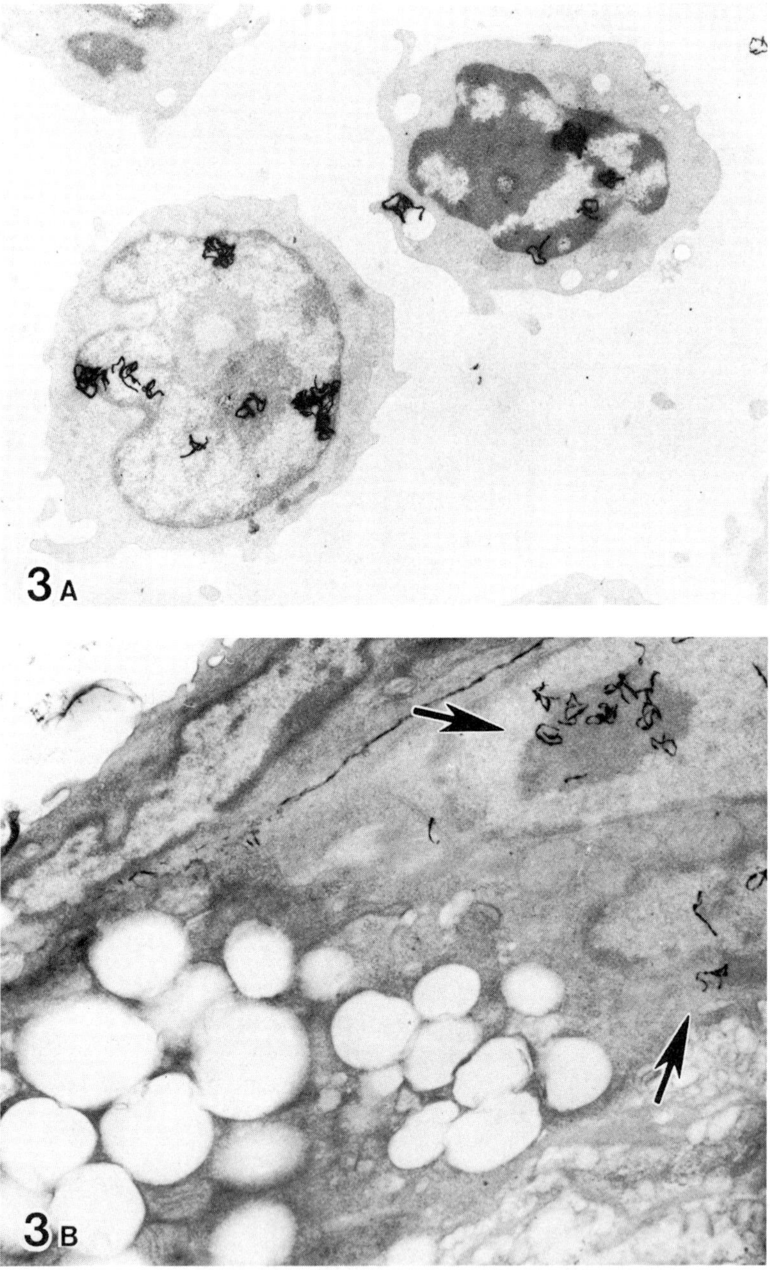

FIGURE 3. Autoradiographs of blood cells and the artery wall following thymidine infusion. A. Leukocytes harvested from a donor bird for infusion into a recipient animal. As anticipated, all silver grains are in the nuclei prior to infusion. (×10,500). B. Select region of a foam cell lesion illustrating thymidine label (arrows) in the nucleus of a lipid filled macrophage-like cell. (×16,000).

TABLE 2. ^{3}H-Thymidine Distribution in Lesions

	Grain Distribution by Percent	Grain Density (grains/cell section)
Foam Cells	66	7.9
Smooth Muscle	21	1.6
Endothelium	13	2.5

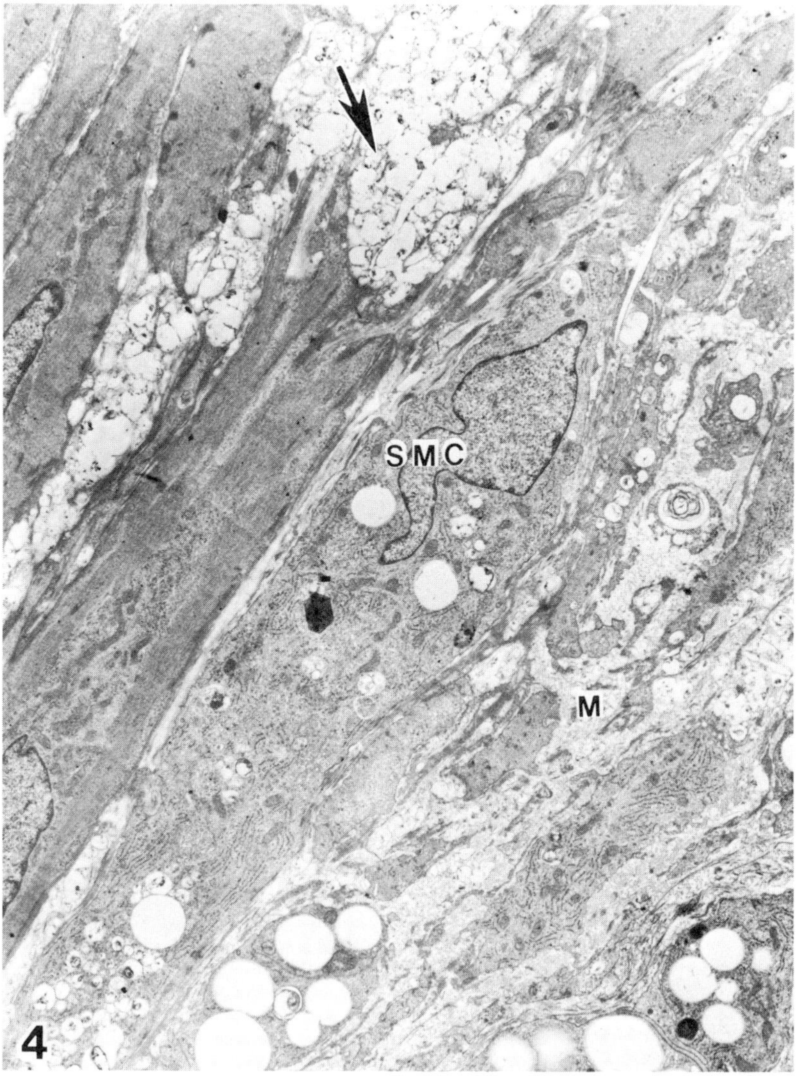

FIGURE 4. Select region of an advance lesion in the hypercholesterolemic pigeon. Note that in addition to the macrophage foam cells illustrated in FIGURE 2, the more advanced lesions contain lipid filled smooth muscle cells (SMC) and extensive extracellar lipid (arrow) enmeshed in a complex matrix (M). (×6500).

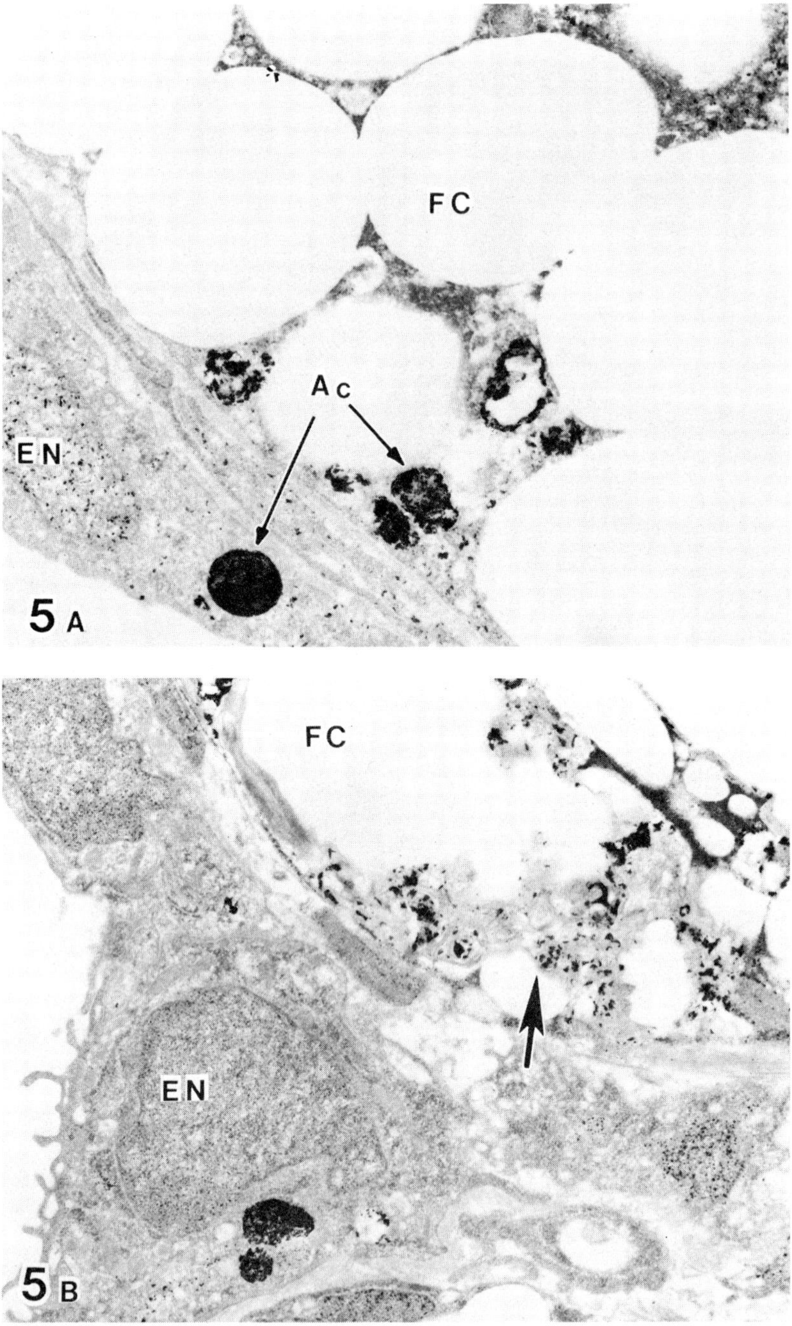

FIGURE 5. Acid phosphatase reaction in atherosclerotic pigeon coronary arteries. A. Early foam cell region of a lesion with lipid, primarily cytoplasmic. Acid phosphatase reaction produce (Ac) is restricted to discrete lysosomes in both the foam cell (FC) and the endothelium (EC). (×14,000). B. Advanced lesion region with foam cell (FC) lipid contained in a complex acid phosphatase positive lysosome (arrow). Reaction product in the endothelium (EN) is contained within discrete lysosomes. (×17,500).

This suggestion is consistent with *in vitro* studies documenting lipid accumulation in cultured monocytes,[15] and with the numerous observations of monocytes penetrating the endothelial surface.[2,3,6] Although several lines of investigation have implicated monocytes as foam cell precursors, direct evidence linking the two has been limited. Spraragen and associates reported, in 1966, a pioneering experiment in which radiolabeled leukocytes were tracked into developing lesions in the hypercholesterolemic rabbit.[16] An approach similar to that reported by these earlier workers was used in the present study, which established a monocyte identity for foam cells in early hypercholesterolemic lesions in the pigeon.

The involvement of monocytes appears to continue as lesions progress, but with more advanced lesions, blood cell adherence and probably penetration into the intima was greatest at the lesion edge. In the aorta, the area of greatest leukocyte interaction was the superior edge, which has been established in two separate studies as the primary region of lesion development.[17,6] Interestingly, the area of leukocyte adherence corresponds to that in which enhanced endothelial turnover has been identified in the pigeon.[19] The relationship between these two events, though, has not been established. However, recent *in vitro* studies have demonstrated enhanced monocyte adhesion to the wound edge of experimentally disrupted endothelial monolayers,[20] and Ooi *et al.* have recently reported monocyte modulation of human endothelial cell proliferation *in vitro*.[21] Conceivably, alterations in endothelial cells at the lesion edge result in focally enhanced adhesion, which could in turn contribute as a modulator of subsequent endothelial proliferation. Alternatively, the blood monocytes may be responding to chemoattractants produced by the artery wall. Such activity has been isolated from aortic lesions of hypercholesterolemic swine,[22] and preliminary studies in our laboratory suggest a similar activity from aortic lesions in the White Carneau pigeon.[23] Lesion derived chemoattractants would explain monocyte penetration into the intima, but they will not explain the highly focal nature of monocyte adhesion as noted in the present and previous reports.[6,7,19]

Whatever the nature of monocyte involvement at the luminal surface, it is clear that these cells contribute significantly to early lesion foam cells. This contribution, though, appears to be less significant in more advanced lesions. Based upon serial section analysis, as summarized in the present report, the composition of more advanced regions is complex, involving both macrophage and smooth muscle foam cells.[24] The time frame for this transition is relatively short; for in the studies reported, the animals had been hypercholesterolemic for only twelve weeks at the time of necropsy. Morphometric analysis of aortic lesions has established the rate of lesion progression at 100–150 μM per week.[6,17,18] Using this estimate, total lesion expansion during the course of the present study was approximately 1.0 mm, indicating that, as in the case of time, very little size change was needed to shift the cellular and ultrastructural composition of lesions. Both the complex cellularity and the alteration in locale of intracellular lipid reported in this study are consistent with reports of others.[11,12] This suggests, at the cellular level, that atherosclerotic arteries are undergoing constant cellular as well as biochemical change.

REFERENCES

1. GERRITY, R. G., H. K. NAITO, M. RICHARDSON & C. J. SCHWARTZ. 1979. Dietary induced atherogenesis in swine. Morphology of the intima in pre-lesion stages. Am. J. Pathol. **95:** 775–792.
2. POOLE, J. C. & H. W. FLOREY. 1958. Changes in the endothelium of the aorta and the behavior of macrophages in experimental atheroma of rabbits. J. Pathol. Bacterol. 75:245–251.

3. JORIS, I., T. ZAND, J. J. NUNNARI, F. J. KROLIKOWSKI & G. MAJNO. 1983. Studies on the pathogenesis of atherosclerosis. I. Adhesion and emigration of mononuclear cells in the aorta of hypercholesterolemic rats. Am. J. Pathol. **113:** 341–358.
4. STARY, H. C. 1976. Coronary artery fine structure in rhesus monkeys: The early atherosclerotic lesion and its progression. Primates Med. **9:** 359–395.
5. LEWIS, J. C., R. G. TAYLOR, N. D. JONES & D. GRIMES. 1979. Vascular endothelium in pigeon coronary atherosclerosis. Scan. Electron Microsc. **3:** 823–828.
6. JEROME, W. G. & J. C. LEWIS. 1984. Early atherogenesis in White Carneau pigeons. I. Leukocyte margination and endothelial alterations at the celiac bifurcation. Am. J. Pathol. **116:** 56–68.
7. LEWIS, J. C., R. G. TAYLOR, N. D. JONES, R. W. ST. CLAIR & J. F. CORNHILL. 1982. Endothelial surface characteristics in pigeon coronary artery atherosclerosis. I. Cellular alterations during the initial stages of dietary cholesterol challlenge. Lab. Invest. **46:** 123–138.
8. THOMAS, W. A., J. M. REINER, R. A. FLORENTIN, R. F. SCOTT, K. T. LEE & K. JANAKIDEVI. 1980. Population dynamics of arterial cells in atherogenesis. Biochem. of Disease **9:** 111–119.
9. GEER, J. C., H. C. MCGILL, JR. & J. P. STRONG. 1961. The fine structure of human atherosclerotic lesions. Am. J. Patho. **38:** 263–287.
10. GATON, E. & M. WOLMAN. 1977. The role of smooth muscle cells and hematogenous macrophages in atheroma. J. Pathol. **123:** 123–128.
11. SHIO, H., N. J. HALEY & S. FOWLER. 1978. Characterization of lipid-laden aortic cells from cholesterol-fed rabbits. II. Morphometric analysis of lipid-filled lysosomes and lipid droplets in aortic cell populations. Lab. Invest. **39:** 390–397.
12. SHIO, H., N. J. HALEY & S. FOWLER. 1979. Characterization of lipid-laden aortic cells from cholesterol-fed rabbits. III. Intracellular localization of cholesterol and cholesteryl ester. Lab. Invest. **41:** 160–167.
13. BASS, D. A., J. C. LEWIS, P. SZEJDA, L. COWLEY & C. E. MCCALL. 1981. Activation of lysosomal acid phosphatase of eosinophil leukocytes. Lab. Invest. **44:** 403–409.
14. LEWIS, J. C. 1979. 5-hydroxytryptamine storage in pigeon thrombocytes: A biochemical and electron microscopic autoradiography study. J. Submicrosc. Cytol. **11:** 345–352.
15. VAN LENTEN, B. J., A. M. FOGELMAN, M. M. HOKOM, L. BENSON, M. E. HABERLAND & P. A. EDWARDS. 1983. Regulation of the uptake and degradation of β -very low density lipoprotein in human monocyte macrophages. J. Biol. Chem. **258:** 5151–5157.
16. SPRARAGEN, S. C., A. R. GIORDANO, T. P. POON & H. HAMEL. 1969. Participation of circulating mononuclear cells in the genesis of atheromata. Circulation **39–40**(Suppl.): III–24.
17. BUSOWSKI, J. D. 1980. Aortic endothelial surface changes during initiation and progession of atheroclerosis. Master's Thesis, Bowman Gray School of Medicine of Wake Forest Univeristy.
18. HUBBARD, K. L. 1979. The time course of diet-exacerbated atherogenesis in a strain of White Carneau pigeon bred for enhanced susceptibility to atherosclerosis. Master's Thesis, Bowman Gray School of Medicine of Wake Forest University.
19. JEROME, W. G., J. C. LEWIS, R. G. TAYLOR & M. S. WHITE. 1983. Concurrent endothelial cell turnover and leukocyte margination in early atherosclerosis. Scan Electron Microsc. **3:** 1453–1459.
20. DICORLETO, P. E. & C. A. DELAMOTTE. 1984. Characterization of the adhesion of the human monocyte cell line U9377 to cultured endothelial cells. Arteriosclerosis **4:** 536a.
21. OOI, B. S., E. P. MACCARTHY, H. ANGELA & Y. M. OOI. 1983. Human mononuclear cell modulation of endothelial cell proliferation. J. Lab. Clin. Med. **102:** 428—433.
22. GERRITY, R. G. & J. A. GOSS. 1983. A monocyte chemotactic factor from lesion-prone areas of swine aorta. Circulation **68:** III-301.
23. DENHOLM, E. M., J. C. LEWIS, R. G. GERRITY & W. G. JEROME. 1983. Monocyte (MC) migration induced by lesion homogenates from atherosclerotic aortas of White Carneau (WC) pigeons. J. Cell Biol. **97**(Pt 2): 423a.
24. JEROME, W. G. & J. C. LEWIS. 1985. Early atherogenesis in White Carneau pigeons. II. Ultrastructural and cytochemical observations. Am. J. Pathol. **119:** 210–222.

Role of Macrophages in Regression of Atherosclerosis

ASSAAD S. DAOUD, KATHERINE E. FRITZ, JOHN JARMOLYCH, AND ADRIENNE S. FRANK

Department of Pathology
Albany Medical College
and
VA Medical Center
Albany, New York 12208

There is only a small body of experimental work pertaining to the prevalence and activities of macrophages during a regression regimen. The presence of macrophages during regression was reported by several investigators including Drs. Wissler, Stary, Tucker, and our group. Stary[1] reported that, in early, fatty streak-like atherosclerotic lesions of the rhesus monkey, there was a rapid decrease in the number of "macrophage-derived foam cells" within four to six months after imposition of a regression diet. He attributed this decrease to death of these cells. Tucker *et al.*[2] showed, electron microscopically, a dramatic decrease in the number of "lipid-laden macrophages" in the aortic intimal lesions after a four-month regression regimen. Our interest in macrophages in regression stems from an experiment,[3,4] in which we sequentially studied a number of morphological and biochemical changes occurring in swine aortic atherosclerosis during the course of a 14-month regression regimen.

MORPHOLOGICAL AND BIOCHEMICAL CHANGES OF ATHEROSCLEROTIC LESIONS DURING REGRESSION

Advanced aortic atherosclerosis was produced in Yorkshire swine by a hyperlipidemic diet following denudation of the abdominal aorta with a balloon catheter. The reference group was sacrificed after six months of cholesterol feeding. The regression groups were killed at six weeks, five months, and 14 months after withdrawal of the atherogenic diet. There were also mash-fed controls for each of the above groups. The morphologic features of the baseline lesions consisted of central necrosis, often with calcification and a fibrous cap. In and around the necrosis, there were large numbers of foam cells. Also present around and within the necrotic foci were round or oval mononuclear cells, with eosinophilic cytoplasms. Electron microscopy of these round, mononuclear cells disclosed many of the features of macrophages, including microvilli, a large Golgi apparatus, and lysosome-like structures.

The six-week regression lesions differed from the corresponding reference group lesions in that they were characterized by a somwhat thicker fibrous cap, more calcification, a decrease in the number of foam cells, and a marked increase in the number of macrophage-like cells. In many instances, the latter formed sheets of cells that filled the entire necrotic portion of the atheroma.

In the five-month regression lesions, there was a marked decrease in the number of foam cells and a thick fibrous cap was present. The macrophage-like cells were much less numerous than at six weeks of regression; their number was below that of the reference group. In these lesions, macrophages were also associated with necrosis or calcification. Necrosis had either disappeared, being replaced by loose fibrous stroma, or had markedly decreased, when compared with the reference or six-week regression lesions. The residual necrosis was mainly present around calcium deposits, which were more extensive and dense than in the above two groups. The lesions from the 14-month regression group appeared more flattened than in the other groups. Histologically, there was a virtual absence of foam cells, a further decrease in the size of the necrotic foci, and an increase in the thickness and density of the fibrous caps. The macrophage-like cells were present only around the necrotic or calcified areas. Calcium deposits appeared more dense than those of the other groups.

Quantitative assessments showed that there was a significant decrease in both sudanophilia and necrosis in the aortas of the five- and 14-month regression swine. There was also a gradual decrease in the number of foam cells of the reference lesions compared to those of the 14-month regression group. The macrophage-like cells were most abundant in the six-week regression lesions; subsequently, they decreased in

TABLE 1. Morphologic and Biochemical Results from Swine Sequential Study

Features Studied	Reference	6 Wks Regression	5 Mos Regression	14 Mos Regression
Lesion Thickness / Media Thickness	1.27	1.27	0.88	1.22
Cholesterol Concentration (μg/mg dry wt.) Total / Esterified	107.8 / 74.5	63.5 / 50.0	53.0 / 26.1[a]	55.8 / 27.6
DNA Concentration (μg/mg dry wt.)	3.3	3.6	2.7	2.4[a]
DNA Synthesis DPM ^{3}H-Thymidine / μg DNA	2,302	3,776	1108	290[a]
Calcium (μg/mg dry wt.)	9.1	55.5	87.2[a]	128.6[a]

[a]Significantly different from reference value.

number. There was no significant change in the ratio of the thickness of the lesion to the average thickness of the media (TABLE 1).

Biochemically (TABLE 1), there were no significant differences between the reference group lesions and those of the six-week regression animals, although a considerable numerical drop in free, esterified and total cholesterol was noted at this time. By five months, DNA concentration and esterified cholesterol concentration and synthesis had significantly decreased; the concentrations, esterified and free cholesterol, were approximately equal. Collagen synthesis, however, was increased. By fourteen months, synthesis of DNA and total protein had reached mash-fed control levels, but the concentrations of cholesterol, phospholipids, and triglycerides were still substantially elevated. Calcium concentration showed a gradual and significant increase from the reference to the 14-month regression swine.

In summary, this sequential study demonstrated that among the earliest changes during regression are the gradual disappearance of necrosis, decrease in cholesteryl ester and DNA concentration, and increase in calcification. These changes were accompanied by changes in the number of macrophages which were mainly present around necrotic areas or calcific foci.

MACROPHAGE FUNCTIONS WHICH MAY RELATE TO REGRESSION

The documented functions of macrophages are numerous, varied, and wide-ranging. For example, they are "professional phagocytes" and, as such, can be actively involved in the removal of particulate matter such as necrotic debris. They will even phagocytize mineralized calcium.[5] Under varying circumstances, they have been known to synthesize collagen and glycosaminoglycans (GAG),[6] as well as proteinases which will degrade the major extracellular components of the artery wall.[7] They secrete an impressive array of other substances: complement components and acid hydrolases,[8] peroxidase, superoxide dismutase, enzyme inhibitors, and chemotactic factors.[9] Of special interest, with respect to their role in atherosclerosis, is their secretion of a growth factor which stimulates proliferation of both smooth muscle cells (SMC) and endothelial cells,[10,11] and of fibronectin,[12] a protein involved in cell adhesion and in nonimmune opsonization of particles for phagocytosis.

Also important in atherogenesis, is the macrophage's assumed role as a major source of foam cells by entering the arterial wall carrying a large complement of plasma-derived lipid,[13–16] or as suggested by Gerrity,[17] that blood-borne monocytes migrate into lesion-prone areas of the blood vessels in the early phase of hypercholesterolemia and become foam cells by accumulating large amounts of lipid by phagocytosis. Also, of possible importance in the transformation of macrophages to foam cells, is the fact that β-VLDL and chemically-modified lipoproteins are capable of delivering large quantities of cholesteryl esters to macrophages via a high affinity, receptor-mediated uptake process.[8,21]

In considering the contribution of macrophages to the regression process, it is obvious that many of the same potential functions must be considered. Because of their phagocytic capacity, they may be acting as scavengers of particulate matter, whether of cellular or extracellular origin. They may even be involved in the resolution of calcium deposit, since it has been reported that they will phagocytize mineralized calcium.[5] This function may be enhanced by the macrophage's own production of fibronectin, which, with its affinity sites for collagen, fibrin, glycosaminoglycan, and cell membranes, serves as an effective "nonspecific" opsonin.[22,23] The internalized debris may be removed from the arterial wall or digested by the macrophage lysosomal enzymes. Gerrity[24] has shown that "lipid-laden" foam cells, presumably macrophages which became phagocytic and accumulated lipid, migrate back into the blood stream by crossing the arterial endothelium. However, Stary[25] has not found any evidence of macrophage migration during regression. It should be remembered here that this phagocytic capability may be a cause of lipid accumulation and formation of foam cells.

The extensive complement of hydrolytic enzymes may also aid in the resolution of necrosis by degradation of cellular and extracellular substance-derived debris to soluble, and thus diffusible, components. Yet this same hydrolytic capacity, if directed toward normal arterial wall components, might equally contribute to their disorganization and degradation typical of lesion development.

The overall effect of the production of collagen and GAG may be debatable. The accumulation of collagen is viewed by some as an unfortunate sequela of atherogenesis, but by others as part of a healing process. Likewise, the secretion of GAG may help restore normal arterial composition. On the other hand, depending on the type and quantity of GAG produced, there may be an enhanced retention of low density lipoprotein in the lesion through the documented affinity of this lipoprotein for several species of GAG.[26] In addition, the overproduction of the extracellular substance can add to the volume of the lesion. The same is true for the production of the endothelial and smooth muscle cell mitogens. In appropriate amounts, they may speed the repair of denuded endothelium and the healing of necrosis within the lesion, while an excess of the SMC mitogen can add to the lesion volume.

The possible effects of the macrophage in its role as an effector cell in the immune response have not been considered. Yet, it is well established that active immunization, as with *Bacillus Calmette-Guerin* (BCG), will result in nonspecific enhancement of many of the previously mentioned functions of macrophages. This can occur on a systemic basis, or in localized areas of antigen accumulation. The degree of such enhancement of "activation" of lesion macrophages is not known. Yet, they may, indeed, reflect the immune status of the host. The possibility of manipulating the overall immune reactivity of an individual as a means of modulating the activity of lesion macrophages is intriguing. It should be noted that such an approach has been reported to be effective in cancer therapy.[27] On a more localized level, an activation of lesion macrophages could result from the presence of immune complexes. The demonstration, in experimental lesions, of the components of circulating immune complexes resulting from a single episode of serum sickness,[28] raises the possibility of macrophage activation via binding of the Fc fragment of the immunoglobulin, perhaps through the involvement of C_3 derived either from the plasma or secreted by the lesion macrophages themselves. Perhaps an even more likely source of an immune complex within a lesion would be an altered arterial wall component to which a plasma-derived autoantibody had been bound. The presence of autoantibodies which bind selectively to aortic lesions, but not to adjacent normal aortic tissue, has been reported.[29] Such insoluble complexes, with C_3, might prove to be chemotactic, as well as activators for macrophages.

So far, we have been considering only functions of macrophages for which a relatively direct association with lesion components can be postulated. However, other products, such as peroxidase, superoxide dismutase, chemotactic factors,[9] and complement components[8] may affect the regression process.

From the above, it is obvious that the role of macrophages in regression may be very complex and a comprehensive study of such is unattainable by a single experiment by one or a small group of investigators. However, the results of the sequential study in swine[3,4] suggest that the contribution of these cells during the regression process may be both positive and negative. The fact that macrophages were present in large numbers concomitantly with a biochemically defined decrease in cholesterol concentration and a decrease in the number of foam cells indicates that they may be responsible for the removal of cholesterol from the atheroma. Their prominence when necrosis was most marked and their proximity to necrotic areas, combined with the parallel decrease in their number and amount of necrosis, suggest a role for them in the resolution of necrosis. On the other hand, the close association of macrophages and calcification during the regression period suggests that these cells may be responsible, at least in part, for the deposition of calcium within the atheroma, in spite of their reported capability of phagocytizing this mineralized element.

For the last few years, our laboratory has been involved in studying the role of macrophages in calcification and in the removal of necrosis. As far as the latter is concerned, our working hypothesis was that macrophages are responsible for the removal of necrotic debris by either phagocytosis or hydrolytic enzymatic digestion, or both. In other words, the hypothesis depicts the macrophage as a "friend." For this hypothesis to be valid, macrophages in the regressing lesion should be actively phagocytic and they should be, at least, the major source of hydrolytic enzymes.

To establish the phagocytic activity of the lesion macrophages, the technique of releasing lesion cells by mechanical teasing, as described by Schaffner *et al.*,[30] was adapted to swine lesions. We have been able to isolate macrophages from well-minced lesions, allow them to adhere to glass, and demonstrate their ability to phagocytize yeast by incubating them at 37°C in the presence of *Saccharomyces cerevisiae,* which has been opsonized by exposure to either fresh human or fresh swine sera. The glass adherent cells were found to internalize varying numbers of yeast cells (FIGURE 1). Attempts to quantitate the phagocytic potential of cells derived from lesions of animals under various regimens, using the principle of dye exclusion by vital cells at the termination of the incubation period, proved unsatisfactory for two reasons. First, the heavily lipid-laden cells proved both fragile and, in most cases, failed to adhere to glass.

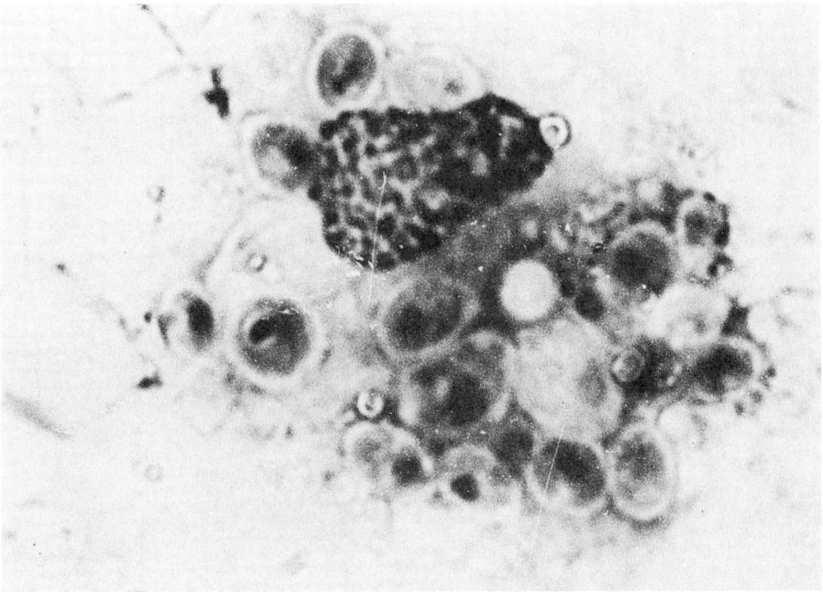

FIGURE 1. A glass-adherent cell, presumably a macrophage, from our experimentally-diet-injury–induced atheroma of the abdominal aorta of swine, showing phagocytosis of a large number of yeast cells.

Secondly, the assay depended on the presence of unstained yeast internalized by the cells, most of which also contained large unstained fat globules, which proved to be indistinguishable from the unstained yeast.

To establish the extent to which macrophages of atherosclerotic lesions serve as the source of hydrolytic enzymes, we carried out histochemical studies at the light and electron microscopic levels. Two enzymes were chosen for study. Nonspecific esterase (NSE) was chosen because of its demonstrated capability of hydrolyzing cholesteryl ester, among many other substrates. It also has been considered to be a "marker enzyme" for macrophages.[31] The second enzyme chosen was β-glucuronidase, an important enzyme involved in the degradation of GAG.

The localization and pattern of NSE activity was studied at the light and electron

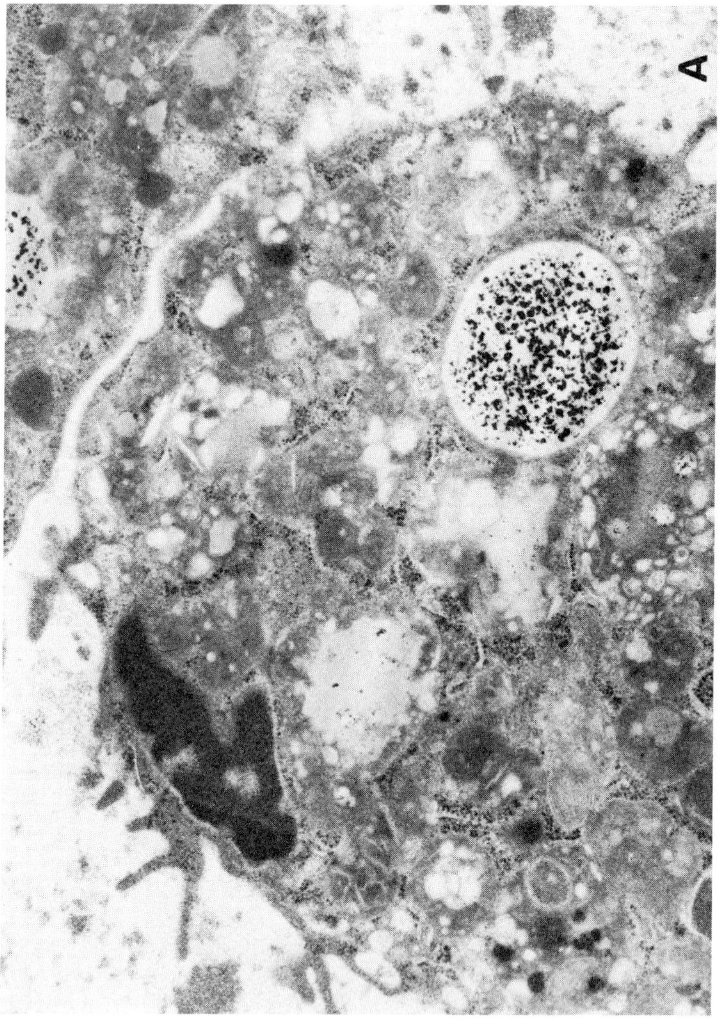
A

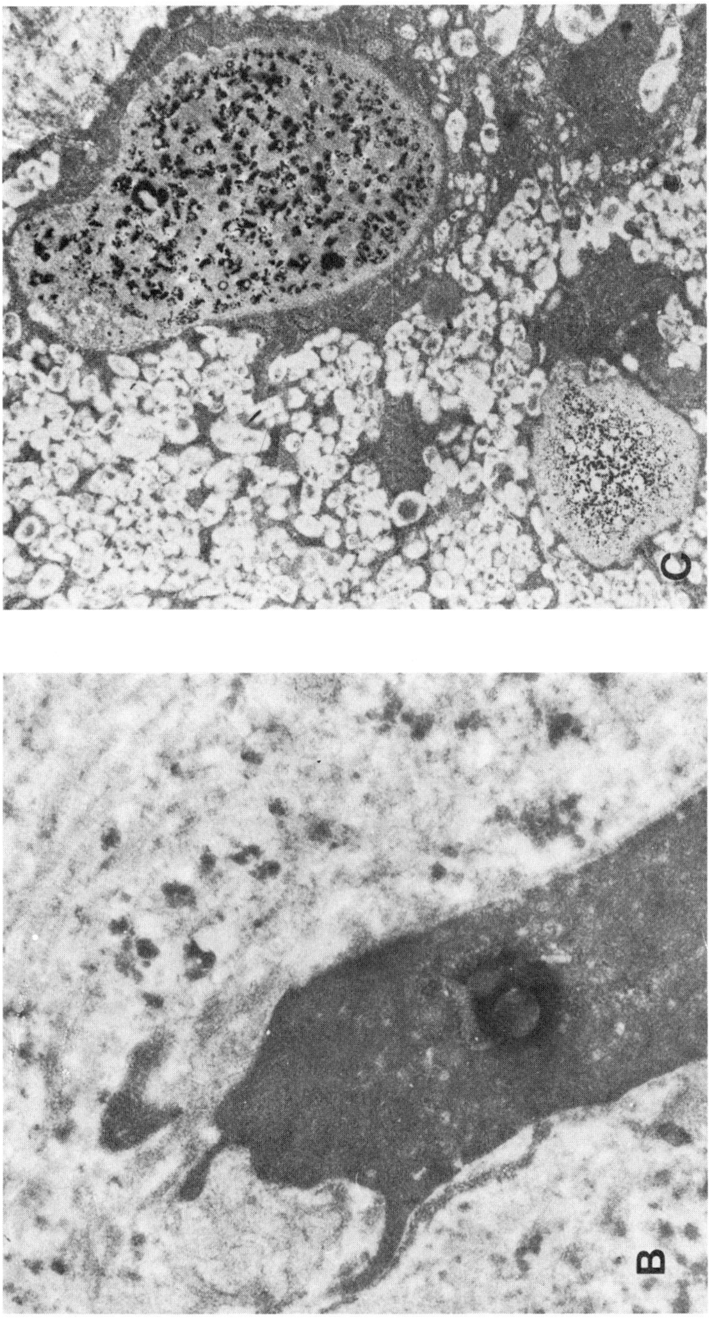

FIGURE 2. Portions of a macrophage (A), a smooth muscle cell (B), and a foam cell (C) showing reaction products of nonspecific esterase. Note the granular appearance of the products within vacuoles, probably secondary lysosomes, in macrophages and foam cells, and the linear appearance at the periphery of a primary lysosome in the smooth muscle cell.

microscopic levels during the progression and regression phases of atherosclerosis. With the methods we employed, no activity was detected in normal arterial wall. The SMC of the media and non-lesion areas of the intima were negative in animals on either high fat or mash diets. In lesions, however, at the light microscopic levels, the cells containing the reaction product of NSE were of various shapes and sizes; some were round, mononuclear, with eosinophilic cytoplasm resembling macrophages; others were foam cells or elongated fusiform cells. Most of the cells containing reaction products were present within or around necrotic foci. Electron microscopy showed that there were three types of positive cells (FIGURE 2).[32] One cell type had the ultrastructural characteristics of macrophages and contained large amounts of enzyme, SMC, which had occasional linear accumulations associated with the membranes of primary lysosomes, and foam cells of indeterminate origin, which showed reaction product associated with numerous membranous vesicles. Although enzyme histochemical methods are not appropriate for precise quantitation, light and electron microscopic studies indicate that the bulk of the enzymatic activity demonstrable in the lesions was associated with macrophages. The presence of reaction products in SMC, only in lesion tissue, indicates that the atherosclerosis process causes induction of NSE in smooth muscle cells.

The hydrolytic enzyme, β-glucuronidase, exhibits reactivity similar to that of NSE. By light microscopy, the most intensely reactive cells in the lesion were found to be large, round mononuclear macrophage-like cells, with eosinophilic cytoplasm. Also, within the lesions, there was a lesser amount of reaction product in foam cells and elongated fusiform cells, presumably SMC. The positive cells were mostly within or around necrosis. In contrast to NSE, β-glucuronidase reaction products were occasionally found in the media of both normal arteries and that subjacent to lesions. Here also, one has the unmistakable impression that macrophages were providing the greatest component of the β-glucuronidase activity.

Foam cells in the atheroma are not of a homogenous cell type. Some are recognizable as of SMC origin, while others are macrophage in origin. However, the origin of a considerable number of these cells cannot be determined even with the so-called marker enzyme, structural proteins, or electron microscopy. However, most investigators[13,17,24,33] believe these unidentified cells originate from macrophages. Since many of these unidentified cells contain enzyme reaction products, we are now carrying out, in conjunction with Dr. Kenji Adachi, monoclonal antibody studies in order to establish the origin of these cells. Elicited peritoneal cells were harvested from swine, allowed to adhere to glass, and the glass-adherent cells, presumably macrophages, were used as antigens in immunizing mice. The spleen cells from the immunized mice were fused with myeloma cells, and antibody-producing cells were cloned using standard techniques. Of six lines producing antibody reactive with "macrophages," two were exceptionally strong and were further characterized and used as primary antiserum in the avidin-biotin-horseradish peroxidase procedure for localizing antigen. Preliminary studies were carried out on suspensions of swine peritoneal cells, and by either light or electron microscopy, no definite positive reaction with lymphocytes or polymorphonuclear leukocytes was demonstrated. There was considerable variation in the amount of antibody binding to the surface of the macrophages, and this variation was not related to size. In experiments designed to see if the antigen was related to phagocytic capability, glass-adherent peritoneal cells were incubated with opsonized yeast prior to the antibody reaction. The results showed no relation between phagocytosis and presence, absence, or amount of antigen.

The next step was the application of the antiserum to tissue sections. As a positive control, a section of spleen was processed on the same slide as an aortic lesion section. Adjacent sections were also stained for NSE activity. Results have been somewhat unexpected. On slides where apparently appropriate spleen cells in sections had been stained by the anti-macrophage antibody, no reaction was detectable in aortic sections, even though the NSE-stained control suggested the presence of macrophages in considerable numbers. The implications of this finding are not clear. One interpretation is that the antigenic determinant, present in varying degrees, on peritoneal macrophages as recovered in suspension, is lost in the milieu. This concept is not without precedent, since many surface markers either appear or disappear during maturation or culture. However, before one can accept this, the possibility of technical failure as the basis for the inability to demonstrate the antigenic determinant must be rigorously explored. Nonetheless, it seems that this monoclonal antibody approach may not be the most productive one for identifying unclassified foam cells because of

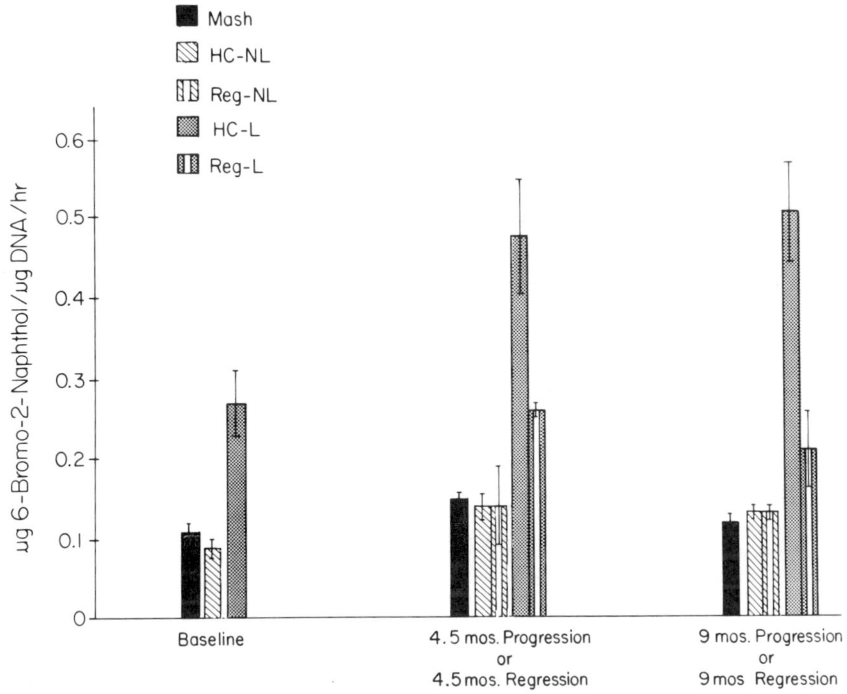

FIGURE 3. β-Glucuronidase activity of different types of swine aortic tissue. HC-high cholesterol; Reg-regression; L-lesion; NL-non-lesion.

the marked variation in reaction among cells presumed to be macrophages, including some very large, actively phagocytizing cells. Although at present the true origin of many of the foam cells containing the reaction product remains uncertain if we assume, as many do, that the foam cells are of macrophage origin, our study indicates that the great proportion of hydrolytic enzymes in the lesion are derived from macrophages and, hence, the activity of these enzymes in the lesion reflects that of the macrophages.

We are now following changes in lesion β-glucuronidase activity during the progression and regression phases of atherosclerosis. This enzymatic part is just one section of a comprehensive experiment involving swine. Although not all of the animals have been sacrificed at this time, the data at hand shows some definite trends. The

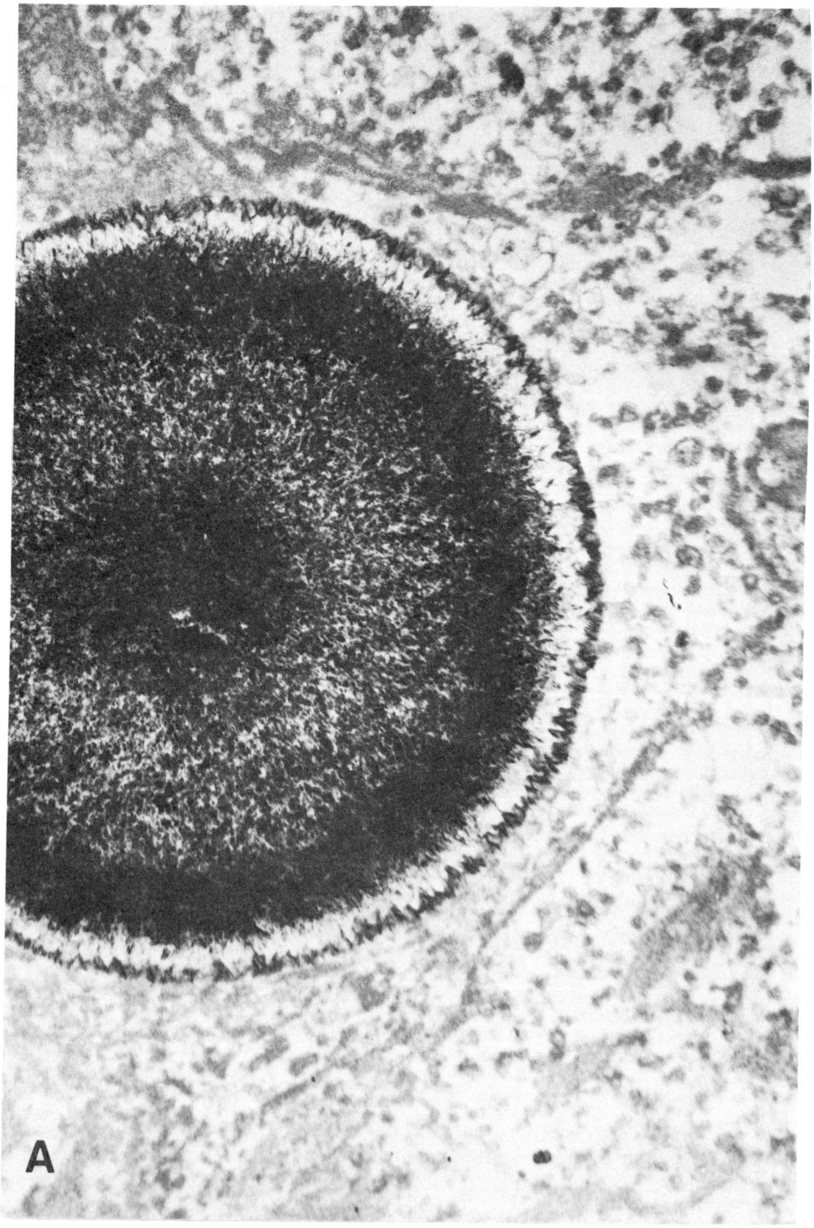

FIGURE 4A. Electron-dense body from a calcified atheroma before exposure to EDTA. The removal of the electron-dense material by this complexing agent supports its calcium identity. Note that a limiting membrane-like structure, similar in configuration to the outline of the "calcific" body, remained after EDTA exposure.

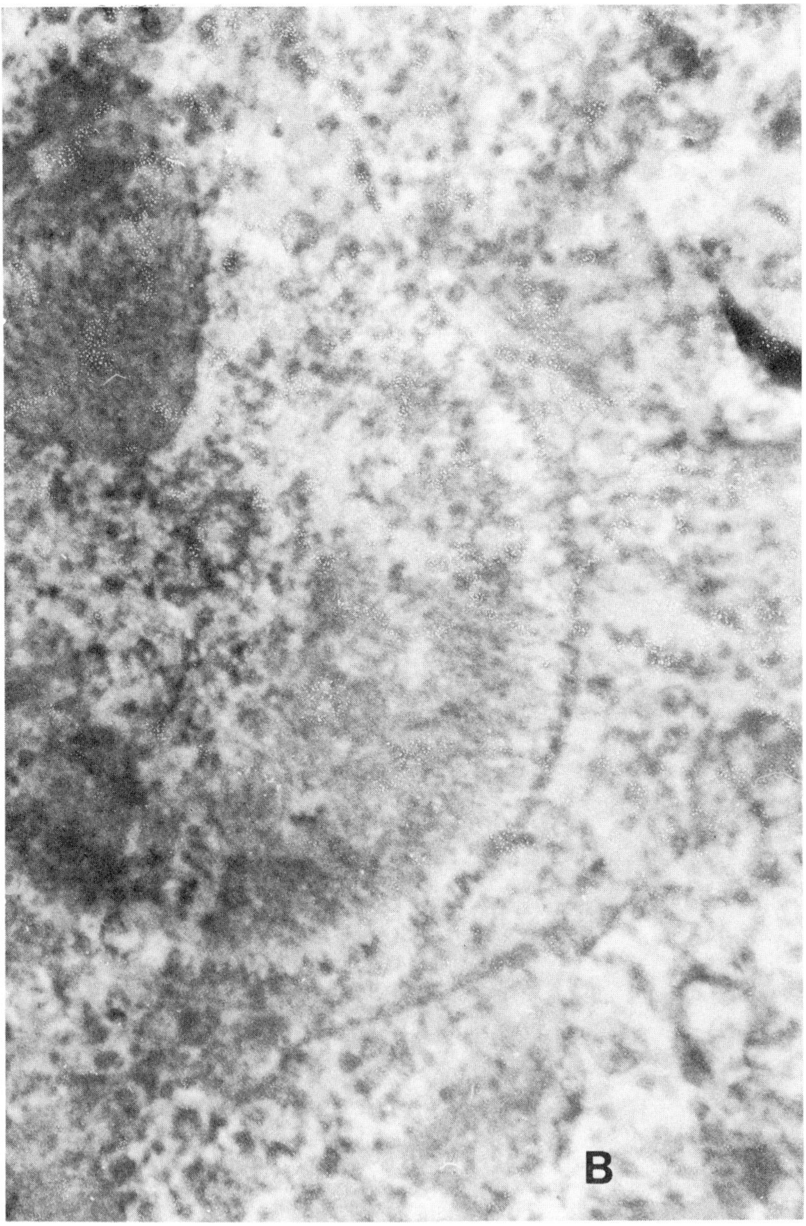

FIGURE 4B. Electron-dense body from a calcified atheroma after exposure to EDTA. The removal of the electron-dense material by this complexing agent supports its calcium identity. Note that a limiting membrane-like structure, similar in configuration to the outline of the "calcific" body, remained after EDTA exposure.

experimental design called for swine to be fed a semisynthetic diet for nine months, at which time some would be sacrificed as a baseline group, while others would be maintained on the diet for another four and a half or nine months (progression groups), or shifted to a mash diet for four and a half or nine months (regression groups). Parallel groups of animals which had been fed only mash for the appropriate periods were also included as controls.

The β-glucuronidase activities (FIGURE 3) of the non-lesion tissues of diet-fed baseline animals are the same as those of the comparable mash controls in every instance, suggesting that something other than an elevated serum cholesterol level is required for normal arterial tissue to respond with increased activity of this enzyme. It should be noted that macrophages were not observed in normal tissue,[3] which may help to explain the low levels of activity. However, the baseline lesion activity was significantly elevated over either type of non-lesion tissue. In the four and a half month progression groups, the lesion activity continued to rise to nearly twice that of the baseline lesion activity, whereas, the activity in the four and a half month regression lesions remained the same as in the baseline lesions. This indicates that return of serum cholesterol level to normal did not alter the activity of the enzyme since it remained high during this period. After nine months of added atherogenic diet, the lesion activity had plateaued at a level slightly above the previous progression level, which was still significantly higher than the baseline or nine-month regression lesions, while the activity of the latter had decreased so that, although numerically still higher than the non-lesion tissue, it was no longer significantly different from it. These results indicate that the activity of the hydrolytic enzyme β-glucuronidase remained high during a long period in which the animals were on regression regimen. The relationship of this enzymatic activity to the removal of necrosis and the presence of macrophages is being studied.

ROLE OF MACROPHAGES IN CALCIFICATION

As was mentioned earlier, the swine sequential study indicated a tremendous increase in lesion calcification during 14 months on regression diet. It also showed a close spacial association between macrophages and calcification. The increase in calcification occurred in lesion areas without any increase in calcium concentration in the adjacent non-lesion tissue, which remained comparable to tissue from mash-fed controls. Energy dispersive analysis of the grossly calcified atherosclerotic lesions revealed that the two major elements present were calcium and phosphorus. Line profile analysis showed a close association between calcium and phosphorus, suggesting that the deposit is a calcium phosphate. By select area electron diffraction, these deposits were identified as hydroxyapatite crystalline material.

Light microscopy with special staining for calcium (Von Kossa and alizarin red S) showed that, in addition to the dense aggregate in the necrotic center, there were granular deposits in the surrounding tissue not visible in the hematoxylin and eosin stained sections. Electron microscopic studies of the granular deposits revealed round and/or oval electron-dense bodies, often folded or shrunken, measuring up to several microns in greatest dimensions. They sometimes contained a central core of amorphous electron-dense particles and needle-shaped crystals—the latter often associated with smaller vesicular inclusions. There were also spherical aggregates of granular or amorphous electron-dense precipitates. In support of the calcium identity of these electron-dense structures, is the fact that they were removed by one and a half hours exposure to bis(aminoethyl)glycolether-N,N,N′,N′-tetraacetic acid (EGTA) or ethylene-diaminetetraacetic acid (EDTA). After removal of the electron-dense material, a limiting membrane-like structure, similar in configuration to the outline of the "calcific" body, remained (FIGURE 4). This vesicular structure also contained a matrix of unspecified nature. Almost all of the "calcific" bodies, examined within the atheroma, appear to be of this nature. Very few were associated with elastic tissue or collagen. In many instances, intracellular dense bodies, similar to those seen extracellularly and also removable by EGTA, were observed. These structures were present within cells showing varying degrees of degeneration. The occurrence of calcification on membrane-like structures resembling cellular degradation products and their presence within degenerating cells suggests that cell necrosis may be, in large part, responsible for the calcification of the atheroma.

Kim *et al.*[34] have observed similar structures in the aging aortic valve and have suggested that calcification of the human valves takes place on products of cellular degeneration. In an extensive study of various pathological calcification in humans, Kim[34,35] found that calcification occurred at the cellular degradation product regardless of the tissue involved. It appears, from our work and that of Kim, that most calcification of the atheroma occurs on cell degradation products. Macrophages and macrophage-derived foam cells are the most likely candidates to generate such products because of their numbers and short life span.

SUMMARY

The exact role of macrophages in regression is still not clear. It appears that some of their functions are beneficial, while others are detrimental. Among their beneficial functions are: (1) their ability to phagocytize cellular and extracellular debris and remove them outside the arterial wall. This function may be enhanced by the macrophage's own secretion of fibronectin; (2) their ability to solubilize necrotic debris by their complement of hydrolytic enzymes, thus, rendering them diffusible through the arterial wall; and, (3) their secretion of SMC mitogen and components of the arterial wall. Our work supports the role of macrophages in the removal of necrotic debris by the mechanisms cited in (1) and (2) above.

On the other hand, macrophages may be detrimental to regression if they secrete an excess of the same hydrolytic enzymes, mentioned above as being beneficial, and if directed towards normal arterial wall components. This can result in disorganization and degradation of these components, and in more necrosis, as was seen at the six-week regression period in our sequential study.[3] Cell debris resulting from necrosis of SMC and from death of macrophages themselves may form nidi for calcific bodies to occur. Our work suggests this may be the case during regression. Finally, excess stimulation of SMC, mitogen, and the secretion of the arterial wall components may contribute to the lesion growth and could explain the lack of regression in some species and under certain conditions.

In conclusion, our hypothesis that the macrophage is a "friend" during regression appears to be only partially true, and their presence at this phase of the disease may be a "two-edged sword." On one hand, they may help in the removal of necrosis, while on the other hand, they may accelerate calcification.

REFERENCES

1. STARY, H. C., J. P. STRONG & D. A. EGGEN. 1980. *In* Atherosclerosis V. A. M. Gotto, L. C. Smith & B. Allen, Eds.: 753–756. Springer-Verlag. Berlin, Heidelberg, New York.

2. TUCKER, C. F., C. CATSULIS, J. P. STRONG & D. A. EGGEN. 1971. Am. J. Pathol. **65:** 493–502.
3. DAOUD, A. S., J. JARMOLYCH, J. M. AUGUSTYN & K. E. FRITZ. 1981. Arch. Path. Lab. Med. **105:** 233–239.
4. FRITZ, K. E., J. M. AUGUSTYN, J. JARMOLYCH & A. S. DAOUD. 1981. Arch. Path. Lab. Med. **105:** 240–246.
5. RIFKEN, B. R., R. L. BAKER, M. J. SOMERMAN, S. E. POINTON, S. J. COLEMAN & W. Y. W. AU. 1980. Cell Tiss. Res. **210:** 493–500.
6. KULONEN, E. & M. POTILA. 1980. Acta Path. Microbiol. Scand. Sect. **C:** 7–13.
7. WERB, Z., M. J. BAND & P. A. JONES. 1980. J. Exp. Med. **152:** 1340–1357.
8. UNANUE, E. R. 1976. Am J. Pathol. **83:** 396–417.
9. ROSS, R. 1981. Arteriosclerosis **1:** 293–311.
10. MARTIN, B. M., M. A. GIMBRONE, JR., E. R. UNANUE & R. S. COTRAN. 1981. J. Immuno. **126:** 1510–1515.
11. GLENN, K. C. & R. ROSS. 1981. Cell **25:** 603–615.
12. ALITALO, K., T. HOVI & A. VAHERI. 1980. J. Exp. Med. **151:** 602–613.
13. STILL, W. J. S. & R. M. O'NEAL. 1962. Am. J. Pathol. **40:** 21–35.
14. SUZUKI, M. & R. M. O'NEAL. 1964. J. Lipid Res. **5:** 624–627.
15. SUZUKI, M. & R. M. O'NEAL. 1967. Arch. Path. Lab. Med. **83:** 169–174.
16. MARSHALL, J. R. & R. M. O'NEAL. 1966. Exp. Mol. Pathol. **5:** 1–11.
17. GERRITY, R. G., H. K. NAITO, M. RICHARDSON & C. J. SCHWARTZ. 1979. Am. J. Path. **95**(3): 775–785.
18. MAHLEY, R. W. & T. L. INNERARITY. 1983. Biochim. Biophys. Acta **737:** 197–222.
19. MAHLEY, R. W., T. L. INNERARITY, K. H. WEISGRABER & S. Y. OH. 1979. J. Clin. Invest. **64:** 743–750.
20. GOLDSTEIN, J. L., Y. K. HO, S. K. BASU & M. S. BROWN. 1979. Proc. Natl. Acad. Sci. USA **76:** 333–337.
21. FOGELMAN, A. M., I. SHECHTER, J. SEAGER, M. HOKOM, J. S. CHILD & P. A. EDWARDS. 1980. Proc. Natl. Acad. Sci. USA **77:** 2214–2218.
22. PEARLSTEIN, E., L. I. GOLD & A. GARCIA-PARDO. 1980. Mol. Cell Biochem. **29:** 103–128.
23. YAMADA, K. M., D. W. KENNEDY, K. KIMATA & R. M. PRATT. 1980. J. Biol. Chem. **255:** 6055–6063.
24. GERRITY, R. G. 1981. Am. J. Pathol. **103**(2): 191–200.
25. STARY, H. C. 1979. Virchows Arch. A. Pathol. Anat. Histol. **383:** 117–134.
26. BIHARI-VARGA, M. 1965. Acta Clin. Acad. Sci. Hung. **45:** 219–229.
27. MCKNEALLY, M. F., C. MAVER, H. W. KAUSEL & R. D. ALLEY. 1976. J. Thor. Cardiovasc. Surg. **72:** 335–338.
28. LAMBERSON, H. V., JR. & K. E. FRITZ. 1974. Fed. Proc. **33:** 235.
29. HARPER, G. R. & K. E. FRITZ. 1974. Circulation **50** (Suppl. III): 264.
30. SCHAFFNER, T., K. TAYLOR & E. J. BARTUCCI. 1980. Am. J. Pathol. **100:** 57–80.
31. YAM, L. T., C. Y. LI & W. H. CROSBY. 1971. Am. J. Clin. Pathol. **55:** 283–290.
32. FRITZ, K. E., A. S. DAOUD & J. JARMOLYCH. 1980. Artery **7:** 352–366.
33. FOWLER, S., H. SHIO & N. J. HALEY. 1979. Lab. Invest. **41**(4): 372–378.
34. KIM, K. M., J. M. VALIGORSKY, W. J. MERGNER, R. T. JONES, R. E. PENDERGRASS & B. F. TRUMP. 1976. Human Pathol. **7:** 47–60.

Atherosclerosis as an Inflammatory Process

The Roles of the Monocyte-Macrophage[a]

COLIN J. SCHWARTZ, ANTHONY J. VALENTE,
EUGENE A. SPRAGUE, JIM L. KELLEY,
C. ALAN SUENRAM, AND MARIUS M. ROZEK

Department of Pathology
University of Texas Health Science Center
San Antonio, Texas 78284

INTRODUCTION

The advanced human atherosclerotic plaque is characterized by the frequent presence of granulomatous foci[1,2] and a prominent adventitial cellular infiltrate, predominantly lymphocytic.[3] Both features are consistent with an inflammatory component in plaque pathogenesis. Further, in both human and experimental atherosclerosis,[4–14] an enhanced monocyte-macrophage recruitment to the arterial intima has been reported. In this presentation, selected facets of monocyte-macrophage participation in atherogenesis are discussed, with particular emphasis on intimal blood monocyte recruitment and the spectrum of pathobiological roles of monocyte-derived intimal macrophages. Specific attention is devoted to the nature and possible roles of a monocyte chemoattractant synthesized by cultured arterial smooth muscle cells (SMC),[15,16] and the monocyte-derived macrophage as a progenitor of cholesteryl ester-rich foam cells.[13,17,18]

THE NATURE OF THE PROBLEM

Although this presentation focuses on only certain aspects of plaque pathogenesis, namely the roles of the monocyte-macrophage, it seems important to emphasize that the essential components of atherogenesis involve complex cascades of interactions among arterial endothelium, platelets, peripheral blood monocytes, smooth muscle cells, lipoproteins, connective tissue elements, and the patterns of blood flow. Within this broad conceptual framework, we are inclined to the view that the enhanced endothelial permeability, together with the intimal accumulation of plasma constituents and blood derived cells, notably monocytes, are consistent with the view of atheroma as an inflammatory process. Some aspects of this process are described below.

MECHANISMS IN INTIMAL MONOCYTE RECRUITMENT

TABLE 1 summarizes the mechanisms which on general principles should participate in the phenomenon of intimal monocyte recruitment. Circulating blood monocytes

[a]This work was supported by NHLBI grant nos. HL-26890 and HL-07446.

TABLE 1. Mechanisms in Intimal Monocyte Recruitment

A.	Endothelial contact—Blood flow
B.	Endothelial attachment
C.	Locomotion—Migration
D.	Presence of chemotactic gradients
E.	Recognition of chemotactic gradients
F.	Immobilization in intima—Migration inhibition

must of necessity make contact with the vascular endothelium as a prelude to attachment, and this is most likely to occur in areas of disturbed blood flow. Attachment itself, may involve changes in the surface properties of the monocytes, the endothelium, or both. In this regard, the cellular glycocalyx and surface charge, certain chemoattractants, and the nature of proteins adsorbed to the cell surfaces, including native and glycosylated fibrinogens,[19] may all be of considerable importance. Furthermore, activation of the monocyte by various modalities enhances attachment and spreading, and this may be an additional component of the attachment or "margination" process. It should be noted, however, that many monocytes attached to the arterial endothelial surface are rounded,[13] with little or no evidence of spreading, as indicated by the absence of cytoplasmic aprons, leaving the role of intravascular activation uncertain. When monocytes, however, attach to foreign or abnormal surfaces such as plastic, the attachment is associated with activation as measured by enzyme release.[20]

Our studies,[13] and those of others,[7] indicate that blood monocytes enter the subendothelial space (SES) mainly, but not exclusively, via the endothelial cell junctions. This migration across the endothelium implies that the cells must be capable of locomotion, and further, that as the migration is directed to the SES, chemotactic gradients must exist across the endothelium and intima which the monocytes must have the ability to recognize. The nature of these chemoattractants originating within the intima or media is of considerable interest, and subsequently, we shall describe a monocyte-specific chemoattractant synthesized and released by cultured aortic medial smooth muscle cells, which may serve as a mediator in the recruitment process.[15,16]

The phenomenon of intimal monocyte recruitment is enhanced in experimental hyperlipidemia.[7,9,13] This may result from an enhanced production of chemoattractant(s) in the intima-media, and/or an altered responsiveness of the circulating monocytes to chemoattractants. It is also feasible that hyperlipidemia will influence the attachment process itself, by modifying surface properties of either the monocytes or the endothelial cells.

There is clearly much to be done before the phenomenon of monocyte recruitment to the arterial intima in atherogenesis is fully understood. It is also of relevance to explore further those factors regulating intimal monocyte activation and their subsequent differentiation into intimal macrophages.

PUTATIVE ROLES OF THE MONOCYTE-MACROPHAGE IN ATHEROGENESIS

The diversity of roles which the monocyte-macrophage might play in atherogenesis is in part summarized in TABLE 2. The monocyte-macrophage, because of its phagocytic capacity, can clearly serve as a scavenger cell, thus, ensuring intimal debridement, and perhaps providing a cellular basis for arterial remodeling. One tends to forget the role that macrophages play in thrombolysis, not only via their phagocytic functions, but also in fibrinolysis. Furthermore, the phagocytosis of platelets or platelet debris in organizing thrombi can result in the development of lipid-rich foam cells,[21-24] a process that deserves clarification. As processors of antigen and in lymphocyte activation,[25,26] the intimal macrophages will clearly play a key role in vascular immunologic processes and in one or more components of the atherogenic sequence.

Activated monocytes and macrophages secrete a broad spectrum of hydrolytic and proteolytic enzymes which may modify components of the arterial wall such as collagen and elastin, or proteins within the interstitium. The secretion of the mitogen macrophage-derived growth factor (MDGF) is of particular interest,[27] in that it might mediate SMC and EC proliferation, and vascular angiogenesis.[28] Lipoprotein lipase (LPL), an enzyme actively involved in the catabolism of triglyceride-rich lipoproteins, is also secreted by the macrophages.[29,30] In addition to the secretion of LPL, it appears likely that macrophages may modify lipoproteins, including low density lipoproteins (LDL), within the intimal interstitium, either enzymatically or via an oxidative pathway, resulting in their recognition by cellular receptor pathways other than the classical LDL receptor. Further, macrophages are clearly important in the uptake and catabolism of lipoproteins from the tissues, and they can accumulate considerable amounts of cholesteryl ester as they assume the morphologic features of plaque foam cells.[17,18]

Finally, some comments on the macrophage generation of superoxide anion and hydrogen peroxide. Membrane lipid peroxidation could feasibly alter membrane compliance, and may prove to be an important mechanism contributing to cellular injury and in particular endothelial ulceration. The latter possibility is supported by the close topographical association of endothelial ulceration and underlying clusters of macrophage-foam cells, which we have observed in nonhuman primate lesions.[14]

TEMPORAL EVOLUTION OF THE MONOCYTE-DERIVED FOAM CELL

We have recently reported the development of an experimental granuloma model for the extravascular development of foam cells in modestly hypercholesterolemic (HC) rabbits.[17] In this model, monocyte-derived macrophages are recruited subcutaneously in response to injection of the long chain sulfated polysaccharide, carrageenan. In normocholesterolemic (NC) rabbits, no lipid accumulation in the macrophages is observed, in striking contrast to HC animals in which the granuloma macrophages avidly accumulate Oil-Red-O stainable lipid as early as four days after granuloma induction. Macrophages from HC rabbits progressively accumulate increasing quantities of lipid, and at 28 days, some 70% of the granuloma cells are morphologically indistinguishable from the foam cells characteristic of the atheromatous plaque. This lipid accumulation is, we believe, the result of the uptake and metabolism of the

TABLE 2. Roles of the Monocyte-Macrophage in Atherogenesis

A. Scavenger—Phagocytic
B. Immunologic–process antigen; Lymphocyte activation
C. Secretion of hydrolytic and proteolytic enzymes
D. Secretion of mitogen–MDGF
E. Secretion of lipoprotein lipase–LPL
F. Lipoprotein catabolism—Cholesterol esterification
G. Membrane injury—Superoxide anion and hydrogen peroxide generation

cholesteryl ester-rich, very low density lipoprotein (VLDL). A complete sequence of transition from the monocyte to the fully developed nonspecific esterase (NSE) positive macrophage foam cell was observed.

Lipid inclusions in the granuloma foam cells were seen both within lysosomes, and also free with no limiting membranes within the cytoplasm. It is notable that at 28 days, the cholesteryl ester content of the granuloma foam cells from HC rabbits had increased some 180-fold compared to macrophages from NC animals.

These granuloma experiments have established that monocyte-derived macrophages, when exposed *in vivo* to elevated circulating levels of cholesteryl ester-rich VLDL, assume both the morphologic and biochemical characteristics of plaque foam cells. Just how interstitial lipoproteins may be modified by the secretory products of macrophages, and how such modifications may influence their cellular uptake and catabolism, are questions currently being evaluated.

AN ARTERIAL SMC-DERIVED CHEMOATTRACTANT FOR PERIPHERAL BLOOD MONOCYTES

In two earlier reports,[15,16] we have established that cultured aortic medial SMC synthesize and release a powerful chemoattractant for human peripheral blood

TABLE 3. Properties of Cultured Baboon Aortic Medial Smooth Muscle Cell-Derived Chemotactic Factor (SMC-CF)

A. Low molecular weight (10–12 kilodaltons)
B. Cationic
C. Heat stable
D. More active for monocytes than polymorphonuclear leukocytes
E. Both chemotactic and chemokinetic
F. Cycloheximide and protease sensitive

monocytes. Such a chemoattractant could, we believe, be an important mediator in the recruitment of blood monocytes to the arterial intima in atherogenesis. This chemoattractant's features are summarized in TABLE 3.

Briefly, it is relatively heat stable, and of high specific activity. Its synthesis is significantly inhibited by the protein synthesis inhibitor, cycloheximide, and its activity is destroyed by the bacterial protease, subtilisin, indicating that it is protein in nature. The SMC-CF activity has been shown by gel filtration to elute in the 10–12,000 dalton region. Furthermore, chromatofocusing studies indicate that the chemoattractant is a cationic protein with a pI > 10.5. Finally it is of some interest that the SMC-CF exhibits a significant degree of target-cell specificity, with little or no influence on polymorphonuclear leukocytes.

Studies examining the influence of the SMC-derived chemoattractant on various biologic phenomena, including monocyte activation, superoxide anion generation, and monocyte attachment to endothelium, are in progress. Factors regulating the production of SMC-CF are also being explored with a particular emphasis on the influence of lipoproteins and the cyclic endoperoxides. Whether the SMC-CF shares any homology with platelet-derived growth factor is also a question of some interest and importance.

SUMMARY

In this brief review, we have addressed the roles of the monocyte-macrophage in atherogenesis, with emphasis on the recruitment to the arterial wall. We have presented summary data on the SMC-derived chemoattractant protein and also on the temporal evolution of monocyte-derived macrophages into cholesteryl ester-rich foam cells. The concept of atheroma as an inflammatory process has also been discussed.

REFERENCES

1. Schwartz, C. J. & J. R. A. Mitchell. 1962. The morphology, terminology, and pathogenesis of arterial plaques. Postgrad. Med. J. **38:** 25–34.
2. Mitchell, J. R. A. & C. J. Schwartz. 1965. Arterial Disease. Chapter 2. Blackwell Scientific Publications. Oxford, UK.
3. Schwartz, C. J. & J. R. A. Mitchell. 1962. Cellular infiltration of the human arterial adventitia associated with atheromatous plaques. Circulation **26:** 73–78.
4. Stary, H. C. 1980. The intimal macrophage in atherosclerosis. Artery **8:** 205–207.
5. Schaffner, T., K. Taylor, E. J. Bartucci, K. Fischer-Dzoga, J. H. Beeson, S. Glagov & R. W. Wissler. 1980. Arterial foam cells with distinctive immunomorphologic and histochemical features of macrophages. Am. J. Pathol. **100:** 57–80.
6. Gerrity, R. G., H. K. Naito, M. Richardson & C. J. Schwartz. 1979. Dietary induced atherogenesis in swine. Am. J. Pathol. **95:** 775–792.
7. Gerrity, R. G. 1981. The role of the monocyte in atherogenesis: 1. Transition of blood-borne monocytes into foam cells in fatty lesions. Am. J. Pathol. **103:** 181–190.
8. Still, W. J. S. & R. M. O'Neal. 1962. Electron microscopic study of experimental atherosclerosis in the rat. Am. J. Pathol. **40:** 21–35.
9. Joris, I., T. Zand, J. J. Nunnari, F. J. Krolikowski & G. Majno. 1983. Studies on the pathogenesis of atherosclerosis: 1. Adhesion and emigration of mononuclear cells in the aorta of hypercholesterolemic rats. Am. J. Pathol. **113:** 341–358.
10. Lewis, J. C., R. G. Taylor, N. D. Jones, R. W. St. Clair & J. F. Cornhill. 1982. Endothelial surface characteristics in pigeon coronary artery atherosclerosis: 1. Cellular alterations during the initial stages of dietary cholesterol challenge. Lab Invest. **46:** 123–138.
11. Duff, G. L., G. C. McMillan & A. C. Ritchie. 1957. The morphology of early atherosclerotic lesions of the aorta demonstrated by the surface technique in rabbits fed cholesterol. Am. J. Pathol. **33:** 845–873.
12. Barbolini, G., G. A. Scilabra, A. Botticelli & S. Botticelli. 1969. On the origin of foam cells in cholesterol-induced atherosclerosis of the rabbit. Virchows Arch. (Cell Pathol.) **3:** 24–32.
13. Schwartz, C. J., E. A. Sprague, J. L. Kelley, A. J. Valente & C. A. Suenram. 1985. Aortic intimal monocyte recruitment in the normo- and hyper-cholesterolemic baboon (*Papio cynocephalus*): An ultrastructural study. Implications in atherogenesis. Virchows Arch. **405:** 175–191.
14. Kelley, J. L., E. A. Sprague, K. D. Carey, A. J. Valente, C. A. Suenram & C. J. Schwartz. 1985. Atherosclerosis in vervet monkeys (*Cercopithecus aethiops*) after a seven-year dietary challenge. In preparation.
15. Jauchem, J. R., M. Lopez, E. A. Sprague & C. J. Schwartz. 1982. Mononuclear cell chemoattractant activity from cultured arterial smooth muscle cells. Exp. Mol. Pathol. **37:** 166–174.
16. Valente, A. J., S. R. Fowler, E. A. Sprague, J. L. Kelley, C. A. Suenram & C. J. Schwartz. 1984. Initial characterization of a peripheral blood mononuclear cell chemoattractant derived from cultured arterial smooth muscle cells. Am. J. Pathol. **117:** 409–417.
17. Schwartz, C. J., J. J. Ghidoni, J. L. Kelley, E. A. Sprague, A. J. Valente & C. A.

SUENRAM. 1985. Evolution of foam cells in subcutaneous rabbit carrageenan granulomas: 1. Light microscopy and ultrastructure. Am. J. Pathol. **118:** 134–150.
18. KELLEY, J. L., C. A. SUENRAM, A. J. VALENTE, E. A. SPRAGUE, M. M. ROZEK & C. J. SCHWARTZ. 1985. Evolution of foam cells in subcutaneous rabbit carrageenan granulomas: II. Tissue and macrophage lipid composition. Am. J. Pathol. In press.
19. VALENTE, A. J., E. A. SPRAGUE, M. R. NASSIRI, S. WADDINGHAM, J. L. KELLEY, C. A. SUENRAM & C. J. SCHWARTZ. 1984. Influence of plasma proteins on blood monocyte adherence to vascular endothelium. Arteriosclerosis **4:** 540a.
20. ROZEK, M. M., J. L. KELLEY, C. A. SUENRAM, A. J. VALENTE, E. A. SPRAGUE & C. J. SCHWARTZ. 1985. Activation of human blood monocytes by adherence to tissue culture plastic. In preparation.
21. ARDLIE, N. G. & C. J. SCHWARTZ. 1968. A comparison of the organization and fate of autologous pulmonary emboli and of artificial plasma thrombi in the anterior chamber of the eye, in normocholesterolemic rabbits. J. Path. Bact. **95:** 1–18.
22. ARDLIE, N. G. & C. J. SCHWARTZ. 1968. The organization and fate of autologous pulmonary emboli in hyperchoesterolemic rabbits. J. Path. Bact. **95:** 19–29.
23. CRAIG, I. H. & C. J. SCHWARTZ. 1972. Contribution of thrombus free and esterified cholesterol to atherosclerotic plaques. Pathology **4:** 303–306.
24. CRAIG, I. A., F. P. BELL, C. H. GOLDSMITH & C. J. SCHWARTZ. 1973. Thrombosis and atherosclerosis: The organization of pulmonary thromboemboli in the pig. I. Macroscopic observations, protein, DNA, and major lipids. Atherosclerosis **18:** 277–300.
25. UNANUE, E. R. 1979. The macrophage as a regulator of lymphocyte function. Hosp. Practice. **Nov:** 61–74.
26. PIERCE, C. W. 1980. Macrophages: Modulators of immunity. Am. J. Pathol. **98:** 10–28.
27. MARTIN, B. M., M. A. GIMBRONE, E. R. UNANUE & R. S. COTRAN. 1981. Stimulation of nonlymphoid mesenchymal cell proliferation by a macrophage-derived growth factor. J. Immunol. **126:** 1510–1515.
28. THAKRAL, K. K., W. H. GOODSON III & T. K. HUNT. 1979. Stimulation of wound blood vessel growth by wound macrophages. J. Surg. Res. **26:** 430–436.
29. KHOO, J. C., E. M. MAHONEY & J. L. WITZUM. 1981. Secretion of lipoprotein lipase by macrophages in culture. J. Biol. Chem. **256:** 7105–7108.
30. CHAIT, A., P. H. IVERIUS & J. D. BRUNZELL. 1982. Lipoprotein lipase secretion by human monocyte-derived macrophages. J. Clin. Invest. **69:** 490–493.

The Problems and the Promise of Prostaglandin Influences in Atherogenesis

S. MONCADA AND M. W. RADOMSKI[a]

Wellcome Research Laboratories
Langley Court, Beckenham, Kent BR3 3BS England
[a]Department of Pharmacology
Copernicus Academy of Medicine
Grzegorzecka 16
31-531 Cracow, Poland

INTRODUCTION

Prostaglandins (PGs) are made by all mammalian cells. They are released easily by perturbation of the cell membrane, either induced mechanically or by chemicals. In 1964, it was demonstrated that prostaglandins are biosynthesized from polyunsaturated fatty acids. Arachidonic acid (AA), the main precursor of prostaglandins in man, is the most common fatty acid present in cellular phospholipids and can be obtained by desaturation and chain elongation from dietary linoleic acid (C18:2ω6) or directly from the diet.

Much of the earlier work in this field concentrated on prostaglandins E_2 and $F_{2\alpha}$, as these possessed potent and diverse biological activities and were available in pure form. Since 1973, other important derivatives of arachidonic acid have been discovered, including the prostaglandin endoperoxides (PGG_2 and PGH_2), thromboxane A_2 (TXA_2), and prostacyclin (PGI_2). These are all chemically unstable, but they have potent biological activities. Investigations into the sites of production of these compounds and their differing and, in some cases, opposing biological activities have led to the development of new concepts in vascular homeostasis, as well as a better understanding of the nature of several pathological conditions. In this review, we will discuss some of the most relevant biological activities of prostacyclin in relation to atherogenesis.

FORMATION AND PROPERTIES OF PROSTACYCLIN

Prostacyclin is the main product of arachidonic acid in all vascular tissues so far tested, including those of man. The ability of the large vessel wall to synthesize prostacyclin is greatest at the intimal surface and progressively decreases toward the adventitia.[1] Production of prostacyclin by cultured cells from vessel walls also shows that endothelial cells have the greatest capacity to produce prostacyclin.[2,3]

Prostacyclin relaxes isolated vascular strips and is a strong hypotensive agent through vasodilation of all vascular beds studied, including the pulmonary and cerebral circulations (for review, see reference 4). Several authors have suggested that prostacyclin generation participates in, or accounts for, functional hyperemia.[5,6]

Prostacyclin is the most potent endogenous inhibitor of platelet aggregation yet discovered. This effect is short-lasting *in vivo,* disappearing within 30 minutes of cessation of intravenous administration. Prostacyclin disperses platelet aggregates *in vitro*[7,8] and in the circulation of man.[9] Moreover, it inhibits thrombus formation in models using the carotid artery of the rabbit[8] and the coronary artery of the dog,[10] protects against sudden death induced by intravenous arachidonic acid in rabbits,[11] and inhibits platelet aggregation in pial venules of the mouse when applied locally.[12]

In blood at 37°C, the activity of prostacyclin (as measured by bioassay on vascular smooth muscle) has a half-life of 3 min,[13] although there have been various reports of a stabilizing effect of plasma.[14] Alkaline pH increases the chemical stability of prostacyclin,[15] so that at pH 10.5 at 25°C, it has a half-life of 100 h. It is stabilized as a pharmaceutical preparation (Epoprostenol) by freeze drying. (For reviews, see Moncada[16] and Vane.[17]).

Prostacyclin inhibits platelet aggregation by stimulating adenylate cyclase, leading to an increase in cAMP levels in the platelets.[18,19] In this respect, prostacyclin is much more potent than either PGE_1 or PGD_2, and its effect is longer-lasting. In contrast to TXA_2, prostacyclin enhances Ca^{++} sequestration in platelet membranes.[20] Moreover, inhibitory effects on platelet phospholipase[21,22] and platelet cyclo-oxygenase[23] have been described. All these effects are related to its ability to increase cAMP in platelets. Prostacyclin, by inhibiting several steps in the activation of the arachidonic acid metabolic cascade, exerts an overall control of platelet aggregability.

Prostacyclin increases cAMP levels in cells other than platelets (for review, see reference 16), raising the possibility that in these cells a balance with the thromboxane system exerts a similar homeostatic control of cell behavior to that observed in platelets. Thus, the prostacyclin/TXA_2 system may have wider biological significance in cell regulation. An example is that prostacyclin inhibits white cell adherence to the vessel wall,[24,25] to nylon fibers, and to endothelial monolayers *in vitro.*[26] Prostacyclin increases cAMP in the endothelial cell itself, suggesting a possible negative feedback control for prostacyclin production by the endothelium.[27,28]

One of the functional characteristics of the intact vascular endothelium is its nonreactivity to platelets. Clearly, prostacyclin generation contributes to this property as a defense mechanism of the vascular endothelium against thrombosis. Prostacyclin inhibits platelet aggregation (platelet-platelet interaction) at much lower concentrations than those needed to inhibit adhesion (platelet-collagen interaction).[29] Thus, prostacyclin may permit platelets to stick to damaged vascular tissue and to interact with it, so allowing platelets to participate in the repair, while at the same time preventing or limiting thrombus formation. In addition, platelets adhering to a site where prostacyclin synthetase is present could well feed the enzyme with endoperoxide, thereby producing prostacyclin and preventing other platelets from clumping onto the adhering platelets, limiting the cells to a monolayer.

In addition to its well-known vasodilator and anti-aggregating actions, prostacyclin shares with other prostaglandins a "cytoprotective" activity. This term arose from studies, mainly in the rat, of the protective effects of prostaglandins on the gastric mucosa subjected to chemical and physical traumas. Prostacyclin also shares this activity and we have suggested[30] that this third property may be important in explaining certain therapeutic effects of prostacyclin. In some models of myocardial infarction, prostacyclin reduces infarct size[31–33] and arrhythmias,[34] and also decreases oxygen demand[33] and the release of enzymes from infarcted areas.[35] In sheep, prostacyclin protected the lungs against injury induced by endotoxin.[36] A beneficial effect of prostacyclin has also been reported in endotoxin shock in the dog[37] and in the cat,[38] where it improves splanchnic blood flow and reduces the formation and release of lysosomal hydrolases (cathepsin D). The effects of hypoxic damage in the cat isolated perfused liver are also substantially reduced by prostacyclin.[39] Canine livers can be preserved *ex vivo* for up to 48 hours and then successfully transplanted, using a combination of refrigeration, Sacks' solution, and prostacyclin.[40]

All these are related to "cytoprotection," another example of which occurs in platelets when prostacyclin is added to them during their separation from blood and subsequent washing. This procedure substantially improves their immediate functionality *in vitro*. In addition, whereas normal *in vitro* platelet survival time is about 4 to 8 h, platelets prepared with the addition of prostacyclin remain functional for more than 72 h.[41] This effect is not accompanied by a prolonged increase in cAMP level in platelets, thus separating it from the classical anti-aggregating effect.[42] Interestingly, a prostacyclin analogue shows a dissociation between anti-aggregating and "cytoprotective" effects in a model of acute myocardial ischemia.[43] All these results suggest that some of the therapeutic effects of prostacyclin might be related to the "cytoprotective" property, and they point to even wider indications for prostacyclin in cell or tissue preservation *in vivo* and *in vitro*.

High doses of prostacyclin infused intravenously in dogs induce significant fibrinolytic activity in plasma.[44] In man, however, two studies using smaller doses have produced contradictory results.[45,46] More recent results, however, suggest that the induced fibrinolytic activity is short-lasting, reaching a peak three hours after the start of the infusion and disappearing at 24 h in spite of continuation of the infusion.[47] The mechanism by which this fibrinolytic effect is induced is not yet understood, but experiments *in vitro*[48] suggest that prostacyclin and PGE_1 induce the release of a plasminogen activator probably through a cAMP-mediated effect.

PROSTACYCLIN AND ATHEROSCLEROSIS

Platelet activation, accumulation of lipid peroxides, accretion of cholesterol and cholesteryl esters, migration of phagocytes, and proliferation of smooth muscle cells are some of the hallmarks of the pathogenesis of atherosclerosis. Platelets from rabbits made atherosclerotic by dietary manipulation[49] and from patients who have survived myocardial infarction[50] are abnormally sensitive to pro-aggregating agents and produce more TXB_2 than those from controls. Several lipid peroxides occur in advanced atherosclerotic lesions.[51] Lipid peroxides, including 15-hydroperoxy arachidonic acid (15-HPAA), are potent (IC_{50} 0.48 μg/ml) and selective inhibitors of platelet generation by vessel wall microsomes or by fresh vascular tissue.[52,53] Thus, accumulation of lipid peroxides in, for example, atheromatous plaques could predispose to thrombus formation by inhibiting generation of prostacyclin by the vessel wall, without affecting TXA_2 production by platelets. A decrease in prostacyclin formation by atherosclerotic vascular tissue has been demonstrated both in experimental animals[54] and in man.[55] Moreover, smooth muscle cells obtained from atherosclerotic lesions and cultured *in vitro* consistently produce less prostacyclin than normal vascular smooth muscle cells.[56]

It is also noteworthy that the process of ageing seems to be connected with an impaired ability of cells in culture to produce prostacyclin. Human diploid fibroblasts which produce prostacyclin lose the ability to do so during ageing, while their production of the other arachidonic acid metabolites such as PGE_2, $PGF_{2\alpha}$, and TXA_2 increases.[57] In addition, aortic smooth muscle cells obtained from old rats produce less prostacyclin in culture than those obtained from young animals. Deleterious effects of lipid peroxides on prostacyclin production may also be related to an endogenous deficiency of natural anti-oxidants. In rats, a diet deficient in vitamin E leads to an increase in peroxide levels in the aorta and to a decrease in prostacyclin production *in vitro*.[58] The empirical use of vitamin E in atherosclerosis may be endorsed by the fact that platelet aggregation is decreased following pretreatment of platelet suspensions with α-tocopherol.[59]

A raised concentration of low density lipoprotein (LDL) is regarded as one of the risk factors associated with ischemic heart disease,[60] whereas high density lipoproteins (HDL) protect against the disease.[61] LDL reduces the release of a prostacyclin-like substance by human endothelial cells.[62] Furthermore, LDL inhibits, whereas HDL stimulates prostacyclin synthesis.[63] An interesting link between lipid peroxides and LDL was discovered by Gryglewski & Szczeklik.[64] The LDL fraction (but not the HDL) of lipoproteins taken from a group of hyperlipidemics contained lipid peroxide concentrations several times higher than those in the total serum. However, the concept that atherosclerosis is invariably associated with reduced generation of prostacyclin has recently been challenged,[65] for in human patients suffering from severe diffuse atherosclerosis, excretion of 2,3-dinor-6-keto-prostaglandin $F_{1\alpha}$, a major urinary metabolite of prostacyclin, was significantly higher than in healthy volunteers. The mechanism for this enhancement may be the release from activated platelets of factors with potential prostacyclin-releasing properties, such as platelet-derived growth factor, 5-hydroxytryptamine, and platelet-activating factor. Thus, a reduction in capacity of the atherosclerotic arterial wall to produce prostacyclin might coexist with an enhanced rate of its synthesis when stimuli which promote vascular prostacyclin release are produced *in vivo.*

As an atherosclerotic lesion progresses, cholesterol and cholesteryl esters are deposited in the extracellular matrix of the aortic smooth muscle cells as well as in lysosomal and cytosolic compartments of these cells.[66] Biochemical processes associated with cholesteryl ester accumulation in the arterial wall during atherogenesis include altered activity of the major enzymes responsible for cholesteryl ester hydrolysis and synthesis. Hydrolysis of cholesteryl ester via acid and neutral cholesteryl ester hydrolase activity (ACEH, NCEH) and esterification of cholesterol via a cholesterol-O-acyltransferase (ACAT) have been identified as major mechanisms by which these sterols are metabolized.[66] In cultured smooth muscle cells from the thoracic aorta of rabbits, prostacyclin increases the activity of ACEH and NCEH at low concentrations,[67,68] whereas in contrast, PGE_2 inhibits cholesteryl ester synthetic activity. The stimulatory effect of prostacyclin on the hydrolysis of cholesteryl ester is thought to be mediated via an increase in adenylate cyclase activity since dibutyryl cAMP mimics the prostacyclin-induced increase in cholesteryl ester degradation. These findings suggest that prostacyclin has an important regulatory role in aortic cholesteryl ester metabolism.[69]

Proliferation of smooth muscle cells migrating into the intima is an early manifestation of atherosclerosis. Platelet-derived growth factor,[70] as well as 12-lipoxygenase products,[71] stimulate proliferation and migration of smooth muscle cells. A decrease in cAMP levels occurs in zones of aortic lesions of rabbits with experimentally-induced atherosclerosis.[72] Dibutyryl cAMP decreases by two to fivefold the uptake of labeled thymidine into the intimal cells isolated from atherosclerotic aorta.[73] Based on this discovery, the same authors demonstrated that two stable prostacyclin analogues, 6β-PGI_1 and carbacyclin, also inhibit the proliferation of intimal smooth muscle as measured by ^{3}H-thymidine uptake into aortic cells.[69] In human atherosclerotic cells in culture, cholesteryl ester metabolism is enhanced by these prostacyclin analogues via a cAMP-dependent mechanism, confirming the work of Hajjar and Weksler.[67,68] These results, in addition to their physiological and pathophysiological interest, suggest that it may be possible to develop prostacyclin analogues with potential anti-atherosclerotic effects.

The role of white cells in myocardial infarction[74] or in vascular damage during arteritis[75] or atherosclerosis[76,77] has become an area of great interest during the last few years. Because of this, we decided to study the effect of cell migration on prostacyclin production in a model of experimental arteritis.

Injections of heterologous serum into the circulation of experimental animals and of man result in the development of a disorder most commonly described as serum sickness. Since vascular injury consequent to white cell migration plays an important role in the pathophysiology of this model, we studied the prostacyclin-synthesizing

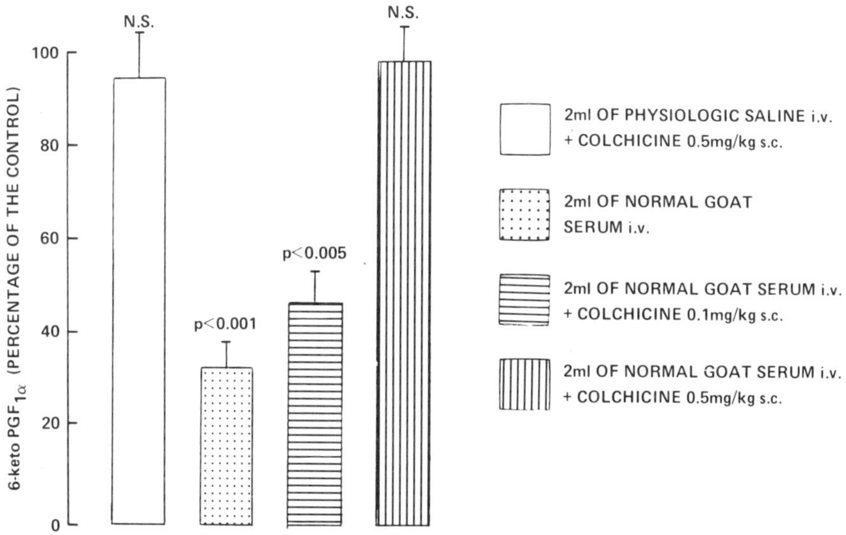

FIGURE 1. New Zealand white male rabbits were injected daily with 2 ml of goat serum i.v. At day 7, the animals were sacrificed, and prostacyclin (measured as 6-keto-$PGE_{1\alpha}$ by radioimmunoassay) generation by rings of the mesenteric arteries incubated *in vitro* was measured. Injection of colchicine alone did not alter significantly the production of prostacyclin by vascular tissue when compared with normal control animals (N.S.). Goat serum induced a significant ($p < 0.001$) reduction in prostacyclin generation, which recovered when animals were treated with increasing concentrations of colchicine.

capacity of arteries of rabbits treated for several days with goat serum. Intravenous daily injections of heterologous goat serum (0.5–2 ml) into rabbits resulted in a substantial reduction in 6-keto-$PGF_{1\alpha}$ production by incubates of rings of mesenteric artery as measured by specific RIA. Concomitant treatment of animals with colchicine (0.1–0.5 mg/kg/day subcutaneously), a drug which inhibits inflammatory cell migration, prevented this decrease in the production of prostacyclin by arterial tissue (FIGURE 1). These findings suggest that activated mononuclear phagocytes entering the vessel wall inhibit prostacyclin formation. The mechanisms of this inhibition remain to be investigated, but it is likely that free radicals or oxygenated products of the migrating cells might play a role.

MODIFICATION OF FATTY ACID PRECURSORS

Eicosapentaenoic acid (EPA) is a polyunsaturated fatty acid like arachidonic acid, but has a higher degree of unsaturation. It gives rise to prostaglandins of the '3' series and, when incubated with vascular tissue, leads to the release of an anti-aggregating substance.[78] Synthetic Δ^{17}-prostacyclin (PGI_3) is as potent an anti-aggregating agent as prostacyclin. In contrast, thromboxane A_3 has a weaker pro-aggregating activity than TXA_2.[78,79] Phospholipids in cell membranes, such as platelets, from Greenland Eskimos contain 8% EPA compared with 0.5% in Danes.[80] Similarly, the AA in phospholipids of Eskimos is approximately one-third of that in Danes. These differences may explain why Eskimos have a low incidence of acute myocardial infarction, low blood cholesterol levels, and an increased tendency to bleed. This prolonged bleeding time is related to a reduction in *ex vivo* platelet aggregability.[80] The plasma concentrations of cholesterol, triglyceride, and low and very low density lipoprotein are low in Eskimos, whereas that of high density lipoprotein is high.[81]

Eicosapentaenoic acid inhibits platelet aggregation in platelet-rich plasma stimulated by ADP, collagen, AA, and a synthetic analogue of PGH_2.[78] Also, EPA inhibits aggregation in aspirin- and imidazole-treated platelets,[82] and inhibits thrombin-induced aggregation.[83] It is clear, therefore, that both prostaglandin dependent and independent pathways of platelet aggregation are inhibited by EPA *in vitro. In vivo,* however, EPA is incorporated into platelet phospholipids, to some extent replacing arachidonic acid and exerting an anti-thrombotic effect either by competing with remaining arachidonic acid for cyclo-oxygenase and lipoxygenase,[84,85] or by being converted to the less pro-aggregatory PGH_3 and TXA_3.[78] Studying seven Caucasians who had been on a mackerel diet for one week, Seiss *et al.*[86] showed a reduced sensitivity of platelets to collagen, associated with a reduced ability to produce TXB_2, which was dependent on the ratio of EPA/AA in platelet phospholipids. ADP-induced aggregation was significantly reduced in some subjects and platelet aggregation to exogenously added AA was unchanged, indicating normal cyclo-oxygenase activity. Similarly, Sanders *et al.*[87] showed a significant increase (40%) in bleeding time in volunteers who had taken cod liver oil (equivalent to 1.8 g EPA) daily for six weeks. This was consistent with a decrease in AA and an increase in EPA in the platelet phospholipids.

Under normal peroxide levels *in vivo,* EPA is a poor substrate for the cyclo-oxygenase enzyme, but increasing peroxide tone in an incubate containing purified cyclo-oxygenase considerably increases the conversion of EPA.[84] Incubation of platelet-rich plasma with EPA does not induce the generation of a thromboxane-like material; indeed, it prevents the formation of TXA_2 induced by AA or by collagen.[78] Conversely, in human umbilical vasculature, Dyerberg *et al.*[88] demonstrated that EPA did not influence the conversion of AA to prostacyclin, but gave rise to additional synthesis of prostacyclin-like material. Aortic microsomes readily convert PGH_3 to Δ^{17}-6-keto-$PGF_{1\alpha}$.[89] Formation of Δ^{17}-2,3 dinor 6-keto-$PGF_{1\alpha}$ (a metabolite of Δ^{17}-prostacyclin) has been detected in the urine of volunteers fed with EPA.[90]

Fish oil feeding increased the amount of C20:5 (ω3) fatty acids present in heart and liver of cats and in the platelets of dogs.[91,92] Brain infarct volume after experimentally induced cerebral ischemia and the neurological deficit were less in cats fed fish oil than in a corresponding control group.[91] In dogs fed fish oil, thrombosis and subsequent infarct size (3% compared with 25% in a control group) induced by electrical stimulation were reduced, with less than 30% ectopic beats after 19 hours compared with 80% after 19 hours in the control group.[92]

The prolonged bleeding time in Eskimos is reduced after aspirin ingestion,[80] suggesting a decreased thromboxane synthesizing capacity coupled with a normal or possibly elevated prostacyclin production. Feeding spontaneously hypertensive male weanling rats a diet containing fish oil as the main source of fat resulted in significantly lower blood pressure 22 weeks after the diet was started compared with rats fed corn oil.[93] The precise mechanism of this effect is still to be elucidated.

More recently, studies in man suggest that a diet supplemented with EPA decreases whole blood viscosity, reduces triglyceride plasma concentration,[94] increases cutaneous bleeding time, reduces platelet aggregability, and reduces blood pressure.[95] In addition, long-term supplementation of the diet with EPA reduces plasma triglyceride and cholesterol levels, and decreases platelet aggregability in patients with cardiovascular disease.[96]

CLINICAL APPLICATIONS OF PROSTACYCLIN

Prostacyclin is available as a stable freeze-dried preparation (Epoprostenol) for administration to man. Intravenous infusion of prostacyclin in healthy volunteers leads to a dose-related inhibition of platelet aggregation, dispersal of circulating platelet aggregates, arteriolar vasodilatation, increases in skin temperature, and facial flushing (for review, see reference 16). Headache has been reported as a common side effect with the higher rates of prostacyclin infusion. Infusion of prostacyclin into patients susceptible to migraine or cluster headache induced, in most cases, a headache different from those usually experienced.[97]

The use of prostacyclin in several clinical conditions is now being investigated. In addition to its use in extracorporeal circulation systems such as cardiopulmonary bypass operations, renal dialysis, and charcoal hemoperfusion, prostacyclin is being tested for the treatment of atherosclerotic peripheral vascular disease and Raynaud's syndrome, as well as for the treatment of other thrombotic conditions. Extensive reviews of its clinical applications are available.[30,98,99] What is becoming clear is that the efficacy of prostacyclin, particularly its long-lasting effects, in certain clinical conditions like peripheral vascular disease and Raynaud's syndrome, cannot be explained solely in terms of its short-lasting vasodilatory and anti-aggregatory actions. Consequently, interest is being focused on the newly-described actions of prostacyclin such as cytoprotection, fibrinolysis, and stimulation of cholesterol metabolism. A better understanding of these actions might not only explain some of the observed effects, but might also suggest some new clinical applications, as well as clarifying further the role of prostacyclin in physiology and pathophysiology.

REFERENCES

1. Moncada, S., A. G. Herman, E. A. Higgs & J. R. Vane. 1977. Thromb. Res. **11:** 323–344.
2. Weksler, B. B., A. J. Marcus & E. A. Jaffe. 1977. Proc. Nat. Acad. Sci. USA **74:** 3922–3926.
3. MacIntyre, D. E., J. D. Pearson & J. L. Gordon. 1978. Nature (London) **271:** 549–551.
4. Moncada, S. & J. R. Vane. 1979. Pharmac. Rev. **30:** 293–331.
5. Whittle, B. J. R. 1980. *In* Gastro-intestinal Mucosal Blood Flow. Fielding, Ed.: 180–191. Churchill Livingstone. Edinburgh, London.
6. Axelrod, L. & L. Levine. 1981. Diabetes **30:** 163–167.
7. Moncada, S., R. Gryglewski, S. Bunting & J. R. Vane. 1976. Nature **263:** 663–665.
8. Ubatuba, F. B., S. Moncada & J. R. Vane. Thromb. Diath. Haemorrh. 1979. **41:** 425–434.

9. SZCZEKLIK, A., R. J. GRYGLEWSKI, R. NIZANKOWSKI, J. MUSIAL, R. PIETON & J. MRUK. 1978. Pharmac. Res. Commun. **10:** 545–556.
10. AIKEN, J. W., R. R. GORMAN & R. J. SHEBUSKI. 1979. Prostaglandins **17:** 483–494.
11. BAYER, B. L., K. E. BLASS & W. FORSTER. 1979. Br. J. Pharmacol. **66:** 10–12.
12. ROSENBLUM, W. I. & F. EL SABBAN. 1979. Stroke **10:** 399–401.
13. DUSTING, G. J., S. MONCADA & J. R. VANE. 1978. Br. J. Pharmacol. **64:** 315–320.
14. GIMENO, M. J., L. STERIN-BORDA, E. S. BORDA, M. A. LAZZARI & A. L. GIMENO. 1980. Prostaglandins **19:** 907–916.
15. JOHNSON, R. A., D. R. MORTON, J. H. KINNER, R. R. GORMAN, J. C. MCGUIRE, F. F. SUN, N. WHITTAKER, S. BUNTING, J. SALMON, S. MONCADA & J. R. VANE. 1976. Prostaglandins **12:** 915–928.
16. MONCADA, S. 1982. Br. J. Pharmacol. **76:** 3–31.
17. VANE, J. R. 1982. *In* Les Prix Nobel. pp. 176–206. Almqvist & Wiksell International. Stockholm.
18. GORMAN, R. R., S. BUNTING & O. V. MILLER. 1977. Prostaglandins **13:** 377–388.
19. TATESON, J. E., S. MONCADA & J. R. VANE. 1977. Prostaglandins **13:** 389–399.
20. KASER-GLANZMANN, R., M. JAKABOVA, J. GEORGE & E. LUSCHER. 1977. Biochim. Biophys. Acta **466:** 429–440.
21. LAPETINA, E. G., C. J. SCHMITGES, K. CHANDRABOSE & P. CUATRECASAS. 1977. Biochem. Biophys. Res. Commun. **76:** 828–835.
22. MINKES, M., M. STANFORD, M. CHI, G. ROTH, A. RAZ, P. NEEDLEMAN & P. MAJERUS. 1977. J. Clin. Invest. **59:** 449–454.
23. MALMSTEN, C., E. GRANSTROM & B. SAMUELSSON. 1976. Biochem. Biophys. Res. Commun. **68:** 569–576.
24. HIGGS, G. A., S. MONCADA & J. R. VANE. 1978. J. Physiol. (London) **280:** 55–56P.
25. HIGGS, G. A. 1982. *In* Cardiovascular Pharmacology of the Prostaglandins. A. G. Herman, P. M. Vanhoutte, H. Denolin & A. Goossens, Eds.: 315–325. Raven Press. New York.
26. BOXER, L. A., J. M. ALLEN, M. SCHMIDT, M. YODER & R. L. BAEHNER. 1980. J. Lab. Clin. Med. **95:** 672–678.
27. HOPKINS, N. K. & R. R. GORMAN. 1981. J. Clin. Invest. **67:** 540–546.
28. SCHAFER, A. I., M. A. GIMBRONE, JR. & R. I. HANDIN. 1980. Biochem. Biophys. Res. Commun. **96:** 1640–1647.
29. HIGGS, E. A., S. MONCADA, J. R. VANE, J. P. CAEN, H. MICHEL & G. TOBELEM. 1978. Prostaglandins **16:** 17–22.
30. MONCADA, S. 1983. *In* Atherosclerosis: Mechanisms and Approaches to Therapy. N.E. Miller, Ed.: 55–75. Raven Press. New York.
31. JUGDUTT, B. F., G. M. HUTCHINS, B. H. BULKLEY & L. C. BECKER. 1979. Clin. Res. **27:** 177A.
32. OGLETREE, M. L., A. M. LEFER, J. B. SMITH & K. C. NICOLAOU. 1979. Eur. J. Pharmacol. **56:** 95–103.
33. RIBEIRO, L. G. T., T. A. BRANDON, D. G. HOPKINS, L. A. REDUTO, A. A. TAYLOR & R. R. MILLER. 1981. Am. J. Cardiol. **47:** 835–840.
34. STARNES, V. A., R. K. PRIMM, R. L. WOOSLEY, J. A. OATES, & J. W. HAMMON. 1982. J. Cardiovasc. Pharmacol. **4:** 765–769.
35. OHLENDORF, R., E. PERZBORN & K. SCHROR. 1980. Thromb. Res. **19:** 447–453.
36. DEMLING, R. H., M. SMITH, R. GUNTHER, M. GEE & J. FLYNN. 1981. Surgery **89:** 257–263.
37. FLETCHER, J. R. & P. W. RAMWELL. 1980. Circ. Shock **7:** 299–308.
38. LEFER, A. M., J. TABAS & E. F. SMITH III. 1980. Pharmacol. **21:** 206–212.
39. ARAKI, H. & A. M. LEFER. 1980. Am. J. Physiol. **238:** H176–181.
40. MONDEN, M. & J. G. FORTNER. 1982. Ann. Surg. **196:** 38–42.
41. MONCADA, S., M. RADOMSKI & J. R. VARGAS. 1982. Br. J. Pharmacol. **75:** 165P.
42. BLACKWELL, G. J., M. RADOMSKI, J. R. VARGAS & S. MONCADA. 1982. Biochim. Biophys. Acta **718:** 60–65.
43. SCHROR, K., R. OHLENDORF & H. DARIUS. 1981. J. Pharmac. Exp. Ther. **219:** 243–249.
44. UTSUNOMIYA, T., M. M. KRAUSZ, C. R. VALERI, D. SHEPRO & H. B. HECHTMAN. 1980. Surgery **88:** 25–30.

45. HOSSMAN, V., A. HEINEN, H. AUEL & G. A. FITZGERALD. 1981. Thromb. Res. **22:** 481–490.
46. DEMBINSKA-KIEC, A., E. KOSTKA-TRABKA & R. J. GRYGLEWSKI. 1982. Thromb. Haem. **47:** 190.
47. SZCZEKLIK, A., M. KOPEC, K. SLADEK, J. MUSIAL, J. CHMIELEWSKA, E. TEISSEYRE, G. DUDEK-WOJCIECHOWSKA & M. PALESTER-CHLEBOWCZYK. 1983. Thromb. Res. **29:** 655–660.
48. CRUTCHLEY, D. J., L. B. CONANAN & J. R. MAYNARD. 1982. J. Pharmacol. Exp. Ther. **222:** 544–549.
49. SHIMAMOTO, T., M. KOBAYASHI, T. TAKAHASHI, Y. TAKASHIMA, M. SAKAMOTO & M. MOROOKA. 1978. Jap. Heart J. **19:** 748–753.
50. SZCZEKLIK, A., R. J. GRYGLEWSKI, J. MUSIAL, L. GRODZINSKA, M. SERWONSKA & E. MARCINKIEWICZ. 1978. Thromb. Diath. Haem. **40:** 66–74.
51. GLAVIND, J., S. HARTMANN, J. CLEMMESEN, K. E. JESSEN & H. DAM. 1952. Acta Pathol. Microbiol. Scand. **30:** 1–6.
52. MONCADA, S., R. J. GRYGLEWSKI, S. BUNTING & J. R. VANE. 1976. Prostaglandins **12:** 715–733.
53. SALMON, J. A., D. R. SMITH, R. J. FLOWER, S. MONCADA & J. R. VANE. 1978. Biochim. Biophys. Acta **523:** 250–262.
54. DEMBINSKA-KIEC, A., T. GRYGLEWSKA, A. ZMUDA & R. J. GRYGLEWSKI. 1977. Prostaglandins **14:** 1025–1034.
55. ANGELO, V. D., S. VILLA, M. MYSLIWIEC, M. B. DONATI & G. DE GAETANO. 1978. Thromb. Diath. Haem. **39:** 535–536.
56. LARRUE, J., M. RIGAUD, D. DARET, J. DEMOND, J. DURAND & H. BRICAUD. 1980. Nature **285:** 480–482.
57. MUROTA, S. I., Y. MITSUI & M. KAWAMURA. 1979. Biochim. Biophys. Acta **574:** 351–355.
58. OKUMA, M., H. TAKAYAMA & H. UCHINO. 1980. Prostaglandins **19:** 527–536.
59. WHITIN, J. C., R. K. GORDON, L. M. CORWIN & E. R. SIMONS. 1982. J. Lipid Res. **23:** 276–282.
60. MEDALIE, J. H., H. A. KAHN, H. N. NEUFELD, E. RISS & U. GOULDBOURT. 1973. J. Chron. Dis. **26:** 63–84.
61. STREJA, D., G. STEINER & P. O. KWITEROVICH. 1978. Ann. Intern. Med. **89:** 871–880.
62. NORDOY, A., B. SVENSSON, D. WIEBE & J. C. HOAK. 1978. Circ. Res. **43:** 527–534.
63. BEITZ, J. & W. FORSTER. 1980. Biochim. Biophys. Acta **620:** 352–355.
64. GRYGLEWSKI, R. J. & A. SZCZEKLIK. 1981. *In* Clinical Pharmacology of Prostacyclin. P.J. Lewis & J. O'Grady, Eds.: 89–95. Raven Press. New York.
65. FITZGERALD, G. A., B. SMITH, A. K. PEDERSEN & A. R. BRASH. 1984. New Eng. J. Med. **310:** 1065–1068.
66. ST. CLAIR, R. W. 1976. Atheroscler. Rev. **1:** 61.
67. HAJJAR, D. P., B. B. WEKSLER, D. J. FALCONE, J. M. HEFTON, K. TACK-GOLDMAN & C. R. MINICK. 1982. J. Clin. Invest. **70:** 479–488.
68. HAJJAR, D. P. & B. B. WEKSLER. 1983. J. Lipid Res. **24:** 1176–1185.
69. OREKHOV, A. N., V. V. TERTOV & V. N. SMIRNOV. 1983. Lancet **ii:** 521.
70. ROSS, R. & A. VOGEL. 1978. Cell **14:** 203–210.
71. NAKAO, J., T. OOYAMA, H. ITO, W-C. CHANG & S-I. MUROTA. 1982. Atherosclerosis **44:** 339–342.
72. NUMANO, F. 1980. *In* Atherosclerosis, vol. 5. A.M.J. Gotto, L.C. Smith & B. Allen, Eds.: 537. Springer-Verlag. New York, Heidelberg, Berlin.
73. TERTOV, V. V., A. N. OREKHOV, V. S. REPIN & V. N. SMIRNOV. 1982. Biochim. Biophys. Res. Commun. **109:** 1228–1239.
74. MULLANE, K. M. & S. MONCADA. 1983. *In* Mechanism of Drug Action. T.P. Singer, T.E. Mansour & R.N. Ondarza, Eds.: 229–242. Academic Press. New York.
75. HAZEN, P. G. & B. MICHEL. 1979. Arch. Dermatol. **115:** 1303–1306.
76. NAGORNEV, V. A., I. U. V. BOBRISHEV, I. U. V. IVANOVSKI & A. S. KUZNETSOV. 1983. Arkh. Patol. **45:** 19–26.
77. FAGGIOTTO, A., R. ROSS & L. HARKER. 1984. Arteriosclerosis **4:** 323–340.

78. GRYGLEWSKI, R. J., J. A. SALMON, F. B. UBATUBA, B. C. WEATHERLY, S. MONCADA & J. R. VANE. 1979. Prostaglandins **18:** 453–478.
79. RAZ, A., M. S. MINKES & P. NEEDLEMAN. 1977. Biochim. Biophys. Acta **488:** 305–311.
80. DYERBERG, J. & H. O. BANG. 1979. Lancet **ii:** 433–435.
81. BANG, H. O. & J. DYERBERG. 1972. Acta Med. Scand. **192:** 85–94.
82. DYERBERG, J. & K. A. JORGENSEN. 1980. Artery **8:** 12–17.
83. JAKUBOWSKI, J. A. & N. G. ARDLIE. 1979. Thromb. Res. **16:** 205–217.
84. CULP, B. R., B. G. TITUS & W. E. M. LANDS. 1979. Prostaglandins Med. **3:** 269–278.
85. NEEDLEMAN, P., A. RAZ, M. S. MINKES, J. A. FERRENDELLI & H. SPRECHER. 1979. Proc. Nat. Acad. Sci. USA **76:** 944–948.
86. SEISS, W., P. ROTH, B. SCHERER, I. KURZMANN, B. BOHLIG & P. C. WEBER. 1980. Lancet **i:** 441–444.
87. SANDERS, T. A. B., D. J. NAISMITH, A. P. HAINES & M. VICKERS. 1980. Lancet **i:** 1189.
88. DYERBERG, J., K. A. JORGENSEN & T. ARNFRED. 1981. Prostaglandins **22:** 857–862.
89. SMITH, D. R., B. C. WEATHERLY, J. A. SALMON, F. B. UBATUBA, R. J. GRYGLEWSKI & S. MONCADA. 1979. Prostaglandins **18:** 423–438.
90. FISHER, S. & P. C. WEBER. 1984. Nature **307:** 165–168.
91. BLACK, R. L., B. CULP, D. MADISON, O. S. RANDALL & W. E. M. LANDS. 1979. Prostaglandins Med. **3:** 257–268.
92. CULP, B. R., W. E. M. LANDS, B. R. LUCCESI, B. PITT & J. ROMSON. 1980. Prostaglandins **20:** 1021–1031.
93. SCHOENE, N. W. & D. FIORE. 1981. Prog. Lipid Res. **20:** 569–570.
94. WOODCOCK, B. E., E. SMITH, W. H. LAMBERT, W. MORRIS JONES, J. H. GALLOWAY, M. GREAVES & F. E. PRESTON. 1984. Br. Med. J. **288:** 592–594.
95. LORENZ, R., U. SPENGLER, S. FISCHER, J. DUHM & P. C. WEBER. 1983. Circulation **67:** 504–511.
96. SAYNOR, R., D. VEREL & T. GILLOTT. 1984. Atherosclerosis **50:** 3–10.
97. PEATFIELD, R. C., M. J. GAWEL & F. CLIFFORD ROSE. 1981. Headache **21:** 190–195.
98. MONCADA, S. 1983. Stroke **14:** 157–168.
99. VANE, J. R. 1983. Advances in Prostaglandin, Thromboxane, and Leukotriene Research **11:** 449–456.

Pharmacological Analysis of Factors Influencing Platelet Aggregation in Stenosed Coronary Arteries of Dogs

JAMES W. AIKEN

Atherosclerosis and Thrombosis Research
The Upjohn Company
Kalamazoo, Michigan 49001

INTRODUCTION

In vitro studies on platelets, mostly carried out using an aggregometer,[4] have led to the conclusion that a number of naturally occurring substances promote platelet aggregation. These include epinephrine, serotonin, thromboxane A_2 (TXA_2), prostaglandin H_2, adenosine 5′-diphosphate (ADP), collagen, thrombin, and platelet activating factor (AGEPC). However, the relative importance *in vivo* of each of these factors alone or in combination with each other (or with other physical influences, such as shear) is difficult to assess.

Our laboratory has used an *in vivo* experimental approach[5,6] to analyze, pharmacologically, the importance of some of these substances as promoters of coronary artery thrombosis in stenosed vessels in dogs. In the process of this evaluation, the data accumulated pointed to the conclusion that prostacyclin (PGI_2) may play a role as an endogenous inhibitor of platelet aggregation, especially when its activity is enhanced by other pharmacologic means, and that serotonin is of considerable importance as an endogenous promoter of coronary artery thrombosis in this model.

METHODS

Mongrel dogs (17–30 kg) were anesthetized with sodium pentobarbital at a dose of 35 mg/kg i.v. Respiration was maintained in these animals via a cuffed endotracheal tube attached to a Harvard Apparatus respirator. The breathing rate was set at 12 strokes/min with a tidal volume of 20 ml/kg. A cannula placed in the left internal carotid artery was attached to a Gould Statham pressure transducer (P23Db) for the measurement of blood pressure, and a lead II EKG was used to monitor heart rate. All parameters were recorded on multichannel pen recorders.

In Vivo *Platelet Aggregation*

The experimental procedure used to monitor *in vivo* platelet aggregation in anesthetized dogs has been described in detail in several articles.[1–3] In summary, it consists of dissecting free a 20 mm segment of left circumflex coronary artery (CCA) from the surrounding myocardium. Blood flow is constantly measured in this artery by a proximally placed electromagnetic flowprobe. The CCA is then severely stenosed (i.e., about a 90% reduction in lumen size) by placing a Lexan® obstructor around the artery at a point distal to the flowprobe. Under this level of obstruction, blood flow in the isolated CCA will usually begin to decline spontaneously to zero. Histological and pharmacological evidence supports the view that this decline in blood flow is due to platelet aggregation at the obstructed site and not vasospasm.[3] In this model, the intensity of platelet aggregation occurring in the CCA is reflected in the rate of decline in coronary blood flow and the ease at which flow is restored, that is, whether the platelet thrombi are spontaneously shed from the obstructed site (X), or if the thrombi must be shaken loose from the obstructed site by the investigator (SL). A convenient rating system, originally described by Aiken and Shebuski,[2] was used to define the *in vivo* anti-aggregatory efficacy of the different drug doses tested.

Drug Administration

Prostacyclin sodium infusions were given in each experiment to confirm that platelet thrombus formation was occurring in the stenosed coronary arteries of the anesthetized dogs. PGI_2 solutions were freshly prepared daily by dissolving the compound in 50 m*M* tris-saline buffer (pH 9.0), which also served as the infusion vehicle.

Other drugs were dissolved in saline or neutral buffers and administered by i.v. bolus injection. Vehicle controls were done with each solution. In some experiments, drugs were applied topically to the CCA at the site of the obstructor (or just distal to the obstructor as a control) to observe the local effects at the site of stenosis.

RESULTS AND DISCUSSION

The efficacy of several classes of pharmacological agents for inhibiting coronary arterial occlusion in the dog is reviewed in TABLE 1. Three classes of drugs were outstanding in their ability to prevent thrombosis: prostacyclin (and its analogs), serotonin antagonists, and thromboxane synthase inhibitors. All prevented occlusion of the stenosed coronary artery of the dog in over 90% of the experiments.

FIGURE 1 shows the effects of PGI_2 and ketanserin, a serotonin antagonist, which was effective in 11 out of 12 experiments in preventing the cyclical blood flow changes typical of the platelet aggregatory response in this preparation. PGI_2 given by i.v. infusion was the most consistently effective agent. In fact, when occasionally PGI_2 failed to block aggregation (3% of the time), subsequent histological examination

TABLE 1. Efficacy of Anti-Aggregatory Substances for Preventing Coronary Occlusion in Dogs with Severe Coronary Arterial Obstruction

Substance	Efficacy
Prostacyclin (i.v. infusion) (and PGI_2 analogs)	97%
Thromboxane synthase inhibitors (U-63,557A, OKY-1581)	>90%
Serotonin antagonists (Ketanserin, Methysergide, LY53857)	>90%
Alpha-adrenergic antagonists (Yohimbine, Phentolamine)	50%
Cyclooxygenase inhibitors (Aspirin, Indomethacin, Ibuprofen)	50%[a]
Heparin, Dipyridamole, Aminophylline, Theophylline, Nitroglycerine, Hexamethonium	No effect

[a]Efficacy depends on severity of obstruction (Aiken *et al.*, 1981).

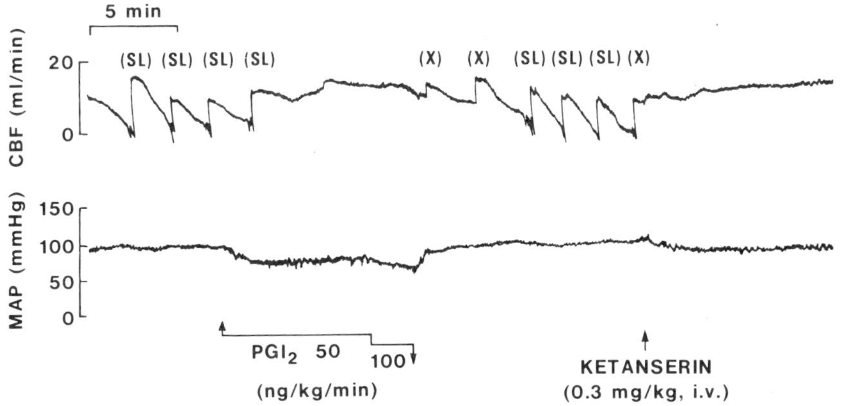

FIGURE 1. Records are of coronary blood flow (CBF; top) and mean arterial pressure (MAP; bottom) in an anesthetized dog. Platelet aggregation in the coronary artery is reflected by the cyclical declines in flow, which were restored by either shaking loose the thrombus manually (SL) or by spontaneous shedding of the thrombus from the obstructed site (X). Platelet aggregation was inhibited by i.v. infusion of prostacyclin (PGI_2) or i.v. injection of the serotonin antagonist ketanserin.

failed to demonstrate a platelet aggregate, suggesting that these rare failures were actually because the artery became obstructed by some other mechanism.

The high efficacy of serotonin antagonists suggests an important role for serotonin in promoting aggregation. Dog platelets, like human platelets, usually do not aggregate to serotonin *in vitro,* but serotonin induces a shape change and potentiates the aggregatory effect on other agonists. This facilitating role for serotonin may be of considerable importance if this model reflects the human situation.

The higher efficacy of thromboxane synthase inhibitors compared to cyclooxygenase inhibitors is because their mode of action is *via* endogenous PGI_2 formation and action.[3] Whereas cyclooxygenase inhibitors are only effective in some experiments, which depend on the severity of the obstruction, TXA_2 synthase inhibitors are equally efficacious to PGI_2 and, like PGI_2, their efficacy is independent of the degree of obstruction. Blocking endogenous PGI_2 synthesis by local topical application of an inhibitor of PGI_2 synthesis at the point of the obstruction, will eliminate the effectiveness of TXA_2 synthesis inhibitors, demonstrating that PGI_2 production in the vessel wall is required for their high efficacy. The mechanisms involved have been discussed in detail elsewhere[3] and suggest that TXA_2 is more important as a promoter of thrombosis than its precursor PGH_2.

The roles of collagen, epinephrine, and ADP in this model are less well-defined. Intentionally damaging the endothelium in the CCA enhances the aggregatory response, but the mechanism could be multifactorial: exposure of collagen, reduced PGI_2 production, release of thrombin, etc. Antagonists of α_2-adrenergic receptors are sometimes effective suggesting that circulating epinephrine has an influence on aggregability. Interestingly, some animals in which there is a moderately high level of hemolysis and whose platelets fail to aggregate to ADP *in vitro* still show the normal aggregation pattern in the CCA, suggesting that desensitization to ADP does not prevent coronary thrombosis *in vivo.*

Although more studies could further define the mechanisms involved, these data suggest that serotonin is an important *in vivo* promoter of thrombosis, and that, under certain circumstances, PGI_2 may be an important endogenous inhibitor and is responsible for the high anti-aggregatory efficacy of TXA_2 synthase inhibitors.

REFERENCES

1. AIKEN, J. W., R. R. GORMAN & R. J. SHEBUSKI. 1979. Prevention of blockage of partially obstructed coronary arteries with prostacyclin correlates with inhibition of platelet aggregation. Prostaglandins **17:** 483–494.
2. AIKEN, J. W. & R. J. SHEBUSKI. 1980. Comparison in anesthetized dogs of chemically stable prostacyclin analog, 6a-carba-PGI_2 (carbacyclin). Prostaglandins **19:** 629–643.
3. AIKEN, J. W., R. J. SHEBUSKI, O. V. MILLER & R. R. GORMAN. 1981. Endogenous prostacyclin contributes to the efficacy of a thromboxane synthetase inhibitor for preventing coronary artery thrombosis. J. Pharmacol. Exp. Ther. **219:** 299–308.
4. BORN, G. V. R. 1962. Aggregation of blood platelets by adenosine diphosphate and its reversal. Nature (Lond.) **194:** 927–929.
5. FOLTS, J. D., E. D. CROMWELL & G. G. ROWE. 1976. Platelet aggregation in partially obstructed vessels and its elimination with aspirin. Circulation **54:** 365–370.
6. GALLAGHER, K. P., J. D. FOLTS & G. G. ROWE. 1978. Comparison of coronary arteriograms with direct measurements of stenosed coronary arteries in dogs. Am. Heart J. **95:** 338–347.

Prostacyclin and Variant Angina

FUJIO NUMANO,[a] SHUZO NOMURA,[a] TADANORI AIZAWA,[b] JUNICHI FUJII,[b] AND MICHIYOSHI YAJIMA[a]

[a]*Department of Internal Medicine*
Tokyo Medical & Dental University
Yushima, Bunkyo-ku, Tokyo 113, Japan
[b]*Cardiovascular Institute*
Roppongi, Minato-ku, Tokyo 106, Japan

Since the first description of the variant form of angina pectoris by Prinzmetal *et al.*,[1] coronary spasm has been considered to play a major role in various clinical manifestations of ischemic heart disease. Evidence has accumulated that coronary spasm is responsible for almost all cases of the variant form of angina, frequently for unstable angina and sometimes, even for acute myocardial infarction.[2–5]

Although coronary spasm has been noted angiographically, clinically, and experimentally,[6–8] the mechanisms responsible are still not well understood and various hypotheses have been put forward.[9,10] The discovery of thromboxane (TXA_2) and prostacyclin (PGI_2) and the clarification of their physiological roles have thrown light on the exquisite balance between the blood flow and the vessel wall.[11–13] Thus, any alteration in this balance would lead to various diseases of vascular systems.[14–17]

Since Ellis *et al.* suggested for the first time the roles of TXA_2 on coronary smooth muscle contraction,[18] prostanoids have gained attention as important local hormonal substances which modulate coronary circulation.[19–23]

Therefore, any unbalance in the levels of these compounds would lead to anginal attacks in patients with coronary heart disease.[24–26]

Tada *et al.* reported increased plasma levels of TXB_2 in patients with variant angina, and stressed that transient coronary vasospasm might be induced by TXA_2, which was locally released in coronary circulation by the aggregating platelets.[27] Lewy *et al.* also reported the high levels of TXB_2 in patients with variant angina, and found statistically increased levels during attack, as compared with findings in patients with coronary arterial disease.[28]

On the other hand, Chierchia *et al.* reported that neither PGI_2 nor TXA_2 blockers prevented clinical vasospastic attacks, thereby suggesting the lack of an important role of prostanoids in coronary vascular spasm.[29,30] Robertson *et al.* found that, despite increased levels of TXB_2 in plasma of patients with variant angina during attack, neither aspirin nor indomethacin had any effect on the frequency or duration of ischemia and suggested that increases in levels of TXB_2 are not the cause, but rather the result of spasm.[31]

We investigated the plasma levels of TXB_2 and 6-keto $PGF_{1\alpha}$ in blood sampled at the coronary sinus and ascending aorta in patients with variant angina, and examined the changes in these levels during coronary spasm which occurred spontaneously or during the ergonovine test. Findings were compared with levels in patients with effort angina and who were free from anginal attack.

MATERIALS AND METHODS

Twenty-one Japanese men and women ranging in age from 46–65 years with the variant form of angina pectoris (VA) and twenty with effort angina (EA) were studied.

All the VA patients had episodes of anginal attacks at rest, and ST elevation in the electrocardiogram was confirmed at the time of attack. Coronary spasm was angiographically confirmed by the ergonovine test or during spontaneous attacks. All patients with EA were diagnosed according to exertional anginal attacks documented in their medical records, positive changes in the electrocardiogram during the treadmill exercise test, and more than 75% obstructive atherosclerotic lesions seen on the angiogram. They were all confirmed "negative" with 0.2 mg of ergonovine maleate injection. Patients with variant angina were subdivided into two groups according to coronary angiographical findings; patients with normal coronary arteries or those with less than 50% luminal diameter narrowing and with greater than 50% fixed narrowing.

Parallel to these two groups of patients, thirteen age-matched patients were studied as controls. They visited our clinic with chest pain and the catheterization studies which were performed under their agreement revealed that they had no coronary disease with normal coronary arteries.

Plasma Levels of TXB_2 and 6-keto $PGF_{1\alpha}$ at Rest

Routine coronary angiography and coronary sinus catheterization were carried out, and 5 ml of blood samples were taken from the coronary sinus (CS) and ascending aorta (AO) through a catheter. The samples were immediately placed into heparinized plastic tubes containing 0.1 volume of 10^{-2} M indomethacin (Merck, Co.) solution and centrifuged at 3,000 rpm for 10 minutes at 0°C. Plasma thus obtained was kept frozen at −80°C until analysis. Plasma levels of TXB_2 and 6-keto $PGF_{1\alpha}$ were radioimmunoassayed using ^{121}I- TXB_2-tyramide or ^{121}I-6-keto $PGF_{1\alpha}$-tyramide[32,33] within one week after the sampling.

Changes in Plasma Levels of TXB_2 and 6-keto $PGF_{1\alpha}$ at Ergonovine Test

To assess the role of prostanoid on the coronary sinus, blood samples were collected from coronary sinus of nine patients with variant angina and from five in the controls before and after the intravenous injection of 0.2 mg of ergonovine maleate (Merck, Co.), and changes of prostanoids in plasma were studied in both groups.

At the time of sampling, coronary spasm was confirmed angiographically to be induced by ergonovine administration in all patients with variant angina.

Plasma Levels of TXB_2 and 6-keto $PGF_{1\alpha}$ at Spontaneous Attack

Plasma levels of TXB_2 and 6-keto $PGF_{1\alpha}$ at spontaneous attack were measured in six coronary sinus blood samples collected at spontaneous attack during the coronary angiography.

RESULTS

Plasma Levels of TXB_2 and 6-keto $PGF_{1\alpha}$ at Rest

Eight of twenty-one patients with VA were confirmed angiographically to have had over a 50% narrowing of lesions in their coronary arteries (VA (+)), and the other

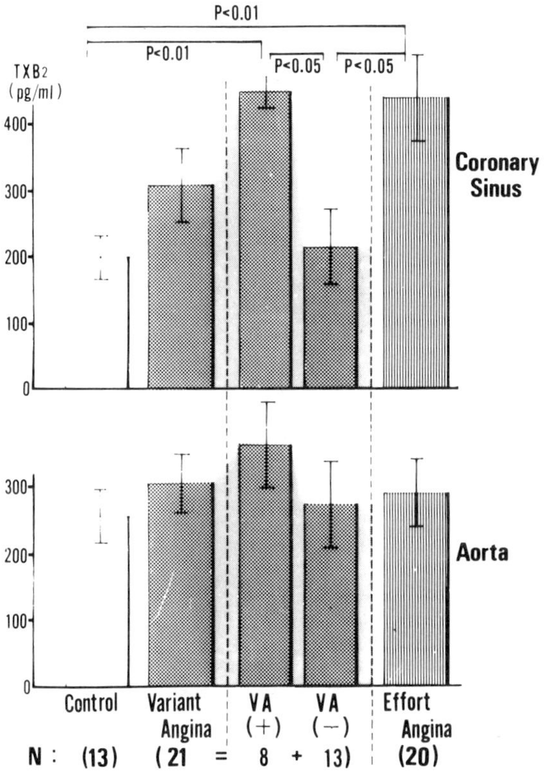

FIGURE 1. Plasma thromboxane B_2 levels (at rest).

thirteen had either normal coronary arteries or less than 50% narrowing of the lesions (VA (−)). FIGURE 1 and TABLE 1 summarize the plasma levels of TXB_2 in three groups. In the coronary sinus samples, both EA and VA groups revealed high levels of TXB_2 in the plasma, the former of which were statistically high, as compared with that in the controls ($p < 0.01$). Though in the VA group as a whole there were no statistically significant high levels of TXB_2, the subgroup VA (+) exhibited statisti-

TABLE 1. Plasma Levels of Thromboxane B_2

Patients/Samples	Plasma TXB_2 (pg/ml) Coronary Sinus	Aorta
Normal controls	200 ± 32	258 ± 44
Variant angina	304 ± 51	307 ± 46
atherosclerotic coronaries VA(+)	453 ± 72[a,b]	364 ± 65
normal coronaries VA(−)	212 ± 58	273 ± 63
Effort angina	438 ± 66[a,b]	290 ± 51

[a] $p < 0.01$, Control versus Angina.
[b] $p < 0.05$, VA(−) versus VA(+) and Effort.

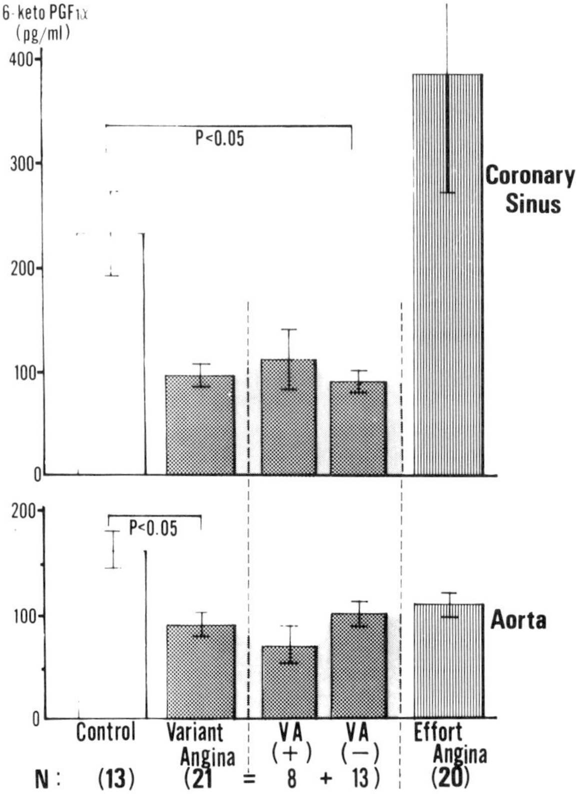

FIGURE 2. Plasma 6-keto $PGF_{1\alpha}$ levels (at rest).

cally significant high levels, as compared with data in normal controls ($p < 0.05$) and the VA (−) subgroup ($p < 0.05$).

On the contrary, in samples taken from the aorta, the same changes observed in coronary sinus blood were recognized, but without any statistical significant difference.

As shown in FIGURE 2 and TABLE 2, plasma levels of 6-keto $PGF_{1\alpha}$ in those with

TABLE 2. Plasma Levels of 6-keto $PGF_{1\alpha}$

		Plasma 6-keto $PGF_{1\alpha}$	
Patients/Samples	No.	Coronary Sinus	Aorta
Normal controls	13	232 ± 59	160 ± 33
Variant angina	21	98 ± 17	90 ± 18[a]
atherosclerotic coronaries VA(+)	8	111 ± 42	67 ± 29
normal coronaries VA (−)	13	90 ± 13[a]	102 ± 23
Effort angina	20	383 ± 120	111 ± 19

[a] $p < 0.05$, Normal control versus VA(−).

TABLE 3. Changes in Plasma Levels of TXB_2 and 6-keto $PGF_{1\alpha}$ in Coronary Sinus Blood during Ergonovine Test

Prostanoids		TXB_2 (pg/ml)			6-keto $PGF_{1\alpha}$ (pg/ml)	
		Ergonovine (0.2 mg I.A.)			Ergonovine (0.2 mg I.A.)	
Patients/Ergonovine Test	N	Before	After	N	Before	After
Normal controls	5	175 ± 23	294 ± 101	5	226 ± 79	213 ± 72
Variant angina	9	293 ± 79	333 ± 50	6	121 ± 28	104 ± 42
atherosclerotic coronaries VA(+)	2	321	406	2	147	159
normal coronaries VA(−)	7	285 ± 101	312 ± 31	4	109 ± 19	77 ± 19

variant angina were very low, as compared with those in normal controls or those with effort angina. It should be noted that, in contrast to TXB_2, both VA(+) and VA(−) revealed low levels of 6-keto $PGF_{1\alpha}$. In particular, a statistically significant low level was confirmed in subgroup VA (−), as compared with findings in the normal control group ($p < 0.05$), and also a statistically significant low level was recognized in aortic samples of variant angina ($p < 0.05$).

Changes in Plasma Levels of TXB_2 and 6-keto $PGF_{1\alpha}$ during the Ergonovine Test

As shown in TABLE 3 and FIGURE 3, during coronary spasm induced by ergonovine injection, plasma levels of TXB_2 in patients with variant angina were increased, albeit without a statistically significant increase, and in turn, almost no changes of 6-keto $PGF_{1\alpha}$ levels were observed. These changes were the same in both subgroups of VA

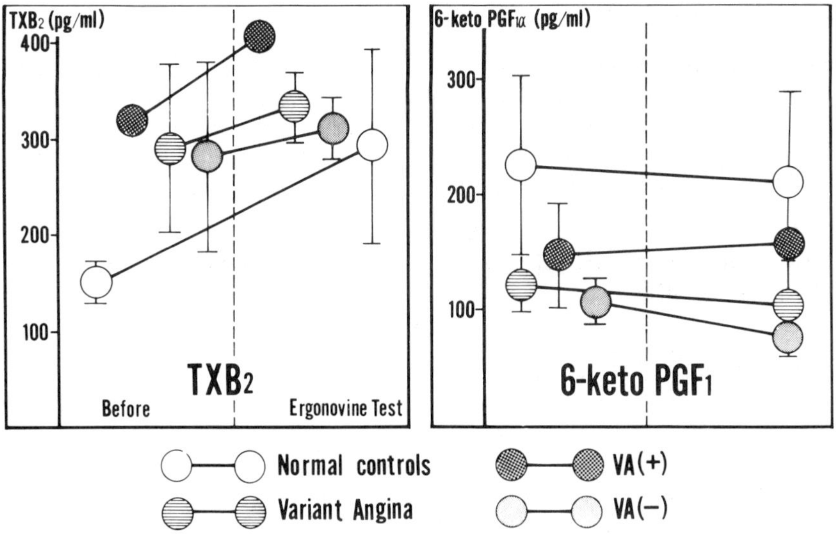

FIGURE 3. Changes in plasma levels of TXB_2 and 6-keto $PGF_{1\alpha}$ of coronary sinus blood during ergonovine test.

(+) and VA (−). More interestingly, the controls revealed the same changes as those in patients with variant angina even though coronary spasm was not induced by ergonovine.

Plasma Levels of TXB_2 and 6-keto $PGF_{1\alpha}$ at Spontaneous Attack

The plasma TXB_2 in patients with variant angina exhibited a statistically significant high level, as compared with those in normal control, and this difference was due to a statistically high level of TXB_2 in the VA (+) group. However, the plasma taken at the time of spontaneous attack revealed a decreased level of TXB_2, as compared with that before attack. (TABLE 4 and FIGURE 4). Low levels of 6-keto $PGF_{1\alpha}$ in plasma of patients with variant angina were again confirmed and no remarkable changes were recognized during spontaneous attack.

DISCUSSION

An association between coronary arterial spasm and atherosclerotic lesions has often been noted since Osler's early description,[9] and extensive studies have been reported on these relationships.[7,34,35] Recently, Shimokawa *et al.* induced coronary spasm at the area of atherosclerotic lesions in miniature pigs fed a high cholesterol diet and after their coronary arteries had been denuded by ballooning.[36] This is the first report in which spasm was angiographically certified in experimental animals. They concluded that atherosclerosis was a primary causative factor of coronary spasm. Kawachi *et al.* observed selective hyper-contraction in the atherosclerotic lesions of the canine coronary artery *in vivo,* and proposed that smooth muscles in atherosclerotic arteries might be hypersensitive to specific agonists such as ergonovine and serotonin.[37] Henry and Yokoyama also reported an increased sensitivity for ergonovine in atherosclerotic aortic strips,[38] while Kishi and Numano observed these same changes when atherosclerotic aortic strips of rabbits were exposed to serotonin.[39] Finally, Nanda and Henry confirmed the increased number of serotonergic and alpha adrenergic receptors in aortas from rabbits fed a high cholesterol diet,[40] and Kalsner and Richards reported that coronary arteries from hearts of cardiac patients contained significantly higher concentrations of histamine, sertonin, and amines than do those from noncardiac patients.[41]

TABLE 4. Changes in Plasma Levels of TXB_2 and 6-keto $PGF_{1\alpha}$ in Coronary Sinus Blood during Angina Attack

Prostanoids / Patients/Attack	TXB_2 (pg/ml) at Rest	TXB_2 (pg/ml) Spontaneous attack	6-keto $PGF_{1\alpha}$ (pg/ml) at Rest	6-keto $PGF_{1\alpha}$ (pg/ml) Spontaneous attack
Normal controls	200 ± 32	—	232 ± 59	—
Variant angina	304 ± 51	193 ± 53 (N:6)	98 ± 17	85 ± 17 (N:6)
atherosclerotic coronaries VA(+)	453 ± 72	240 ± 95 (N:3)	111 ± 42	102 ± 31 (N:3)
normal coronaries VA(−)	212 ± 58	145 ± 50 (N:3)	90 ± 13	68 ± 13 (N:3)

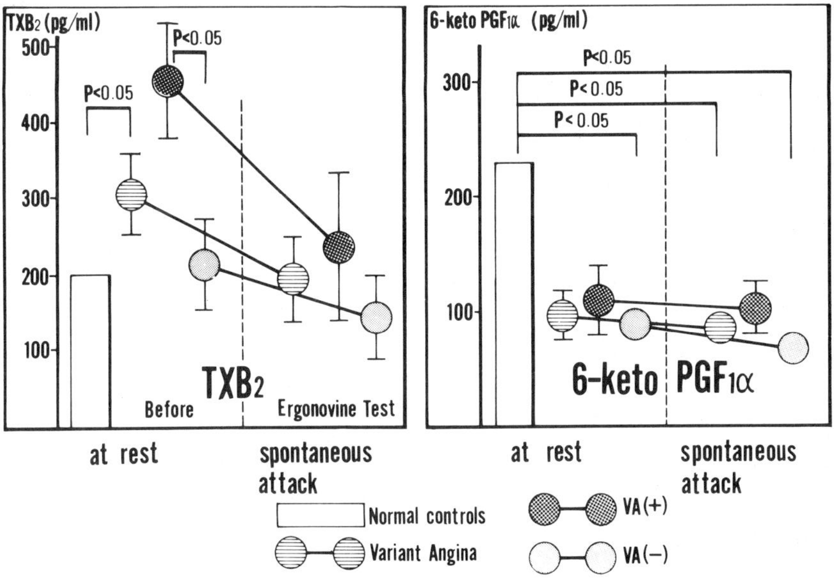

FIGURE 4. Changes in plasma levels of TXB_2 and 6-keto $PGF_{1\alpha}$ of coronary sinus blood during spontaneous attack.

Though these data confirmed that atherosclerotic lesions could be one condition under which spasm is easily induced, this explanation for spasm is not complete. About 10% of all patients with variant angina have no evidence of atherosclerosis.[7,42–44] On the other hand, patients with variant angina are comparatively few, as compared with the number of patients with ischemic heart disease. Furthermore, some authors mentioned that there are many cases of variant angina in Japan and Italy, as compared with countries where coronary atherosclerosis is a relevant disease.[45] The mechanism related to spontaneous remission of spasm and exacerbations of symptoms in the absence of obvious changes in coronary artery is unknown.

We thus studied the mechanism of spasm from the standpoint of prostanoids. From our data, two points should be emphasized. First, thromboxane A_2 may be an important enhancing factor, but not an absolute condition for the occurrence of coronary vascular spasm. Thromboxane A_2 is a potent contracting substance of smooth muscle cells,[28,29] and some authors noted a concomitant increase in plasma TXB_2 levels in patients with ischemic heart diseases during exercise and/or spastic seizure, and insisted on the primary contributing factor of this compound to the spastic changes.[24–26] In our studies, plasma TXB_2 in coronary sinus blood taken from patients with variant angina and during attacks exhibited a comparatively high, but not statistical significance, as compared with levels in normal controls. The plasma levels of TXB_2 in patients with effort angina were high, with a statistical significance.

However, a subgroup of patients with variant angina and in whom the coronary artery was angiographically more than 50% narrowed by atherosclerotic changes revealed statistically significant high plasma levels of TXB_2 and, in contrast, plasma levels of TXB_2 in patients with variant angina with angiographically normal coronaries were as low as in the normal controls. Thromboxane A_2 could be easily activated and released from platelets in atherosclerotic coronaries, which would, in turn, lead to spasm of the vessel wall.[46,47]

However, spasm can be induced in normal coronaries.[42–44] In thirteen of our twenty-one patients with angiographically normal coronary arteries or less than 50% narrowing, the plasma levels of TXB_2 were as low as in the normal controls. Therefore, thromboxane A_2 is probably not an absolute factor related to coronary spasm. Actually, in these patients, the ergonovine test caused a coronary spasm with no increase in the plasma TXB_2 levels.

The second point is the low level of 6-keto $PGF_{1\alpha}$ in patients with variant angina. These characteristic changes are remarkable in patients with normal coronaries. The decrease of PGI_2 in smooth muscle cells is one condition which induces vasospasm.[48,49] Dembinska-Kiék *et al.* reported a decrease of PGI_2 in atherosclerotic coronary arteries of rabbits,[50] and De Angelo *et al.* also confirmed low levels of PGI_2 in the atherosclerotic human aorta, compared with findings in the normal aorta.[51] This may explain why in atherosclerotic portions of coronary arteries spasm is easily provoked. Shimokawa *et al.* also observed that indomethacin intensified coronary spasm as induced by histamine.[36] Miwa *et al.* reported interesting clinical cases in which patients with variant angina given 4 g/day of aspirin, readily experienced spastic attacks during the exercise test.[52,53] Thus, a low level of 6-keto $PGF_{1\alpha}$ may be a more important causative factor in coronary spasm than the high levels of TXB_2. It should also be noted that neither TXB_2 nor 6-keto $PGF_{1\alpha}$ levels showed characteristic changes during the ergonovine test or during spontaneous attack when the spasm was angiographically recorded. All these data indicate that low levels of 6-keto $PGF_{1\alpha}$ in coronary arteries may be a required condition for spasm, and that the spasm itself could be directly induced by other substances.

Nevertheless, it remains uncertain why there are such low levels of 6-keto $PGF_{1\alpha}$ in patients with variant angina with normal coronaries. As to variant angina, the frequency among races differs. Recently Mauritson *et al.* gave ergonovine to twenty-four siblings of eleven patients with variant angina. In no individual was spasm provoked, and they concluded that coronary spasm is an acquired disease.[45]

We have also done HLA studies on twenty-three patients with variant angina and noted a statistically significant high association of Bw-52 and B-40 antigens in these patients,[54] as compared with frequencies among 152 healthy Japanese. Genetic and biopharmacological studies are ongoing in our clinic.

SUMMARY

Plasma levels of thromboxane B_2 (TXB_2) and 6-keto $PGF_{1\alpha}$ in the blood samples taken at the coronary sinus and ascending aorta from twenty-one Japanese patients with variant angina and twenty with effort angina were measured by radioimmunoassay, the objective being to search for the contribution of prostanoids in coronary spasm. The data were compared with data on thirteen subjects free from coronary artery diseases. In coronary sinus blood, plasma TXB_2 in patients with effort angina exhibited statistically significant high levels, as compared with data in the controls. These with variant angina also had high levels, albeit without a statistically significant difference.

Eight patients with variant angina and for whom the coronary angiogram showed more than 50% of narrowing had statistically significant high levels of TXB_2, and the other thirteen with variant angina and normal coronaries or less than 50% of narrowing had the same plasma levels of TXB_2 as the controls.

In contrast to TXB_2, the plasma levels of 6-keto $PGF_{1\alpha}$ in both coronary sinus and aortic blood of patients with variant angina were very low, as compared with normal controls. Statistically significant low levels of 6-keto $PGF_{1\alpha}$ were noted in the coronary sinus blood of patients with variant angina with normal coronaries and in the aortic blood of those with variant angina, as compared with data on the normal controls. Neither ergonovine test nor spontaneous attacks in patients with variant angina revealed characteristic changes in levels of TXB_2 and 6-keto $PGF_{1\alpha}$ in the coronary sinus.

These data suggest that high levels of TXB_2 in patients with atherosclerotic coronaries may be one factor leading to spasm, while low levels of PGI_2 may be a contributing factor.

ACKNOWLEDGMENT

Gratitude is extended to Mariko Ohara, Kyushu University, for critical reading of the manuscript.

REFERENCES

1. PRINZMETAL, M., R. KENNAMER, R. MERLISS, T. WADA & N. BOR. 1959. Angina pectoris. I. A variant form of angina pectoris; preliminary report. Am. J. Med. **27:** 375–388.
2. OLIVA, P. B., D. E. POTTS. & R. G. PLUSS. 1972. Coronary arterial spasm in Prinzmetal's variant form of angina with angiographic evidence of coronaary arterial spasm. Am. J. Cardiol. **30:** 902–905.
3. WIENER, L., H. KA SPARIAN, P. R. DUCA, P. WALINSKY, R. S. GOTTLIEB, F. HANCKEL & A. N. BREST. 1971. Spectrum of coronary arterial spasm. Clinical, angiographic, and myocardial metabolic experience in 29 cases. Am. J. Cardiol. **38:** 945–955.
4. GANZ, W. 1981. Coronary spasm in myocardial infarction. Fact or fiction? Circulation. **63:** 487–489.
5. CONTI, C. R., C. J. PEPINE & R. L. FELDMAN. 1981. Coronary artery spasm. *In* Cardiology Series. H. D. McIntosh, Ed. 1–48.
6. FREEDMAN, B., D. R. RICHMOND & D. T. KELLEY. 1982. Pathophysiology of coronary artery spasm. Circulation **66:** 705–709.
7. MACALPIN, R. N. 1980. Relation of coronary spasm to sites of organic stenosis. Am. J. Cardiol. **46:** 142–153.
8. CREA, F., G. DAVIES, F. ROMEO, S. CHIERCHIA, R. BUGIARDINI, J. C. KASKI, B. FREEDMAN & A. MASERI. 1984. Myocardial ischemia during ergonovine testing: Different susceptibility to coronary vasoconstriction in patients with exertional and variant angina. Circulation **69:** 690–695.
9. HOPKINS, D. G. & D. C. HARRISON. 1984. Mechanisms of coronary arterial spasm. *In* Hammersmith Cardiology Workshop Series, vol. 1. A. Maser & J. F. Goodwin, Eds.: 137–146. Raven Press. New York.
10. CHIERCHIA, S. 1984. What causes coronary spasm? Theories and Facts. *In* Hammersmith Cardiology Workshop Series, vol. 1. A. Maser & J. F. Goodwin, Eds.: 147–160. Raven Press. New York.
11. GRYGLEWSKI, R. J. 1980. Prostaglandins, platelets, and atherosclerosis. CRC Critical Reviews in Biochemistry. **7:** 291–338.
12. MONCADA, S. 1982. Prostacyclin and arterial wall biology. Arteriosclerosis **2:** 193–207.
13. MONCADA, S. & J. R. VANE. 1980. Interrelationships between prostacyclin and thromboxane A_2. Metabolic Activities of the Lung-Ciba Foundation Symposium '78. Excerpta Medica pp. 165–183. Amsterdam.
14. NUMANO, F. 1981. Thromboxane A_2 and atherosclerosis. *In* Medicinal Chemistry Advances. F. G. De Las Heas & S. Vega, Eds.: 131–140. Pergamon Press. Oxford.

15. VANE, J. R., S. BUNTING & S. MONCADA. 1982. Prostacyclin in physiology and pathophysiology. *In* International Review of Experimental Pathology, vol. 23. G. W. Tichter & M. A. Epstein, Eds. 161–207. Academic Press. New York.
16. MONCADA, S. 1983. Biology and therapeutic potential of prostacyclin. Stroke **14:** 157–168.
17. NUMANO, F. 1984. Cyclic nucleotides, prostaglandins, and ischemic heart disease. *In* Advances in Cyclic Nucleotides and Protein Phosphorylation Research, vol. 17. P. Greengard *et al.*, Eds.: 661–670. Raven Press. New York.
18. ELLIS, E. F., O. OELS, L. J. ROBERTS, N. A. PAYNE, P. J. SWEETMAN, A. S. NICO & T. A. OATES. 1976. Coronary arterial smooth muscle contraction by a substance released from platelets—Evidence that it is thromboxane A_2. Science **193:** 1135–1137.
19. NEEDLEMAN, P., P. S. KALKARNI & A. RAZ. 1977. Coronary tone modulation; formation and action of prostaglandins, endoperoxides, and thromboxanes. Science **195:** 409–412.
20. HOLZMANS, S., W. R. KUKOVETS & K. SCHMIDT. 1980. Mode of action of coronary arterial relaxation by prostacyclin. J. Cyclic Nuc. Res. **6:** 451–460.
21. MEHTA, J. L. 1983. Prostaglandins; regulatory role in cardiovascular system and implications in ischemic heart disease. Internat. J. Cardiology **4:** 249–259.
22. SCHRÖR, K. 1981. Possible role of prostaglandins in the regulation of coronary blood flow. Basic Res. Cardiol. **76:** 239–249.
23. VANE, J. R. 1983. Prostaglandins and the cardiovascular system. Br. Heart J. **49:** 405–409.
24. HIRSCH, P. D., L. D. HILLIS, W. B. CAMPBELL, B. G. FIRTH & J. T. WILLERSON. 1981. Release of prostaglandins and thromboxane into the coronary circulation in patients with ischemic heart disease. New Engl. J. Med. **304:** 685–691.
25. LEWY, R. I., L. WIENER, P. WALINSKY, A. M. LEFER, M. K. SILVER & J. B. SMITH. 1980. Thromboxane release during pacing-induced angina pectoris; possible vasoconstrictor influence on the coronary vasculature. Circulation **61:** 1165–1171.
26. MEHTA, J., P. MEHTA & C. HORALEK. 1983. The significance of platelet-vessel wall prostaglandin equilibrium during exercise induced stress. Am. Heart J. **105:** 895–900.
27. TADA, M., T. KUZUYA, M. INOUE, K. KODAMA, M. MISHIMA, M. YAMADA, M. INUI & H. ABE. 1981. Elevation of thromboxane B_2 levels in patients with classic and variant angina pectoris. Circulation **64:** 1107–1115.
28. LEWY, R. I., L. WIENER, B. SMITH, P. WALINSKY & M. SILVER. 1979. Measurements of plasma thromboxane in peripheral blood of Prinzmetal's angina pectoris. Circulation **60**(Suppl. II): 248.
29. CHIERCHIA, S., R. DE CATERINA, F. CREA, C. PATRONO & A. MASERI. 1982. Failure of thromboxane A_2 blockade to prevent attacks of vasospastic angina. Circulation **66:** 702–705.
30. CHIERCHIA, S., C. PATRONO, F. CREA, G. CIABATTONI, R. DE CATERINA, G. A. CINOTTI, A. DISTANTE & A. MASERI. 1982. Effects of intravenous prostacyclin in variant angina. Circulation **65:** 470–477.
31. ROBERTSON, R. M., D. ROBERTSON, L. J. ROBERTS, R. L. MASS, C. A. FITZGERALD, G. C. FREIGINGER. & J. A. OATES. 1981. Thromboxane A_2 in vasotonic angina pectoris. New Engl. J. Med., **304:** 998–1003.
32. NUMANO, F., K. OMORI, K. NISHIYAMA, Y. KISHI, K. SHIMOKADO, FE. NUMANO, M. YAJIMA & H. MAEZAWA. 1982. Plasma thromboxane B_2 levels and atherosclerotic disorders. Arterial Wall **VII:** 99–106.
33. SEKINE, M., M. YAJIMA & F. NUMANO. 1985. Plasma 6-keto $PFG_{1\alpha}$ levels in patients with vascular disorders. Vascular Med. **3:** 56–65.
34. HELLSTROM, H. R. 1982. The injury-spasm and vascular autoregulatory hypothesis of ischemic disease. Am. J. Cardiol. **49:** 802–810.
35. BERTLAND, M. E., J. M. LABLANCHE, P. Y. TILMANT, F. A. THIEULEUX, M. R. DELFORGE, A. G. CARRE, P. ASSEMAN, B. BERZIN, C. LIBERSA & J. M. LAURENT. 1982. Frequency of provoked arterial spasm in 1809 consecutive patients undergoing coronary arteriography. Circulation **65:** 1299.
36. SHIMOKAWA, H., H. TOMOIKE, S. NABEYAMA, H. YAMAMOTO, H. ARAKI, M. NAKAMURA, Y. ISHII & K. TANAKA. 1983. Coronary artery spasm induced in atherosclerotic miniature swine. Science **221:** 560–562.

37. KAWACHI, Y., H. TOMOIKE, Y. MARUOKA, Y. KIKUCHI, H. ARAKI, Y. ISHII, K. TANAKA & M. NAKAMURA. 1984. Selective hypercontraction caused by ergonovine in the canine coronary artery under conditions of induced atherosclerosis. Circulation **69:** 441–450.
38. HENRY, P. D. & M. YOKOYAMA. 1980. Supersensitivity of atherosclerotic rabbit aorta to ergonovine. J. Clin. Invest. **66:** 306–313.
39. KISHI, Y. & F. NUMANO. 1984. Contraction in normal and atherosclerotic rabbit aortas. Mechanisms of Ageing and Development, **26:** 357–369.
40. NANDA, V. & P. H. HENRY. 1982. Increased serotonergic and alpha adrenergic receptors in aortas from rabbits fed a high cholesterol diet. Clin. Res. **30:** 209A.
41. KALSNER, S. & R. RICHARDS. 1984. Coronary arteries of cardiac patients are hyperreactive and contain stores of amines; A mechanism for coronary spasm. Sci. Marsh **30:** 1435–1436.
42. SELZER, A. S., M. LANGSTON, C. RUGGEROLI & K. COHN. 1976. Clinical syndrome of variant angina with normal coronary arteriogram. New Engl. J. Med. **295:** 1343–1347.
43. HART, N. J., M. E. SILVERMAN & S. B. KING. 1974. Variant angina pectoris caused by coronary artery spasm. Am. J. Med. **56:** 269–274.
44. AIZAWA, T., K. OGASAWARA, K. NISHIMURA, H. SATOH, J. FUJII, A. OHTA & K. KATOH. 1985. The angiographic characteristics of coronary spasm: Relation of coronary spasm to sites, shapes, and severity of organic stenosis. Jap. Circ. J. **49:** 140.
45. MAURITSON, D. R., R. M. PESHOCK, M. D. WINNIFORD, L. STERN, S. M. JOHNSON & L. D. HILLIS. 1983. Prinzmetal's variant angina: It is transmitted genetically? Am. Heart. J. **105:** 1049.
46. ALLY, A. I. & D. F. HORROBIN. 1980. Thromboxane A_2 in blood vessel walls and its physiological significance: Relevance to thrombosis and hypertension. Prostaglandins **4:** 431–438.
47. NERI SERNERI, G. G., G. MASOTTI, G. F. GENSINI, R. ABBATE, L. POGGESI, G. GALANTI & S. FAVILLA. 1981. Prostacyclin, thromboxane, and ischemic heart disease. *In* Atherosclerosis Reviews, vol. 8. R. J. Hegyeli, Ed.: 139–157. Raven Press. New York.
48. MAKITA, Y. 1983. Effects of prostaglandin I_2 and carbocyclic thromboxane A_2 on smooth muscle cells and neuromuscular transmission in the guinea pig mesenteric artery. Br. J. Pharmac. **78:** 517–527.
49. WHITTLE, B. J. R. & S. MONCADA. 1984. Prostacyclin-thromboxane interactions in hemostasis. *In* Cardiovascular Pharmacology. M. Antonaccio, Ed.: 519–534. Raven Press. New York.
50. DEMBINSKA-KIÉK, A., T. GRYGLEWSKA, A. ZMUDA & R. J. GRYGLEWSKI. 1977. The generation of prostacyclin by arteries and by the coronary vascular bed is reduced in experimental atherosclerosis in rabbit. Prostaglandins **14:** 1025–1034.
51. D'ANGELO, V., S. VILLA, M. MYSLIEVIEC, M. B. DONATI & G. DE GAETANO. 1978. Defective fibrinolytic and prostacyclin-like activity in human atheromatous plaques. Thromb. Haemostas. **39:** 535–536.
52. MIWA, K., H. KANBARA & C. KAWAI. 1979. Variant angina aggravated by aspirin. Lancet **II:** 1382.
53. MIWA, K., H. KANBARA & C. KAWAI. 1981. Exercise-induced angina provoked by aspirin administration in patients with variant angina. Am. J. Cardiol. **47:** 1210–1214.
54. NUMANO, F., T. AIZAWA, S. NOMURA, Y. KISHI, M. YAJIMA, J. FUJII & K. KATO. 1985. Coronary spasm, prostaglandin, and HLA factors. Jap. Circ. J. **49:** 119–127.

Thrombosis and Atherogenesis—The Chicken and the Egg

Contribution of Platelets in Atherogenesis

SEAN MOORE

Department of Pathology
McGill University
Montreal, Quebec, Canada H3A 2B4

The topic which I have been asked to address would seem at first sight to be straightforward, but on analyzing the question implicitly posed, some complexity is apparent. One could consider the question quite simply in relation only to the initiation of plaque formation in response to vessel wall injury, but the broader implications are more interesting. Furthermore, it may be useful to break the question into three parts which can be stated as:

Are platelets needed for plaque formation:

in human disease?
in diet-induced disease?
in injury-induced disease?

To each of these questions there are answers, some of which can be given with a degree of scientific support, others to which only tentative answers can be given, indicating the need for further exploration of unresolved questions.

The part played by platelets in atherogenesis is most clearly apparent in relation to atheroma induced by injury. Their role in human disease and in atheroma induced by diet is less clear, the answers which we can now adopt being mainly of the tentative variety. I will first attempt to review what is known in these areas. Then, I will concentrate mainly on the role of platelets in relation to arterial wall injury, and explore the development, progression, and regression of two different forms of vessel wall response to injury.

PLATELETS IN ATHEROSCLEROSIS

While it is clearly established that platelets are the main formed element of the blood involved in thrombosis and embolism complicating atheromatous plaques (thus, leading to recognizable clinical events such as myocardial infarction or transient ischemic attacks), their role in the initiation of plaques is much less clearly defined.[1] It seems also to be well established that plaques may grow or progress by accretion of thrombus material, mainly composed of platelets.[2]

Some authors consider that the occurrence of tiny mural thrombi represents an early lesion of atherosclerosis.[1,3–5] Since most of these are found incidentally on microscopic examination, their real incidence and importance in the process are questionable. Their relationship to the process must be resolved in the context of the significance of other early lesions, such as gelatinous (edematous) lesions and fatty dots and streaks. It is clear that these lesions are morphologically different, which might indicate, at first consideration, a different pathogenesis. It is also possible that they may be different responses or a similar response, seen at different times, to the same stimulus. This is strongly supported by the finding that edematous lesions, fatty streaks, and thrombi are all seen in response to repeated or continuous injury induced by the placement of a polyethylene catheter in the aorta,[6] and to repeated injury caused by immunological damage to the vessel wall.[7] What is the outcome of these early lesions? No definitive answer can be given, but it is relevant that the lesions induced by repeated injury undergo marked regression when the injury stimulus is removed.[8,9] They appear to evolve into fibrous intimal plaques which lack a stainable content of lipid. This raises an obvious question. Is diffuse intimal thickening, which appears to be an almost universal finding in the large musculo-elastic arteries of adult humans,[10] a result of the resolution of such early lesions?

PLATELETS IN DIET-INDUCED DISEASE

Is the role of platelets of key importance, of subsidiary importance, or do they merely have a possible modifying influence? In observations of the lesions developing in response to diet-induced atherosclerosis, the part played by platelets has not been clearly established. They would seem to have, at best, a subsidiary influence on lesion development. Monocytes appear to be involved early[11] and to be seen in all stages of lesion development, whereas platelets are seen only where disruption or loss of the endothelium is observed. There are reports of endothelial injury caused by hyperlipidemic diets.[12–18] If there is significant endothelial injury, then, of course, a role for platelets is indicated.

One of the problems in designing experiments to answer the question is that early endothelial injury is easily confused with artifact induced in the preparation of tissues for electron microscopy. My colleague, Mary Richardson at McMaster University, has been exploring this problem.[19] The outcome of this work is that we will have to look more critically at descriptions of "early" endothelial damage. There is evidence that cholesterol enriched diets may be toxic to cells in the vessel wall, and particular attention has been paid to necrosis of smooth muscle cells.[20] The types of lesions which develop differ according to the composition of the diet as pointed out by Vesselinovitch and colleagues.[21] Some diets induce lesions composed mainly of foam cells, while others produce lesions in which a fibrous component is more evident. Diets containing peanut oil, ethanol, or antioxidants produce this proliferative fibrous lesion in which smooth muscle cells are prominent. My colleague at McGill, Bernard Weigensberg, has been comparing the types of lesions in rabbits fed cholesterol and oleic acid with those in animals fed peanut oil and cholesterol. The cholesterol oleic acid diet induces lesions in which the foam cells seem to be largely of monocytic type, with little evidence of cell proliferation, collagen synthesis, or proteoglycan content. In contrast, the lesions associated with peanut oil have largely myocytic cells, and show evidence of glycoaminoglycans with interstitial, as well as intracellular, lipid. It is possible that the pathogenesis of these two types of lesion is different, in that the type characterized by smooth muscle proliferation and synthesis of connective tissue proteins may be, in part, a response to injury. These two kinds of lesions have some similarity, as we shall see later, to two lesions induced by different forms of injury to the vessel wall.

While it is well established that there is a synergy between various forms of injury and hypercholesterolemia in inducing lesion development,[22,23] it is much less clear what part injury may or may not play in lesions induced by hypercholesterolemia alone. It seems clear from the early reports of dietary atherosclerosis that intimal changes, especially intimal thickening, and a change in the "ground substance" precede the appearance of stainable lipid.[24,25] When the endothelium is removed by a balloon catheter in the presence of diet-induced hypercholesterolemia, no lipid appears in the vessel wall until there is a neointima, which occurs at about four days after the injury.[26] An important question that needs to be answered is whether lipid can accumulate sufficiently in a normal intima to induce the other features of the disease. If, as seems probable from the instances noted above, lipid deposition follows upon the development of a neointima, the part played by injury may well be important. If it is, the relative contribution to the process by platelets, macrophages, and endothelium will need to be further evaluated.

PLATELETS IN ATHEROMA INDUCED BY INJURY

The importance of platelets in lesion development is now a familiar story and it has become, in the last 10–15 years, a much discussed and largely accepted mechanism. The concept is based on biochemical and morphological evidence, and is supported by various examples of arterial wall injury in man.[27] For completeness, I will first briefly review the evidence that platelets play a key part in lesion development, and then discuss two different forms of lesion in which platelets are involved. More knowledge of the biology of these reactions may provide better understanding of lesion formation, progression, and regression.

When an indwelling polyethylene catheter is placed in the aorta of a normal fed rabbit, abundant platelet-fibrin thrombi form at points of repeated contact of the catheter with the vessel wall. These lesions rapidly become lipid rich both by evaluation by oil red O staining[6] and by chemical analysis.[28] Free cholesterol is increased, but the content of cholesterol ester is markedly increased. In other areas, fatty streak-like lesions develop, as well as plaques composed of smooth muscle cells without stainable lipid being present. If the catheter is left in, the raised lesions closely resemble human atheroma with a deeply placed central lipid pool, numerous foam cells, calcification, and eventually ossification characterizing the process. These lesions can be inhibited or even prevented by inducing a severe thrombocytopenia with antiplatelet serum.[29,30] As Dr. Ross will discuss later, the progression and growth of these lesions is an *in vivo* expression of the finding that smooth muscle cells need to be exposed to platelet derived growth factor to proliferate in tissue culture. This factor acts in concert with other factors present in plasma to cause cell proliferation.[31] Platelets release a substance which also causes directed migration of smooth muscle cells.[32] This is most likely platelet derived growth factor.[33] This chemotactic effect on smooth muscle cells acts without the requirement for other factors. The lesions regress markedly in terms of size and lipid content when the catheter is removed.[8] Similar lesions can be induced by placing human serum, which is cytotoxic for rabbit lymphocytes, in a segment of rabbit carotid artery at weekly intervals for four weeks.[7] These lesions also regress with rapid disappearance of lipid, passing through a phase during which fatty streak lesions are prominent.[9]

Both of these types of injury induced atheroma are characterized by abundant formation of platelet-fibrin thrombi. Meuleman and colleagues have shown shortened platelet survival in rats with indwelling aortic catheters.[34]

A very different kind of response of the arterial wall follows upon removal of the endothelium with a balloon catheter. The interaction with the vessel wall of platelets is short-lived, taking the form of a monolayer[35] which covers the whole surface, except for areas distal to branch vessels where very few or no platelets adhere.[36] A second balloon catheter injury is followed by the deposition of platelets and fibrin.[37] Again, the regions just distal to vessel origins are spared.[36] Linear platelet-fibrin thrombi are deposited in the long axis of the vessel, mainly lateral to branch orifices, and extend beyond the confines of the areas which had been covered by regenerated endothelium before the second balloon injury.[36] That fibrin is involved in the response to a second injury indicates that thrombin may be generated when the neointima is injured, as contrasted with the reaction to removal of endothelium from the normal vessel. This is supported by the inhibition of platelet uptake by giving heparin intravenously before the second balloon removal of the endothelium.[37]

The differing reaction of the normal vessel wall from that of the neointima to removal of the surface layer of cells is important in relation to human atheromatous plaques. Disruption or loss of the surface layer from a plaque will result in the formation of platelet-fibrin thrombi, with the implication that drugs which modify or alter platelet function may have little effect on the formation of thrombi.

The lesions which form following balloon removal of the endothelium are progressive in the sense of becoming thicker over time and in continuing to accumulate lipid.[38] The lipid accumulates mainly or preferentially beneath endothelium which has regenerated from branch vessels. Reinjury does not seem to modify the process except to induce lesions that are thicker than those which follow a single injury.[38] We have followed the development of these lesions up to two years following a single injury. Very large amounts of lipid, particularly cholesterol ester, are deposited in the neointima beneath the regenerated endothelium.[39] At six months following injury, the plaques closely resemble human atheromatous lesions being composed of a fibrous cap with a superficially placed layer of foam cells and a deeply placed central lipid pool.[38]

Because lipid accumulates in great quantity in the endothelium covered neointima and to a much lesser extent in the unrecovered neointima, we have investigated the uptake of radioactively labeled lipoprotein into these areas, and efflux from them has been examined in tissue culture of appropriate segments of aorta. These studies, performed by Dr. Zafar Alavi, showed that endothelium covered neointima accumulated considerably more low density lipoprotein (LDL) than control tissues. Removal of LDL from the intima during a 24-hour efflux period, and examined in tissue culture following the initial 48-hour loading period, showed greater removal from normal and de-endothelialized tissues than from the endothelium covered neointima.[40]

Dr. Allan Day, working in our laboratory during a sabbatical leave, has used lipoprotein labeled with ^{3}H and ^{14}C-cholesterol to study the uptake in sham operated and balloon catheter injured rabbit aortas, both those normal fed and those subjected to a hypercholesterolemic diet.[41] The accumulation of ^{3}H-labeled cholesterol and cholesterol ester 72-hours after ingestion of ^{3}H-labeled cholesterol, in both normal and cholesterol fed rabbits, was significantly greater for the re-endothelialized than for the de-endothelialized areas or control. Both entry (mg/day/100 mg wet weight aortic intima) and clearance (μl plasma/day/cm^2) of free and ester cholesterol were increased in the neointima for both normal and cholesterol fed rabbits. Synthesis was minimal in all areas. Hydrolysis of cholesterol ester was greater in the de-endothelialized areas, but less than in the control tissue.

Removal of labeled cholesterol and cholesterol ester from the intima during a 20-hour efflux period, following the 72-hour loading period, showed greater removal from normal intima than either re-endothelialized or de-endothelialized neointima. It was concluded that the accumulation of cholesterol in the neointima after balloon injury must take account of increased permeability to lipoprotein of the neointima, as well as to possible binding of lipoprotein to glycosaminoglycans.

My colleague, Dr. Mary Richardson, has shown in transmission electron microscopy on sections stained with ruthenium red, that there is a greater concentration of large proteoglycan particles in the endothelium covered neointima than in the normal vessel, and a much less concentration than normal in the de-endothelialized areas. We postulated that the reason for the low content of lipid in the de-endothelialized areas might be due to loss or efflux of lipoprotein-GAG complexes from these areas.

Accordingly, Dr. Alavi has been exploring the metabolism and concentration of GAG in the two types of lesion tissue (re-endothelialized and de-endothelialized).[42] Synthesis of GAG as shown by ^{14}C-glucosamine incorporation was twice that of control in de-endothelialized tissue and three times that of control in re-endothelialized tissue. When release of GAG from normal or injured tissue was compared, control and re-endothelialized tissue, both having an endothelial cover, released 25% of the GAG which they synthesized, whereas de-endothelialized tissue, lacking an endothelial cover, released approximately 60% of the GAG it synthesized per day.

The concentration of GAG in the aortic tissue and medium was plotted as a function of time, and patterns similar to synthesis were observed. Although de-endothelialized tissue synthesizes twice as much GAG as control, the concentration of GAG in both was almost equal, reflecting the loss of GAG from de-endothelialized tissue. The amount of GAG released into the medium was related to time and was much greater for de-endothelialized than for re-endothelialized tissue, which was greater than control. The relative distribution of individual GAGs was remarkably altered in the injured tissues. Chondroitin 4-sulfate, which was not measurable in control tissue, appeared in injured tissue, especially re-endothelialized neointima. This tissue also showed a remarkable increase in chondroitin 6-sulfate and in the other GAGs. The GAG released in greatest quantity into the medium from the injured tissue was chondroitin-6-sulfate, more of which was released from de-endothelialized than from re-endothelialized tissue.

The radioactivity incorporated into total GAG was greater for injured than for control tissues, and showed an increasing difference from 12–24 hours. Moreover, the radioactivity of ^{14}C-glucosamine in GAG released into the medium was higher for de-endothelialized than for re-endothelialized tissue, which was in turn higher than for control tissue at all time periods. This supports the notion that the failure of de-endothelialized tissue to accumulate lipid may be related to the loss of LDL-GAG complexes, and this raises the question of a "reverse" barrier function of the endothelium.

Because of the indications that lipid accumulation in the type of arterial wall plaque that follows from removal of the endothelium with a balloon catheter is closely related to the presence of GAG, we have also examined the concentration of GAG in the raised lesions induced by the presence of an indwelling catheter. The examinations were carried out after the catheter had been in place for three weeks, and at four and eight weeks following catheter removal.[43] Large granules, representing dermatan and/or chondroitin sulfate, were increased fivefold in lipid-containing lesions at the time of catheter removal. By four weeks following catheter removal, the concentration of these granules was reduced, although at this time, as estimated morphologically, the lesions had not regressed, showing instead an increase in severity. By eight weeks, however, there was definite regression of lesions in terms of lipid content, at which time the proteoglycan content was at the same level as uninjured control vessel wall. Proteoglycan concentration was reduced in surface parts of the lesion, composed mainly of lipid-containing macrophages in the early phase. It was increased in relation to cells which could be identified as being smooth muscle cells and intermediate in areas where foam cells of indeterminate type made up the bulk of the lesions. Small proteoglycan granules, considered to be heparan sulfate, were increased in the subendothelial zone of lesions containing lipid, and were scanty where endothelial cover was lacking. The findings are again consistent with the hypothesis that the sulfated GAG moieties of the proteoglycan molecule are produced in excess in areas of lipid accumulation, and may trap and retain low density lipoprotein. There may also be an analogy here, worth exploring, to the two kinds of lesion induced by diet, referred to above.

The two types of injury-induced lesion have only a few features in common. Both are associated with the deposition of platelets on the vessel wall, and both can be prevented or inhibited by reducing the circulating platelets to very low levels. Both are characterized by the migration of smooth muscle cells from the media and their proliferation to form a neointima. The type associated with continuing or repeated injury and presumably with repeated or continuing thrombus formation is lipid rich while the injury stimulus is operative, but regresses in size and lipid content when the injury stimulus is removed. The type induced by removal of the endothelial layer has initially a carpet of platelets that is lost over several days, but which results in a lesion that is progressive in terms of smooth muscle cell proliferation and lipid accumulation. In both, the presence of lipid appears to be closely related to the synthesis of proteoglycans by the smooth muscle cells, as well as increased entry of lipoproteins from the blood. The reason or reasons why one type of lesion regresses while the other progresses are not clear. The unraveling of this enigma must await further research on the biology of the arterial wall cells.

REFERENCES

1. HAUST, M. D. 1981. The natural history of atherosclerotic lesions. *In* Vascular Injury and Atherosclerosis. S. Moore, Ed. Marcel Dekker. New York.
2. MOORE, S. 1976. Atherosclerosis: In animal models of thrombosis and hemorrhagic diseases. Department of Health, Education, and Welfare Publication No. (NIH) 72–962. Washington, D.C.
3. MOVAT, H. Z., M. D. HAUST & R. H. MORE. 1969. The morphological element of the early lesions of atherosclerosis. Am. J. Pathol. **35:** 93–103.
4. GEER, J. C. & M. D. HAUST. 1972. Smooth muscle cells in atherosclerosis. S. Karger. Basel.
5. HAUST, M. D. 1971. The morphogenesis and fate of potential and early atherosclerotic lesions in man. Human Pathol. **2:** 1–29.
6. MOORE, S. 1973. Thromboatherosclerosis in normolipemic rabbits: a result of continued endothelial damage. Lab. Invest. **29:** 478–487.
7. FRIEDMAN, R. J., S. MOORE & D. P. SINGAL. 1975. Repeated endothelial injury and induction of atherosclerosis in normolipemic rabbits. Lab. Invest. **30:** 404–415.
8. MOORE, S., R. J. FRIEDMAN & M. GENT. 1977. Resolution of lipid containing atherosclerotic lesions induced by injury. Blood Vessels **14:** 193–203.
9. FRIEDMAN, R. J., S. MOORE, D. P. SINGAL & M. GENT. 1976. Regression of injury-induced atheromatous lesions in rabbit. Arch. Pathol. Lab. Med. **100:** 185–195.
10. TRACY, R. E. & V. TOCA. 1975. Relationship of raised atherosclerotic lesions to fatty streaks in nineteen location race groups. Atherosclerosis **21:** 21–36.
11. GERRITY, R. G. 1981. The role of the monocyte in atherogenesis. I. Transition of blood-borne monocytes into foam cells in fatty lesions. Am. J. Pathol. **103:** 181–190.
12. DAVIES, P. F., M. A. REIDY, T. B. GOUDE & D. E. BOWYER. 1976. Scanning electron microscopy in the evaluation of endothelial integrity of fatty lesions in atherosclerosis. Atherosclerosis **25:** 125–130.
13. MACA, R. D. & J. C. HOAK. 1974. Endothelial injury and platelet aggregation associated with acute lipid mobilization. Lab Invest. **30:** 589–595.
14. NELSON, E., S. D. GETZ, M. L. RENNELS, M. S. FORBES, M. A. KAHN, M. A. MEALD & F. L. EARL. 1975. Endothelial lesions in the aorta of egg yolk-fed miniature swine: a study by scanning and transmission electron microscopy. Circulation **103** (Suppl. 2): 51–62.
15. SVENDSEN, E. 1979. Focal endothelial injury in rabbit aorta: Aggravation of injury by two days of cholesterol feeding. Acta Pathol. Microbiol. Scand. **87:** 123–130.
16. WEBER, G., P. FABRINI & Z. RESI. 1974. Scanning and transmission electron microscopy

observations on the surface lining of aortic intimal plaques in rabbits on a hypercholesteroleric diet. Virchows Arch. Pathol. Anat. (A) **364:** 325–331.
17. Wu, K. K., M. L. Armstrong, J. C. Hoak & M. B. Megan. 1975. Platelet aggregates in hypercholesterolemic monkeys. Thromb. Res. **7:** 917–924.
18. Ross, R. & L. Harker. 1976. Hyperlipidemia and atherosclerosis. Science **193:** 1094–1100.
19. Richardson, M., M. W. C. Hatton, M. R. Buchanan & S. Moore. 1984. Effect of perfusion fixation on the scanning electron microscopy of normal rabbit aorta: Artefact or injury? Presented at the Lofland Conference on Atherosclerosis, San Antonio, Texas, May 23–26, 1984.
20. Imai, H., N. T. Werthessen, B. Taylor & K. T. Lee. 1976. Lofland Conference. Angiotoxicity and atherosclerosis due to contaminants of USP-grade cholesterol. Arch. Pathol. Lab. Med. **100:** 565–572.
21. Vesselinovitch, D., G. S. Getz, R. H. Hughes & R. W. Wissler. 1974. Atherosclerosis in the rhesus monkey fed three food fats. Atherosclerosis **20:** 303–321.
22. Minick, C. R. 1976. Immunological injury in atherogenesis. Ann. N.Y. Acad. Sci. **275:** 210–227.
23. Minick, C. R. 1976. Synergy of arterial injury and hypercholesterolemia in atherogenesis. *In* Injury Mechanisms in Atherosclerosis. S. Moore, Ed. Marcel Dekker. New York.
24. Duff, G. L. 1935. Experimental cholesterol atherosclerosis and its relationship to human atherosclerosis. Arch. Pathol. Lab. Med. **20:** 80–124, 259–304.
25. Duff, G. L., G. C. McMillan & A. C. Ritchie. 1957. The morphology of early atherosclerotic lesions of the aorta demonstrated by the surface technique in rabbits fed cholesterol. Am. J. Pathol. **33:** 845–874.
26. Katocs, A. S., E. E. Largos, L. W. Will, D. K. McClintock & S. J. Riggi. 1976. Sterol deposition in the aortae of normocholesteremic and hypercholesteremic rabbits subjected to aortic de-endothelialization. Artery **2:** 38–52.
27. Moore, S. 1983. Atheroma. *In* Neurology 3: Cerebral Vascular Disease. M.S.G. Harrison & M.L. Dyken, Eds. Medical Rev. Butterworth & Co. London.
28. Day, A. J., F. P. Bell, S. Moore & R. J. Friedman. 1974. Lipid composition and metabolism of thromboatherosclerotic lesions produced by continued endothelial damage in normal rabbits. Circulation Res. **34:** 467–476.
29. Moore, S., R. J. Friedman, D. P. Singal, J. Gauldie, M. A. Blajchman & R. J. Roberts. 1976. Inhibition of injury-induced thromboatherosclerotic lesions by anti-platelet serum in rabbits. Thrombos. Haemostas. **35:** 70–81.
30. Moore, S., L. W. Belbeck & J. Gauldie. 1977. Thrombocytopenia induced by busulfan and antiplatelet serum inhibits aortic lesions caused by injury. Circulation **56:** III–120.
31. Vogel, A., E. Raines, B. Kariya, M. J. Rivest & R. Ross. 1978. Coordinated control of 3T3 cell proliferation by platelet-derived growth factor and plasma components. Proc. Natl. Acad. Sci. USA **77:** 6644–6648.
32. Ihnatowycz, I. O., P. O. Winocur & S. Moore. 1981. A platelet-derived factor chemotactic for rabbit arterial smooth muscle cells in culture. Artery **9:** 316–327.
33. Grotendorst, G. R., H. E. J. Seppa, H. K. Kleinman & G. R. Martin. 1981. Attachment of smooth muscle cells to collagen and their migration toward platelet-drived growth factor. Proc. Natl. Acad. Sci. USA **78:** 3669–3672.
34. Meuleman, D. G., G. M. T. Vogel & A. M. L. van Delft. 1980. Effects of intra-arterial cannulation on blood platelet consumption in rats. Thromb. Res. **20:** 45–55.
35. Groves, H. M., R. L. Kinlough-Rathbone, M. Richardson, S. Moore & J. F. Mustard. 1979. Platelet interaction with damaged rabbit aorta. Lab. Invest. **40:** 194–200.
36. Richardson, M., R. L. Kinlough-Rathbone, H. M. Groves, L. Jorgensen, J. F. Mustard & S. Moore. 1984. Ultrastructural changes in re-endothelialized and non-endothelialized rabbit aortic neointima following re-injury with a balloon catheter. Brit. J. Exp. Pathol. **65:** 597–611.
37. Groves, H. M., R. L. Kinlough-Rathbone, M. Richardson, L. Jorgensen, S. Moore & J. F. Mustard. 1982. Thrombin generation and fibrin formation following injury to rabbit neointima. Studies of vessel wall reactivity and platelet survival. Lab. Invest. **46:** 605–612.

38. MOORE, S., L. W. BELBECK, M. RICHARDSON & W. TAYLOR. 1982. Lipid accumulation in the neointima forms in normal-fed rabbits in response to one or six removals of the aortic endothelium. Lab. Invest. **47:** 32–42.
39. ALAVI, M., C. W. DUNNETT & S. MOORE. 1983. Lipid composition of rabbit aortic wall following removal of endothelium by balloon catheter. Arteriosclerosis **3:** 413–419.
40. ALAVI, M. & S. MOORE. 1984. Kinetics of low density lipoprotein interactions with rabbit aortic wall following balloon catheter de-endothelialization. Arteriosclerosis: **4:** 395–402.
41. DAY, A. J., M. ALAVI & S. MOORE. 1985. Influx of $^{3}H/^{14}$ C-cholesterol labeled lipoprotein into re-endothelialized and de-endothelialized areas of ballooned aortas in normal fed and cholesterol fed rabbits. Atherosclerosis **55:** 339–351.
42. ALAVI, M. & S. MOORE. 1985. Glycosaminoglycan composition and biosynthesis in the endothelium covered neointima of de-endothelialized rabbit aorta. Submitted for publication. Exp. Molec. Pathol. **42:** 389–400.
43. MOORE, S. & M. RICHARDSON. 1985. Proteoglycan distribution in catheter-induced aortic lesions in normolipaemil rabbits—An ultrastructural study. Atherosclerosis **55:** 313–330.

Thrombosis and Atherosclerosis—Some Unresolved Problems[a]

M. DARIA HAUST

Departments of Pathology and Paediatrics
The University of Western Ontario
and
The Children's Psychiatric Research Institute
London, Ontario, Canada

In the foregoing address, Dr. Sean Moore reviewed thoroughly the present status of our knowledge on thrombosis as it relates to atherosclerosis from the aspect of the role of platelets in atherogenesis.

This account reminded us, among others, of Dr. Moore's own contributions to the experimental model of thrombosis by his denuding the aortic surface and investigating the subsequent conversion of thrombi to atherosclerotic plaques. Dr. Moore also summarized data of numerous other experiments, providing evidence that thrombosis is an important factor in atherosclerosis.

Instead of attempting to discuss any aspect of the complete account rendered by Dr. Moore, it would seem desirable, instead, to focus our attention on a few selected areas in this field that either remain controversial or have been largely unexplored.

FOAM CELLS ASSOCIATED WITH THROMBOTIC REMNANTS

Already von Rokitansky,[1] the father of the thrombogenic theory of atherosclerosis, stated clearly over 140 years ago, that the remnants of the unorganized thrombotic substances deposited upon the arterial surface degenerate with the passing of time and give rise to the fatty components of the atherosclerotic plaques. Neither he, nor later the proponents of his theory[2–11] who favored also his explanation of the origin of lipids in lesions provided an explanation of just how the remnants of the proteinaceous matter (largely fibrin) were "converted" to lipids, which were an entirely different biochemical class of substances.

Several investigators tested the role of thrombosis in atherogenesis by means of various experimental models. Mural thrombi produced in rabbit arteries by mechanical means were incorporated into the intima and organized. In this case, the lesions resembled the fibrous atherosclerotic plaques.[12] Similar results were obtained when blood clots or fibrin were introduced into the venous circulation and lodged as emboli in the pulmonary arteries of experimental animals.[13–15] However, in all these experiments the incorporation of the fibrinous substance into the arterial intima and its subsequent organization resulted in the formation of plaques almost entirely devoid of foam cells and the atheromatous core, which were both usually present in the naturally occurring lesions. This was also a feature of plaques produced in hyperlipidemic animals.[16]

Reasoning that in the quoted experiments the failure of producing lesions

[a]This work was supported by a grant-in-aid of research T.3-11 from the Ontario Heart Foundation, Toronto, Ontario, Canada.

containing foam cells and/or an atheroma could be related to utilization of fibrin or clots rather than (true) thrombi, Chandler and Hand carried out similar experiments employing autologous thrombi, instead, and in addition, observed sequentially the degeneration of such thrombi *in vitro*.[17,18] The results of both studies indicated that monocytes phagocytized the platelets contained in the thrombi, thereby transforming themselves to "lipophages" *in vivo* and *in vitro*. In the experimental animal, the lesions produced were lipophages containing fibro-fatty plaques, apparently resembling the naturally occurring lesions. In the discussion of their results, the authors drew attention to the known data that platelets contained several classes of lipids, and thus, could be the source of these substances in the organized thrombi, whereas the other components, e.g., the fibrin, being entirely devoided of lipids, could not.

The explanation that platelets were the source of lipids in atherosclerotic plaques derived from mural thrombi has been widely accepted since then, particularly by those investigators who consider the platelets to be crucial or even the *sine qua non* elements in atherogenesis.

However plausible and attractive the above proposal of lipogenesis in atherosclerotic plaques was, it became increasingly apparent that platelets could not be the single or even the main source of lipids in lesions derived from the organization of mural thrombi (especially those of man). There are several facts and/or observations supporting this contention. First, there are too few monocytes in the circulating blood (and thusly entrapped in the thrombus) to account for all the foam cells present in the lesion. Recognizing this, Hand and Chandler proposed that the monocytes divide amitotically in the lesion, a concept no longer accepted with reference to higher animals.[19] Furthermore, the foam cells illustrated in figure 14 of the publication by Hand and Chandler[17] occupy largely the basal portion of the lesion. However, it has been documented that enzymatically active monocytes do not migrate into or survive at the deep levels of lesions in man or the rabbit.[20,21]

Finally, the most compelling arguments are derived from the observations of human atherosclerotic lesions. It has been observed over a period of almost three decades (see reference 22), that in instances of repeated episodes of sequential mural thrombi deposition upon the arterial wall (aorta; coronary arteries) and their subsequent organization, fibrin (or fibrinoid) that remained unorganized in the deep portions of lesions was consistently associated with foam cells (FIGURE 1). These foam cells were closely applied to the fibrinous remnants and appeared to be "nibbling" on them. This feature is morphologically identical to that observed in the atherosclerotic plaques, initiating and progressing by means of fibrinous insudation into the intima. When such an insudation is superimposed upon a similar intimal change prior to the organization of the previously deposited insudate, foam cells may be seen in close proximity to the condensed masses of the fibrinous remnants (See figure 17–16 in reference 23, figure 6 in reference 11, and figure 2 in reference 24). It should be remembered that no platelets are present in the insudate "entering" the intima, and therefore, the lipid-containing cells could not have derived their fat from disintegrating platelets. Moreover, the close apposition of the foam cells to the fibrinous remnants in all instances suggests some relation between these two components of the lesions.

Despite the close spatial relation between the foam cells and the remnants of the unorganized fibrin in the deep regions of atherosclerotic plaques, it is entirely unknown what that association might be, and indeed, what types of cells are involved, i.e., a monocyte-derived macrophage, a smooth muscle cell, or a myohistiocyte.[25]

In the past, it has been assumed in general that cells with phagocytic properties ingest given substances (or living organisms) in order to digest or alter these appreciably, and in the course of these processes, change their (cellular) appearance. In view of our present-day knowledge relating to true secretory properties of the

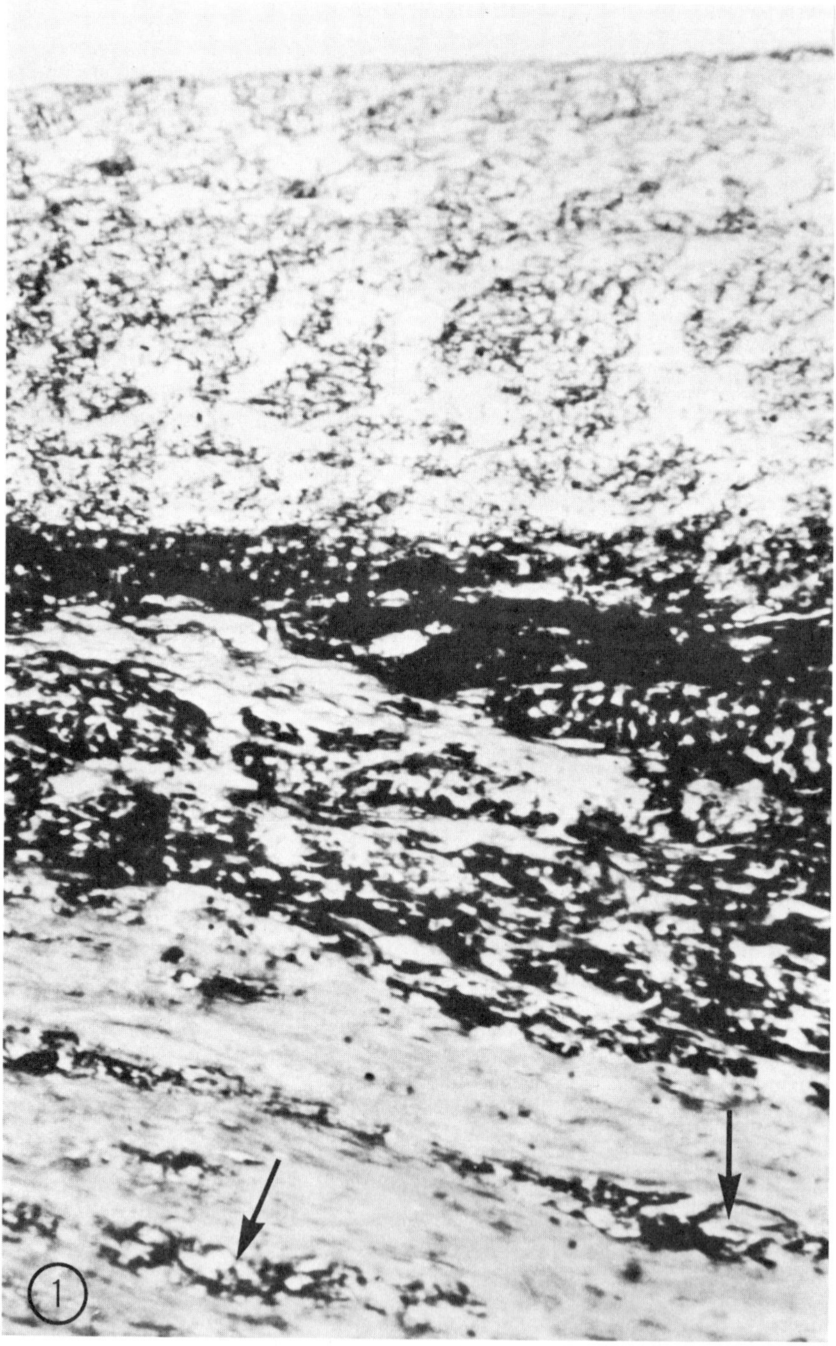

FIGURE 1. A human aortic atherosclerotic plaque is superimposed by several layers of mural thrombi (black) organized to a various degree into connective tissues (grey). The most recent thrombus (top) is recognizable by lines of Zahn. Fibrinous remnants within the plaque are associated with small groups of lipid-containing cells (arrows). Phosphotungstic acid hematein stain; Magnification: ×176.

monocyte-derived macrophages and the intimal smooth muscle cells (see reference 26), it is apparent that the secretory products reaching the cellular environment may effect proteolysis (e.g., fibrinolysis) without internalization of the substrate. Such a mechanism would explain the lytic effect upon the remnants of fibrin, but not the concomitant acquisition of the intracellular fat. Might it be that under the above circumstances the cells themselves undergo a fatty degeneration?

The manifold unclarified facets of the problem as presented must await further investigations designed specifically to answer these outstanding questions.

MICROTHROMBI

Whereas during the past four decades it has been ultimately accepted that large mural arterial thrombi are an important element in the progression of atherosclerotic lesions, there is no such agreement with respect to the role of microthrombi in the inception of the atherosclerotic process. Only some investigators believe that microthrombi represent one form of the early atherosclerotic lesions.[27–32]

The controversy relates largely to two separate, but interrelated questions: do microthrombi occur on unaltered arterial intimal surface, and if so, do they play a role in atherogenesis?

Microthrombi are not apparent on gross inspection of the intimal surface, but are found incidentally on microscopic examination only. This accounts, no doubt, for the difficulty in detecting these tiny lesions and thus, the discrepancy in the findings by different investigators. Microthrombi have been found in several human arteries (aorta; coronary; renal and testicular arteries) at all ages, including young children, and in experimental animals.[27–33] They may be of different size, composition, and shape. Thus, they may consist predominantly of platelets or of fibrin, but most are of a "mixed" variety. They may be covered in part or entirely by endothelium, but not all microthrombi are endothelialized. Therefore, they may be amenable to lytic processes or dislodgment. Some microthrombi may be flat or molded into the intima, and they may extend over a short or a long distance. Others protrude slightly or considerably into the arterial lumen.[27]

Microthrombi may be deposited on the surface of an intima that by all available morphological criteria appears to be normal.[27] In other instances, they were found on an intima containing a slight edema or a tiny fatty dot.[27] In such instances, it would be difficult to state whether the deposition of the microthrombus preceded or followed the development of the other intimal changes.

In support of the contention that microthrombi represent one form of the earliest atherosclerotic lesions are reports that in normal porcine aortae microthrombi are found largely at the bifurcations and at the orifices of the intercostal arteries, arranged in a distribution similar to that of atherosclerotic lesions which develop in the pig.[33] In addition, in swine, the deposition of microthrombi in extracorporeal circulation occurred at sites similar to those of early atherosclerotic lesions.[34]

The main unresolved problem regarding the arterial microthrombi pertains to their incidence relevant to that of atherosclerotic lesions. Even if one accepts the premise that microthrombi represent early lesions of atherosclerosis, do they occur sufficiently often to carry any importance in the overall disease process? Only very few inquiries were undertaken to date to study this problem. In one systematic search of microthrombi at a specific site in aortae of young children, no microthrombi were found.[35] In another study, these tiny lesions were observed in seven serially sectioned segments of left coronary arteries of nine autopsied patients, whose ages ranged from 12 to 30 years.[30–32] Microthrombi were found on normal intima in three instances, and

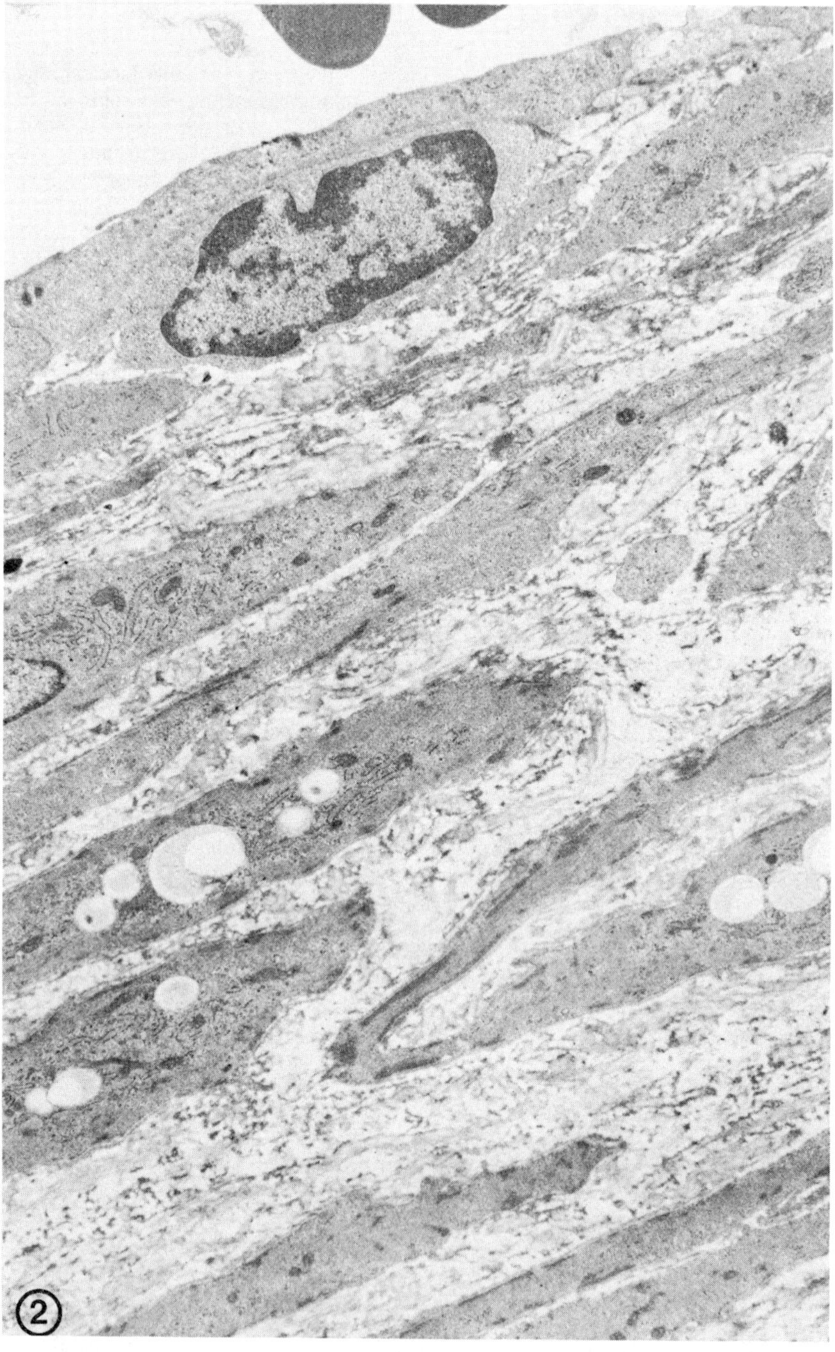

FIGURE 2. Electron micrograph of an organized, small experimentally produced thrombus in a hypercholesterolemic rabbit at 7–9 days. The structure is covered by endothelium (top), and consists of connective tissues and smooth muscle cells. Three of the cells contain a few cytoplasmic lipid droplets. Magnification: ×8200.

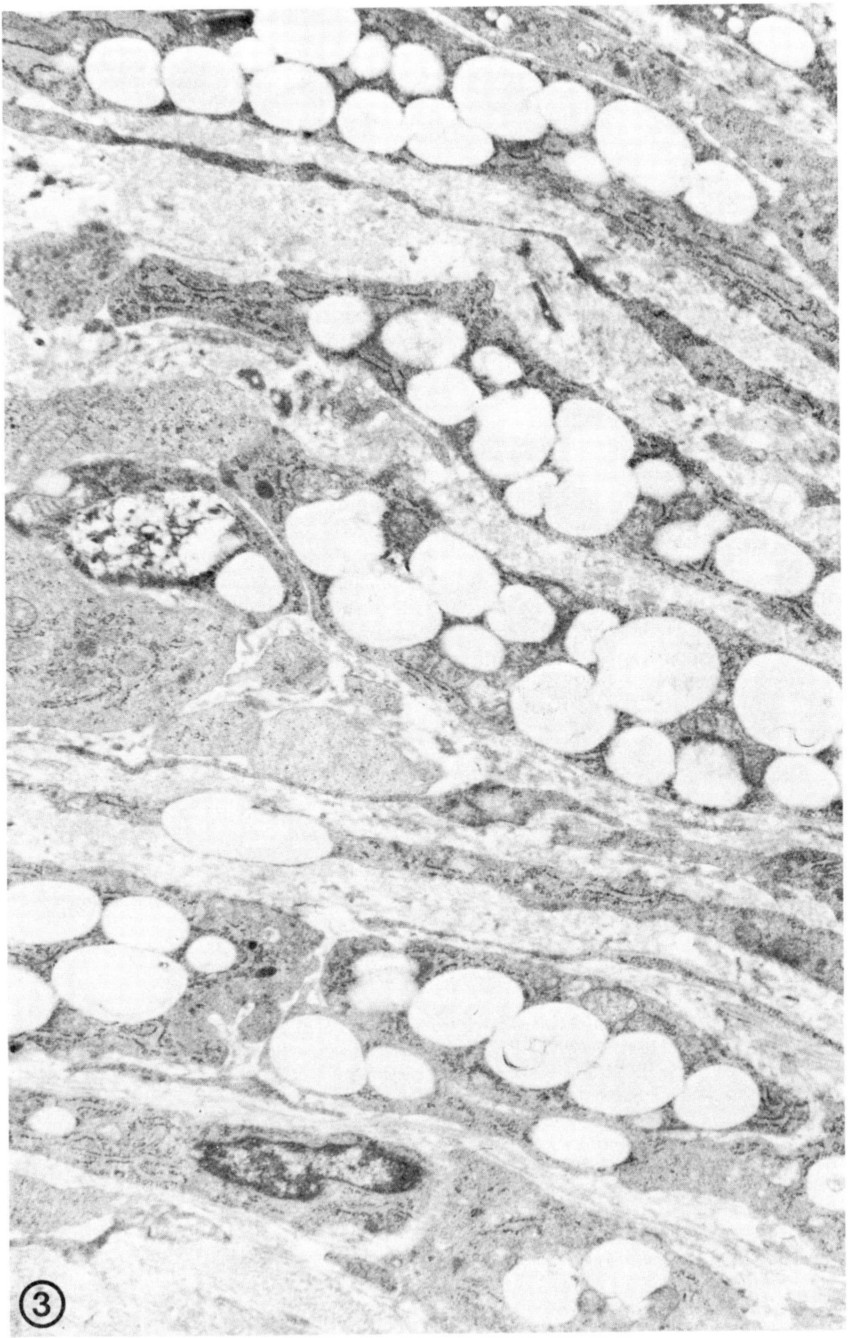

FIGURE 3. Tissues as in FIGURE 2, but at 14–21 days. Numerous cytoplasmic lipid droplets are present in most of the smooth muscle cells. Compare with the appearance of cells in FIGURE 2. Magnification: ×11,500.

in six, they were present on an intima containing another lesion. Therefore, there is a considerable need for large, prospective studies to be undertaken with the aim of a systematic search for arterial microthrombi and an assessment of their incidence.

Another, as yet unknown, aspect of microthrombi relates to some aspects of their organization, that is, the "conversion" of their substances derived from blood to connective tissue elements similar to those of intima. In human tissues, one finds that following endothelialization, such microthrombi are gradually "inhabited" by smooth muscle cells (SMC) migrating from the adjacent intima. These cells elaborate the interstitial connective tissues, gradually converting the thrombus to intima-like tissues. However, in all the human tissues available for study to this author, no intracellular fat was observed in the SMC which had emigrated into the (micro)thrombotic substance, even in patients with a considerable hypercholesterolemia.[36] If one tests this process of organization in experimental animals, a distinct difference becomes apparent: in normolipidemic control rabbits, the microthrombus was organized by normal SMC, but in the hyperlipidemic animals, these SMC contained fat droplets (FIGURE 2). The number of these droplets per SMC and the number of cells affected increased gradually over the time of organization (FIGURE 3).[36] The discrepancy between the SMC-features in human and the above experimental tissues requires elucidation, as do these related questions: do the SMC in hyperlipidemic animals change their metabolic status *prior* to migration into the microthrombus, notwithstanding lack of morphological manifestation of lesions in the intima? Alternatively, do unaltered SMC migrating into the microthrombus of hyperlipidemic animals acquire intracellular fat because considerable amounts of plasma lipids are trapped in the thrombotic substance? These and related problems require further inquiry.

ACKNOWLEDGMENTS

The author wishes to thank Mr. Roger Dewar and Ms. Irena Wojewodzka for their expert technical assistance, and Mrs. Lya Motesharei for efficient typing of the manuscript.

REFERENCES

1. VON ROKITANSKY, K. 1952. Lehrbuch der pathologischen Anatomie. vol. 4. (Vienna). pp. 1841–1846. Translated by G.E. Day. The Sydenham Society. London.
2. MALLORY, F. B. 1912–1913. The infectious lesions of blood vessels. The Harvey Lectures. pp. 150–166. J.B. Lippincott Company. Philadelphia.
3. CLARK, E., I. GRAEF & H. CHASIS. 1936. Thrombosis of the aorta and coronary arteries, with special reference to "fibrinoid" lesions. Arch. Pathol. **22:** 183–212.
4. DUGUID, J. B. 1946. Thrombosis as a factor in the pathogenesis of coronary atherosclerosis. J. Pathol. Bacteriol. **58:** 207–212.
5. DUGUID, J. B. 1948. Thrombosis as a factor in the pathogenesis of aortic atherosclerosis. J. Pathol. Bacteriol. **60:** 57–61.
6. HEARD, B. E. 1949. Mural thrombosis in the renal artery and its relation to atherosclerosis. J. Pathol. Bacteriol. **61:** 635–637.
7. CRAWFORD, T. & C. I. LEVINE. 1952. Incorporation of fibrin in the aortic intima. J. Pathol. Bacteriol. **64:** 523–528.
8. MORE, R. H., H. Z. MOVAT & M. D. HAUST. 1957. Role of mural fibrin thrombi of the aorta in genesis of arteriosclerotic plaques. Arch. Pathol. **63:** 612–620.
9. HAUST, M. D., R. H. MORE & H. Z. MOVAT. 1959. The mechanism of fibrosis in arteriosclerosis. Am. J. Pathol. **35:** 265–273.

10. HAUST, M. D. & R. H. MORE. 1960. The thrombotic basis of arteriosclerosis. The Heart Bulletin **9:** 90–92.
11. MORE, R. H. & M. D. HAUST. 1961. Atherogenesis and plasma constituents. Am. J. Pathol. **38:** 527–537.
12. WILLIAMS, G. 1955. Experimental arterial thrombosis. J. Pathol. Bacteriol. **69:** 199–206.
13. HARRISON, C. V. 1948. Experimental pulmonary arteriosclerosis. J. Pathol. Bacteriol. **60:** 289–293.
14. HEARD, B. E. 1952. An experimental study of thickening of the pulmonary arteries of rabbits produced by the organization of fibrin. J. Pathol. Bacteriol. **64:** 13–19.
15. BARNARD, P. J. 1953. Experimental fibrin thromboembolism of the lung. J. Pathol. Bacteriol. **65:** 129–136.
16. THOMAS, W. A., R. M. O'NEAL & K. T. LEE. 1956. Thromboembolism, pulmonary arteriosclerosis, and fatty meals. Arch. Pathol. (Chicago) **61:** 380–389.
17. HAND, R. A. & A. B. CHANDLER. 1962. Atherosclerotic metamorphosis of autologous pulmonary thromboemboli in the rabbit. Am. J. Pathol. **40:** 469–486.
18. CHANDLER, A. B. & R. A. HAND. 1961. Phagocytized platelets: a source of lipids in human thrombi and atherosclerotic plaques. Science **134:** 946–947.
19. HAM, A. W. & D. H. CORMACK, Eds. 1979. Histology. 8th edition. J.B. Lippincott Company. Toronto, Ontario.
20. ADAMS, C. W. M. & O. B. BAYLISS. 1976. Detection of macrophages in atherosclerotic lesions with cytochrome oxidase. Brit. J. Exp. Pathol. **57:** 30–36.
21. WOLMAN, M. & E. GATON. 1976. Macrophages and smooth muscle cells in the pathogenesis of atherosclerosis. Harefuah **90:** 400–402.
22. HAUST, M. D. 1982. Atherosclerosis;-Lesions and sequelae. *In* Cardiovascular Pathology. Chap. 6. M. D. Silver, Ed. Churchill-Livingstone. New York.
23. HAUST, M. D. 1971. Arteriosclerosis. *In* Concepts of Disease, Textbook of Pathology. Chap. 17. J. G. Brunson & E. A. Gall, Eds. Macmillan Company, New York.
24. HAUST, M. D. 1978. Zur Morphologie der Arteriosklerose. Internist (Berlin) **19:** 621–626.
25. HAUST, M. D. 1980. The nature of bi- and trinuclear cells in atherosclerotic lesions in man. Atherosclerosis **36:** 365–377.
26. HAUST, M. D. 1983. Atherosclerosis and smooth muscle cells. *In* Biochemistry of Smooth Muscle. N. L. Stephens, Ed. CRC Press Inc. Boca Raton.
27. HAUST, M. D. 1971. The morphogenesis and fate of potential and early atherosclerotic lesions in man. Human Pathol. **2:** 1–29.
28. HAUST, M. D. 1978. Light and electron microscopy of human atherosclerotic lesions. Adv. Exp. Med. Biol. **104:** 33–59.
29. MUSTARD, J. F. 1975. Function of blood platelets and their role in thrombosis. Trans. Am. Clin. Climatol. Ass. **87:** 104–127.
30. CHANDLER, A. B. 1972. Thrombosis in the development of coronary atherosclerosis. *In* Atherosclerosis and Coronary Heart Disease. W. Likoff, B. L. Segal, W. Insull & J. H. Moyer, Eds. Grune and Stratton Inc. New York.
31. CHANDLER, A. B. 1974. Mechanisms and frequency of thrombosis in the coronary circulation. Thromb. Res. **4** (Suppl): 3–23.
32. CHANDLER, A. B. & J. T. POPE. 1975. Arterial thrombosis in atherogenesis. A survey of the frequency of incorporation of thrombi into atherosclerotic plaques. *In* Blood and Arterial Wall in Atherogenesis and Arterial Thrombosis. J. G. A. J. Hautvast, R. J. J. Hermus & F. Van der Haar, Eds. E.J. Brill. Leiden, The Netherlands.
33. GEISSINGER, H. D., J. F. MUSTARD & H. C. ROWSELL. 1962. The occurrence of microthrombi on the aortic endothelium of swine. Can. Med. Ass. J. **87:** 405–408.
34. MURPHY, E. A., H. C. ROWSELL, H. G. DOWNIE, G. A. ROBINSON & J. F. MUSTARD. 1962. Encrustation and atherosclerosis: the analogy between early *in vivo* lesions and deposits which occur in extracorporeal circulations. Can. Med. Ass. J. **87:** 259–274.
35. HUDSON, J. & W. T. E. MCCAUGHEY. 1974. Mural thrombosis and atherogenesis in coronary arteries and aorta. An investigation using antifibrin and antiplatelet sera. Atherosclerosis **19:** 543–553.
36. HAUST, M. D. Unpublished observations.

Factors Controlling Thrombus Formation on Arterial Lesions

H.R. BAUMGARTNER AND K.S. SAKARIASSEN

Pharma Research Department
F. Hoffmann-La Roche & Co., Ltd.
CH-4002 Basel, Switzerland

INTRODUCTION

Thrombus formation on arterial lesions involves blood cells, particularly platelets, and the coagulation system. We have tried to mimic the sequence of events observed after endothelial denudation *in vivo,* and thus, we have developed perfusion systems which allow the study of thrombogenesis induced by arterial subendothelium[1-3] or well-defined substrates[4] in flowing anticoagulated blood. These studies have highlighted the crucial role of the blood shear rate at the vessel wall for the rate of platelet adhesion and platelet thrombus growth, as well as given new insight into the mechanism of platelet adhesion.

However, as with most studies with platelets *in vitro,* these investigations neglected the role of the coagulation system in thrombogenesis. We, therefore, modified the perfusion procedure to the use of untreated native blood which is drawn directly from a vein or artery through the perfusion chamber at a preselected flow rate.[5,6] By avoiding anticoagulation of the blood, it became possible to study the relationship between platelet and fibrin deposition on vascular subendothelium at various shear conditions. In addition, by perfusion of blood from patients with defined coagulation defects or after treatment with anticoagulants, the crucial role of thrombin generation and of von Willebrand factor for platelet thrombus growth and stability was established.[7,8]

This short essay restricts itself to a brief presentation of methods used and a description of some results obtained in perfusion systems exposing vascular subendothelium and collagen coated surfaces to flowing anticoagulated and native blood.

MATERIALS AND METHODS

Perfusion Chambers

Annular perfusion chambers were used to expose subendothelium of rabbit aorta[1] and human arteries[9] to flowing blood. These chambers consist of a central rod on which an everted arterial segment is mounted, and they are surrounded by a tube which produces an annular gap space between subendothelial surface and tube. By varying the width of the gap a wide range of shear rates at the subendothelial surface can be obtained.

A variety of parallel plate chambers were constructed to expose flat and translucent surfaces which can be coated with collagens and other proteins. These chambers were described in detail elsewhere.[4,10,11]

Perfusion Procedures

Anticoagulated blood was usually recirculated at 37°C from a reservoir through the chambers at the desired flow rate by a roller pump.[2]

Native blood was directly drawn from an antecubital vein of human volunteers or patients through the annular chamber by means of a roller pump into a calibrated cylinder at the preselected flow rate and 37°C.[5,12] In rabbits, blood was usually recirculated from a carotid artery through the annular chamber into a jugular vein. Blood flow was monitored by a flow meter at the exit of the chamber and was kept constant at the preselected flow rate by a roller pump placed between chamber and jugular vein.[6]

Platelet count and hematocrit were determined in pre- and post-perfusion blood, using coagulation parameters where necessary.

Techniques for Evaluation

Analysis of 0.8 μm thick sections by morphometric techniques yields the most differentiated information. The following parameters were usually determined; % surface coverage with platelets (adhesion), fibrin, and platelet thrombi (arbitrarily defined as mural thrombi > 5 μm in height); thrombus area per surface length ($\mu m^2/\mu m$), which corresponds to the thrombus volume per surface area; and maximum thrombus height (μm), which we arbitrarily defined as the average height of the three highest thrombi.[2,12] Unfortunately, this type of evaluation requires a lot of skill and time.

Densitometry of *en face* preparations is a perfect technique to measure surface coverage with platelets on collagen-coated slides or coverslips.[11] However, it is difficult to obtain absolute values for thrombus dimensions using this technique.

Platelet labeling using ^{51}Cr or ^{111}In is a very useful technique to measure overall platelet deposition on a surace.[13] By using surfaces with low thrombogenicity and/or treating citrated blood with aggregation inhibitors, radiolabeled platelets may also be used to measure platelet adhesion.[9] However, it has not yet been firmly established that full inhibition of aggregation does not interfere with platelet adhesion.

The pressure difference between chamber entrance and exit is a measure of the degree of chamber occlusion by progressively growing thrombotic masses upon perfusion with native blood.[14] This technique has the advantage of yielding a result which can be immediately followed on a recorder. Monitoring of the pressure difference can be combined with morphometric analysis after termination of the experiment.

RESULTS AND DISCUSSION

Perfusion Studies Using Citrated Blood

Platelet Adhesion

Platelet adhesion to vascular substrates is a prerequisite for thrombus growth under arterial blood flow conditions. Our current knowledge about this process shall therefore be briefly summarized.

Rheological considerations and actual measurements in model systems indicate that the concentration of platelets in the boundary layer of the vessel wall increases with the shear rate.[3,15] This is consistent with the experimental observation that the rate of platelet adhesion to vascular subendothelium increases proportionally to the shear rate in a perfusion chamber (FIGURE 1). However, for human platelets and at a citrate concentration of 20 m*M*, this is true only for shear rates up to about 800 s^{-1}; at higher shear rates, there is no further increase of the rate of platelet adhesion.[16] At least two mechanisms may account for these observations: (1) At shear rates up to 800 s^{-1}, the limiting factor for adhesion is platelet transport towards the vessel wall. In other words, a constant fraction of the platelets which encounter the vessel wall adheres. At higher shear rates, adhesion becomes less transport dependent, but more reaction controlled; i.e., an increasingly smaller fraction of those platelets which encounter the vessel wall are able to adhere. (2) Platelet thrombus growth also increases with the shear rate (see below). Thus, as shear rate increases, an increasing fraction of the platelets present in the boundary layer are consumed by the growing thrombi and are no longer available for adhesion. Most likely, both mechanisms are operative, particularly at shear rates above 1300 s^{-1}.

Our currently growing knowledge about the mechanism of adhesion is based on several approaches and their combinations: (1) The perfusion of blood from patients with defects of platelet function;[17–19] (2) The addition of antibodies directed towards specific plasma proteins of platelet membrane glycoproteins to the perfused blood;[20–22] (3) The use of partially reconstituted whole blood as perfusate;[9,23] and, (4)

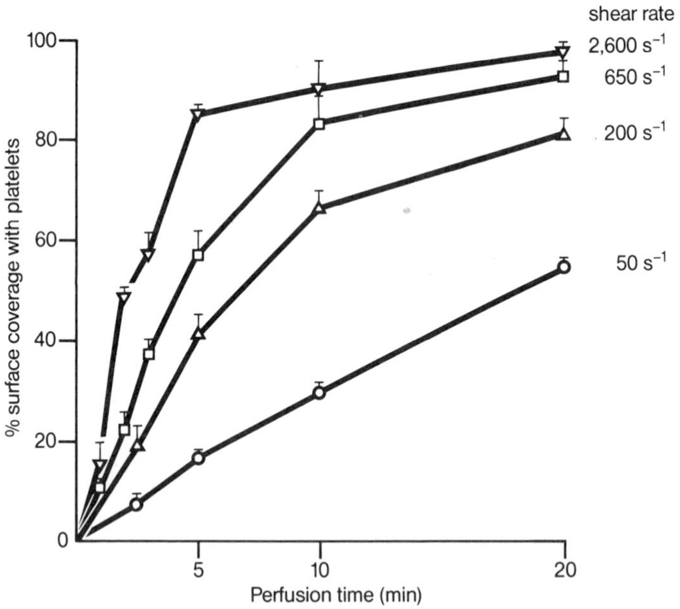

FIGURE 1. Shear rate dependence of platelet adhesion. Rabbit aorta subendothelium was exposed to citrated (~15 m*M*) rabbit blood, which was recirculated through annular chambers at wall shear rates ranging from 50 to 2600 s^{-1}, corresponding to venous and microcirculatory flow conditions, respectively. Values represent means ± SE of 3–7 perfusion experiments.

TABLE 1. Role of Platelet Membrane Glycoproteins and of Adhesive Proteins Present in Plasma, Platelets, and/or the Vessel Wall

	Platelet Membrane Glycoprotein	Adhesive Protein	
	Designation	Designation	Concentration in Plasma [μg/ml]
PLATELET ADHESION			
Initial attachment			
at high shear	Ib	von Willebrand factor	~ 7
at low shear	Ia[a]	Fibronectin[a]	~ 300
Spreading	Ia	Fibronectin	~ 300
		von Willebrand factor[a]	~ 7
PLATELET AGGREGATION (Thrombus formation)	IIb/IIIa	Fibrinogen	~3000
	—[a]	von Willebrand factor[a]	~ 7
	—[a]	Thrombospondin[a]	~ 0.02
	—[a]	Fibronectin[a]	~ 300

[a]Unknown or still not clearly established.

The exposure of surfaces coated with purified components of the vessel wall to flowing blood.[4,10,11,23] The picture emerging from these studies, although in part still incomplete and hypothetical, is summarized in TABLE 1. Basically, certain glycoproteins of the platelet membrane, together with von Willebrand factor and fibronectin, which are both synthesized by vascular endothelial cells, are involved in platelet adhesion at the molecular level. Both proteins appear to have specific domains for binding to platelets and collagen, respectively, and are thus able to act as "glue" between circulating platelets and vessel wall collagen. Von Willebrand factor is essential only at high shear rates, i.e., when the residence time of a platelet at the vessel wall, and thus, the time available for firm attachment, is very short.[21,24] Fibronectin, on the other hand, is probably required for platelet spreading and release, and is thus necessary for optimal adhesion at all shear rates.[19,23] Recent evidence suggests that some adhesive proteins have common recognition sites on activated platelets and may therefore substitute for each other.[25] Preliminary results of our laboratory using purified thrombospondin and antibodies towards thrombospondin indicate that this protein has no important role in platelet adhesion.

Platelet Thrombus Growth and Stability

A platelet which has attached to the subendothelial surface spreads out on it within a few seconds to minutes. The latter process is associated with the release of a number of biologically highly active substances, which are either secreted from intracellular stores (exocytosis of α granules and dense bodies) or are newly synthesized. Amongst the substances released, adenosine diphosphate (ADP), platelet activating factor (PAF), thromboxane A_2, and serotonin are known to activate additional platelets and to induce platelet-platelet cohesion, i.e., thrombus growth. The adhesive proteins released from α granules may be important for further platelet adhesion and/or for function as "glue" in thrombus growth (TABLE 1). In addition, platelet factor 3 made available at the activated platelet membrane may accelerate coagulation at the surface for four to five orders of magnitude. Other released platelet factors may induce vasoconstriction (thromboxane A_2 and serotonin), as well as migration and proliferation of smooth muscle cells (platelet derived growth factors).

Perfusion studies show that platelet thrombus growth is also highly shear rate dependent (FIGURE 2). Thus, mural platelet thrombi grow 30–50 times more rapidly in height, and 600 times more rapidly in area (volume) at 10,000 s^{-1} than at 50 s^{-1} shear rate, respectively. Such an enormous difference was not expected. Even more surprising, was the observation that those thrombi which grew larger and higher were also less reversible (FIGURE 3), despite the increasing and very substantial shear forces which would tend to remove thrombi of similar stability more readily. We thus have to conclude that not only the growth rate, but also the stability of thrombi increases with the shear rate. The mechanisms responsible for thrombus stability at high shear rates have not yet been elucidated. Several possibilities are conceivable: (1) Shear forces could activate platelets and thus, enable them to form stronger bonds between each other; (2) Shear forces could activate other blood cells to release platelet activating substances; and, (3) Rapid thrombus growth, initially primarily due to high platelet concentration in the boundary layer, will cause increasing microturbulence near the vessel wall, which might stimulate, rather than inhibit, further thrombus growth. Interestingly, the largest platelet mass attached to the subendothelial surface was independent of shear rate, and was always observed at 5 min perfusion time (FIGURE 3), suggesting an intrinsic mechanism for platelet thrombus relaxation which is independent of the shear rate. Whether thrombus relaxation is a citrate artifact or not remains to be established.

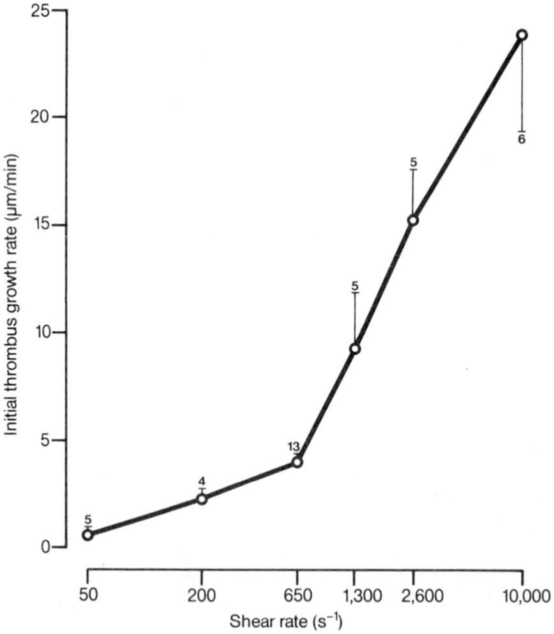

FIGURE 2. Shear rate dependence of platelet thrombus growth induced by rabbit aorta subendothelium in flowing citrated (~15 m*M*) blood of rabbits. Initial (maximal) growth rates were calculated from time curves obtained for maximal thrombus heights. The results shown in FIGURES 1–3 were in part derived from the same set of experiments.

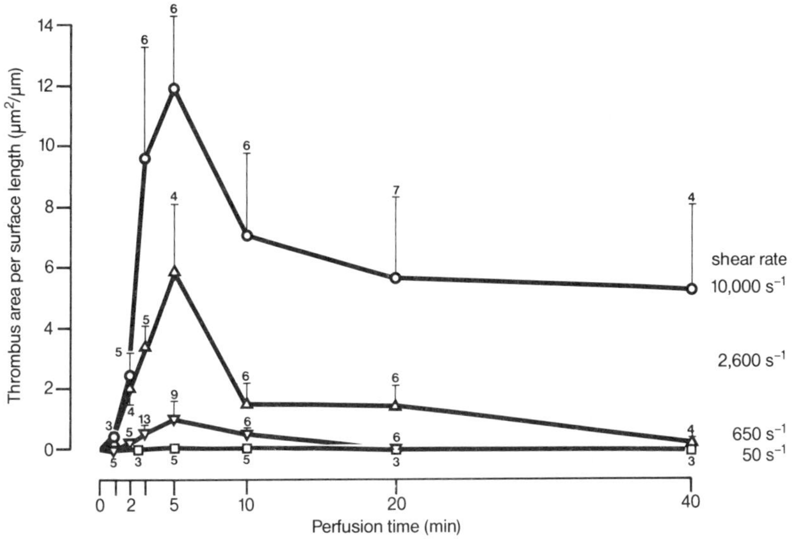

FIGURE 3. Shear rate dependence of platelet thrombus growth and its reversal. Time curves for a few shear rates are shown. The measured thrombus area per surface length corresponds to the thrombus volume per exposed surface area. See legends to FIGURES 1 and 2.

In the context of vascular physiology and pathology, the observations discussed above (FIGURES 2 and 3) may help to explain hemostasis in the microvasculature and thrombosis of stenosed arteries. Under physiologic conditions the highest shear rates of up to 5000 s^{-1} were found in arterioles.[3] Thus, it appears teleologically meaningful that mechanisms exist which cause rapid growth of a stable plug. On the other hand, shear rates are exceedingly high in pathologically stenosed arteries. Our observations suggest that platelet thrombi at such sites will grow more rapidly and will be more stable than those in normal arteries where shear rates between 500–1000 s^{-1} predominate. Thus, clinically relevant thrombotic events or eventually, occlusive thrombosis will most likely occur in stenosed arteries.

Axial Dependence of Platelet Adhesion and Thrombus Growth

Platelet adhesion and thrombus growth and break off are dynamic events. In addition, thrombus growth, release of biologically active substances, and translocation of thrombi along the axis of the flowing blood may greatly influence the result of blood-vessel wall interaction further downstream. Experimental evidence for upstream platelet consumption, translocation of platelets and thrombi, as well as for upstream activation of platelets is briefly summarized below.

Upstream Platelet Consumption. Theoretical considerations predict that platelet adhesion and thrombus growth deplete the boundary layer of platelets.[26] Therefore, adhesion and thrombus growth should decrease along the axis of the flowing blood. Recent results in our laboratory show that this is indeed the case (Sakariassen and Baumgartner, in preparation). The magnitude of the difference between upstream and downstream adhesion and thrombi depends on the thrombogenicity of the exposed surface (i.e., the upstream thrombus growth rate and the wall shear rate). Thus, on a surface such as human umbilical artery subendothelium, which induces only a few small thrombi, downstream platelet deposition is only marginally lower than upstream at an intermediate shear rate of 650 s^{-1} (FIGURE 4). By contrast, on a surface such as fibrillar collagen, which induces rapid thrombus growth, a dramatic axial dependence for adhesion and for thrombi was observed (FIGURE 4). In addition, when the magnitude of axial dependence was investigated at various shear rates, much greater differences between upstream and downstream were observed at low, rather than at

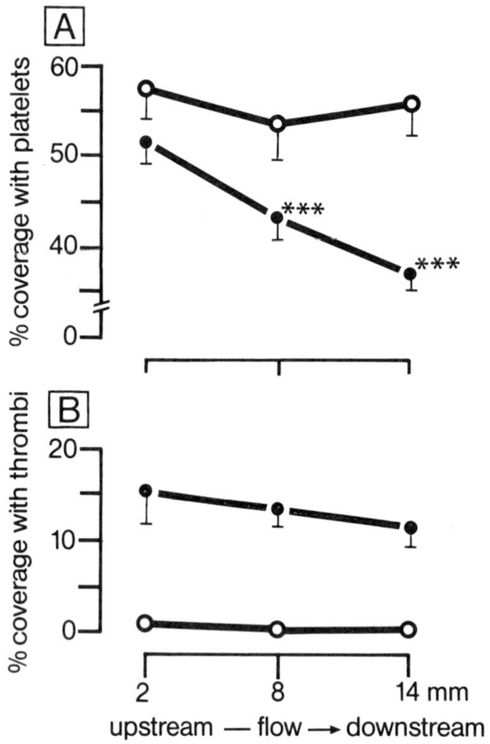

FIGURE 4. Axial dependence of platelet adhesion (A) and platelet thrombi (B). Human umbilical artery subendothelium (○—○, n = 6) and collagen coated cover slips (●—●, n = 9) were exposed to human citrated blood flowing at 650 s^{-1} shear rate for five min. Platelet adhesion and thrombi were determined at three axial positions from the upstream end (=0 mm) of the exposed thrombotic surface. Values at positions 8 and 14 mm were compared with the one at 2 mm; *** indicates $2p < 0.001$ (Student's *t* test).

high shear rate (For example, a 22% versus a 79% decrease in adhesion at shear rates of 2000 and 200 s^{-1}, respectively). These observations underline the importance of the shear rate for the platelet concentration in the boundary layer and its role for platelet thrombus growth and platelet consumption as predicted by theoretical considerations.

Translocation of Platelets and Thrombi. Evidence for this phenomenon can be easily obtained in washout experiments.[27] Thus, when two chambers in series are perfused with blood, very similar values for platelet adhesion and thrombi are obtained on subendothelium in both chambers. If blood perfusion in one of the two chambers is followed by perfusion of platelet-free plasma or blood, then the highest thrombi disappear, and adhesion increases as compared to the other chamber.[2,27] Two mechanisms may account for translocation: (1) break off of single platelets or thrombus fragments with reattachment further downstream, and (2) bending down of thrombi towards the surface in the direction of flow. The latter phenomenon can be directly visualized in longitudinal sections (FIGURE 5).

Upstream Activation. Only a few platelets attach to collagenase digested subendothelium[28] or to an artificial surface, such as epon.[2] Therefore, spreading occurs but very slowly on these surfaces. However, when a thrombogenic surface is placed upstream, spread platelets and platelet thrombi were observed on collagenase digested subendothelium or epon up to 15 mm downstream of the thrombogenic surface.[27] This observation suggests that platelets either were translocated from upstream thrombi, or were activated by platelet release products, which behave differently from platelets of the circulation in that they are able to spread and aggregate on a "non-thrombogenic" surface.

Platelet consumption, translocation, and activation should always be considered when it comes to the interpretation of results obtained in flow systems. It appears advisable to look at time curves and at several axial positions before firm conclusions are drawn.

Perfusion Studies Using Native Blood

Effects of Citrate

Citrate concentrations commonly used in platelet research amount to 15–20 m*M* in plasma. Concentrations around 30 m*M* strongly inhibit platelet aggregation in plasma and thrombus formation in perfusion systems.[6] Still higher concentrations inhibit spreading on subendothelium and thus, adhesion.[6,12,29] The perfusion of native blood (see METHODS) allows a direct comparison with citrated blood. Thus, blood from a donor rabbit was collected into citrate to give a final concentration of approximately 15 m*M*, and was recirculated from a reservoir through an annular chamber. At the same time, blood of the same rabbit was recirculated from a carotid artery through the chamber into a jugular vein at flow conditions and for periods of time which were identical. The result shows that thrombi grew more rapidly in the absence of citrate (FIGURE 6). Already after one minute perfusion, thrombi are higher in native than in citrated blood. In native blood, the highest thrombi grew at a similar rate of about 50 μm/min from one to at least five minutes. At ten minutes, they had reached the outer wall of the annular gap space which has a width of approximately 350 μm. The highest thrombi in citrated blood grew at a maximal rate of 15–20 μm/min only between 1 and 2 min perfusion time, indicating that thrombi begin to break off or bend down toward the surface at a very early stage in the presence of citrate. The analysis of the curve obtained from the measurements of thrombus area per surface length (not shown), which corresponds to the thrombus volume per surface area, revealed interesting differences in comparison to FIGURE 6. Thus, the maximum growth rate was similar in native and citrated blood for about 2 min and amounted to 1.5 $\mu m^2/\mu m/min$. In citrated blood, thrombi continued to grow at a similar rate for another three minutes, and then gradually disappeared. By contrast, in native blood thrombi started to grow at a much higher rate of approximately 14 $\mu m^2/\mu m/min$ from 1 to 10 min. This marked

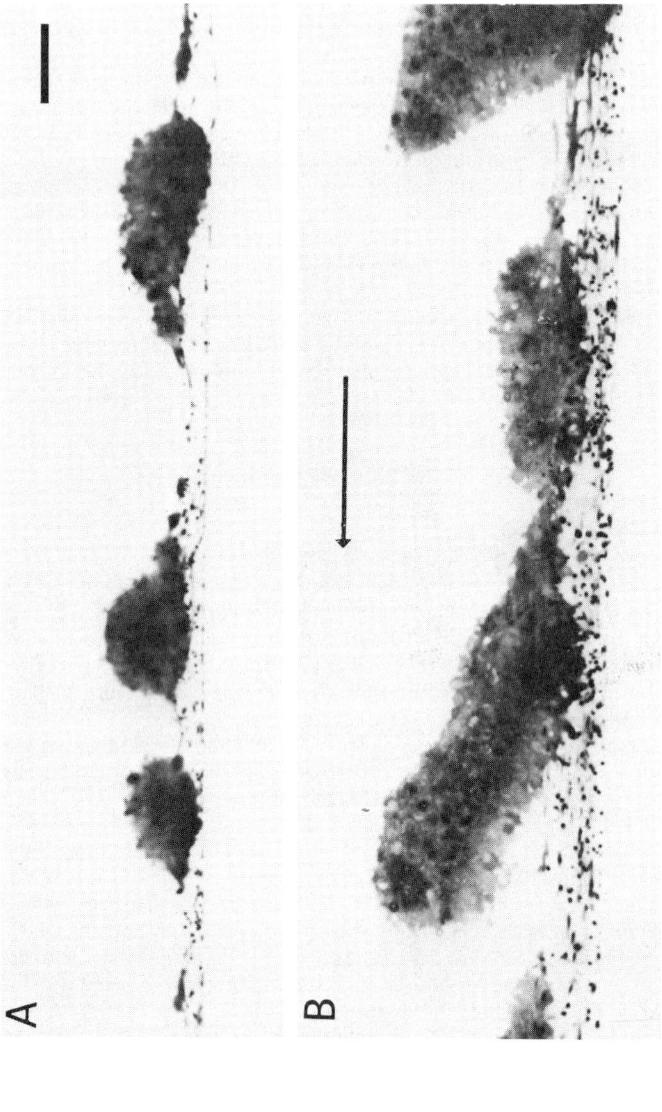

FIGURE 5. Light micrographs of platelet thrombi on a collagen coated coverslip after perfusion of human citrated (~20 m*M*) blood at 650 s^{-1} for five min. A is a cross section (perpendicular to the flow axis); B is a longitudinal section (the arrow indicates the direction of flow). Bar indicates 10 μm.

increase in growth rate may be due to turbulence induced by the growing thrombi in concert with massive activation of the coagulation system.

Interestingly, the time curve for platelet thrombi *in vivo*[1] much more resembles the one in the presence of 15 m*M* citrate *in vitro*, than the one with native blood. This indicates that excessive activation of the coagulation system occurs in the chamber as compared to the *in vivo* situation in rabbits. Whether this is due to activation in the tubing between vessel and exposed subendothelial surface, or whether counter-regulatory mechanisms exist *in vivo* which are no longer operative on the arteries exposed in the chamber remains to be established.

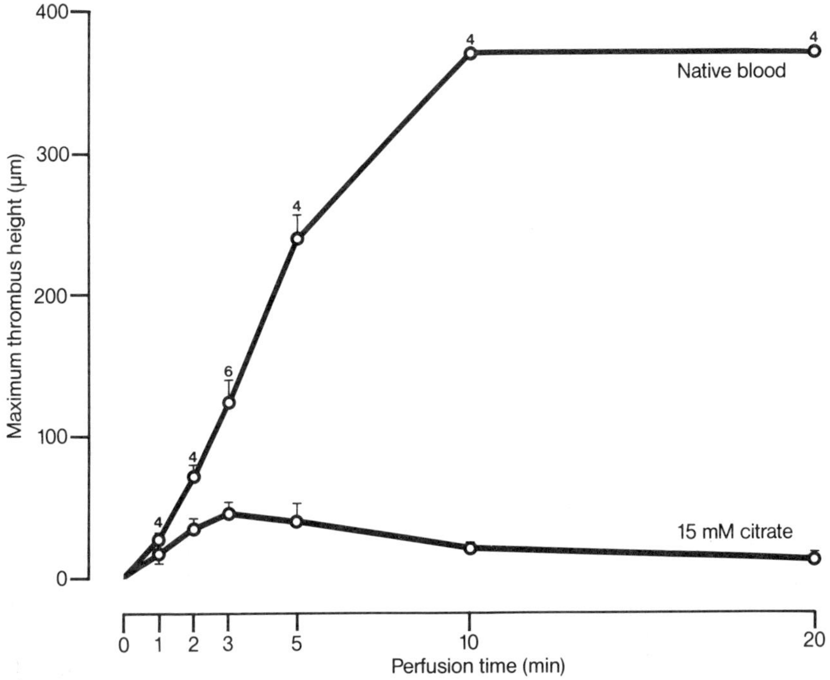

FIGURE 6. Effect of citrate anticoagulation on the growth of platelet thrombi. Native blood (from a carotid artery) and citrated blood (from a reservoir at 37°C) of the same rabbits was perfused through the small annular chamber with exposed subendothelium at 40 ml/min (2600 s^{-1} shear rate) for the times indicated.

Shear Rate Dependence of Fibrin versus Platelet Deposition on Subendothelium

Fibrin formation was never observed in perfusions using citrated blood. However, it was always present on the subendothelial surface after native blood perfusions, except for exposure times of less than 2 min. Time curves for fibrin deposition on subendothelium at various shear rates will be published elsewhere. In FIGURE 7, the result of a morphometric analysis of platelet and fibrin deposition at and in the close vicinity to the subendothelial surface is shown for a wide range of shear rates after 20 min perfusion time. At this time, the subendothelial surface is completely saturated with

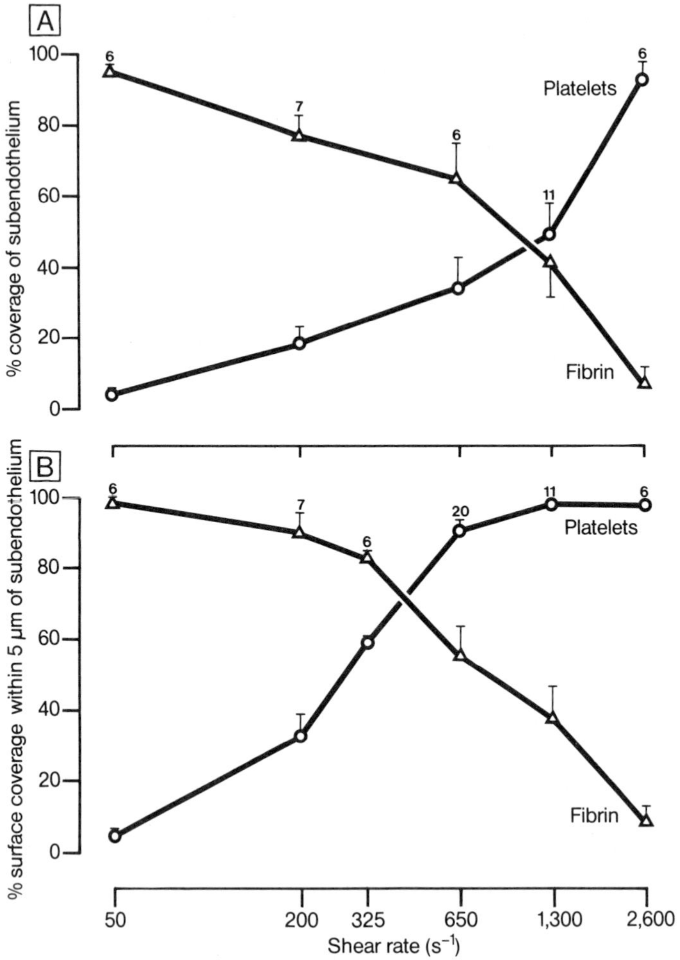

FIGURE 7. Shear rate dependence of fibrin versus platelet deposition on subendothelium. Rabbit aorta subendothelium was exposed to flowing native blood of rabbits for 20 min at the shear rates indicated. Panel A shows the result of the morphometric analysis at the subendothelial surface itself. Panel B shows the result of the morphometric analysis within the boundary area of the subendothelium, thus including platelets on subendothelium and on fibrin, along with fibrin on subendothelium and on platelets.

platelets and/or fibrin. FIGURE 7A shows the percent coverage of the subendothelial surface itself, thus indicating what was deposited first, platelets or fibrin. At shear rates up to about 1000 s^{-1}, a larger fraction of the surface is covered with fibrin; at shear rates >1300 s^{-1}, more than 50% of the surface was covered with platelets before fibrin could form. Analysis for fibrin and platelets within 5 μm of the subendothelial surface reveals that up to a shear rate of 300 s^{-1}, the surface boundary area is virtually saturated with fibrin, while at shear rates >500 s^{-1}, platelets predominate (FIGURE

7B). This analysis also shows that the thrombotic material in the boundary area consists virtually of fibrin only or platelets only at shear rates of 50 and 2600 s^{-1}, respectively. To our knowledge, the shear rate dependence of fibrin deposition has not been demonstrated for such a wide range of shear rates previously. However, these results were to be expected. Finally, at high shear rates, precoagulant activity which is generated is rapidly diluted and swept away by the rapidly flowing blood, and there is not enough time for fibrin monomers to polymerize. Platelets, on the other hand, have the ability to adhere and aggregate within fractions of a second.

Shear Rate Dependence of Thrombus Growth

At 20 min perfusion time with native blood of rabbits, the maximum height of platelet thrombi attached to the subendothelial surface amounted to 46 ± 12, 57 ± 18, 288 ± 40, and 398 ± 25 μm at 50, 200, 650, and 2600 s^{-1} shear rate, respectively; the corresponding values for the thrombus area per surface length were 0.7 ± 0.4, 2.4 ± 1.1, 85 ± 20, and 157 ± 16 $\mu m^2/\mu m$, respectively. To date, the maximum thrombus growth rates have only been determined for shear rates of 650 and 2600 s^{-1}. They amounted to approximately 30 and 50 μm/ min for the maximum heights, and to 10 and 15 $\mu m^2/\mu m/min$ for the thrombus area per surface length, respectively. These morphometric results clearly show that thrombus growth in native blood increases with the shear rate, particularly at shear rates >650 s^{-1}.

The findings described above are supported by measurements of the pressure difference between the entrance and the exit of an annular chamber. When blood is recirculated from a carotid artery into the jugular vein of a rabbit, the pressure at the chamber entrance corresponds to the arterial pressure of the rabbit and usually remains constant throughout the perfusion. At the beginning of a perfusion, the pressure at the chamber exit is (depending on the selected flow rate) only slightly lower than the rabbit's blood pressure, but then, gradually decreases with time to negative values, reflecting progressive occlusion of the chamber by growing thrombotic masses on the subendothelial surface.[14] FIGURE 8 shows the shear rate dependence of the pressure difference between entrance and exit of the same perfusion chamber at 15 min perfusion time. The shape of the curve is similar to the one obtained for initial thrombus growth rates using citrated blood (FIGURE 2) and to the one described above for native blood. The very substantial pressure differences observed at high shear rates, i.e., up to 450 mm Hg at 2600 s^{-1} shear rate and 20 min perfusion time, furthermore support our previous conclusion that rapidly growing thrombi must be very stable.

Thrombus Growth and Stability

Whether a platelet thrombus breaks off as a small aggregate or as a large thrombotic mass, or whether thrombosis eventually becomes occlusive depends on thrombus stability. Our results presented above suggest that the thrombus growth rate and thrombus stability are related. We have discussed several possible explanations, but, in fact, we do not yet understand this positive relationship. Recent evidence from perfusion studies with native blood of patients with various coagulation deficiencies and of heparinized rabbits indicates that thrombin generation is essential for thrombus stability, particularly at intermediate to low shear rates. In addition, von Willebrand factor plays a role in thrombus stability, whereas the formation of fibrin for plasma fibrinogen appears not to be crucial for stability during the first 20 min of thrombus growth. The evidence supporting these conclusions is briefly summarized below.

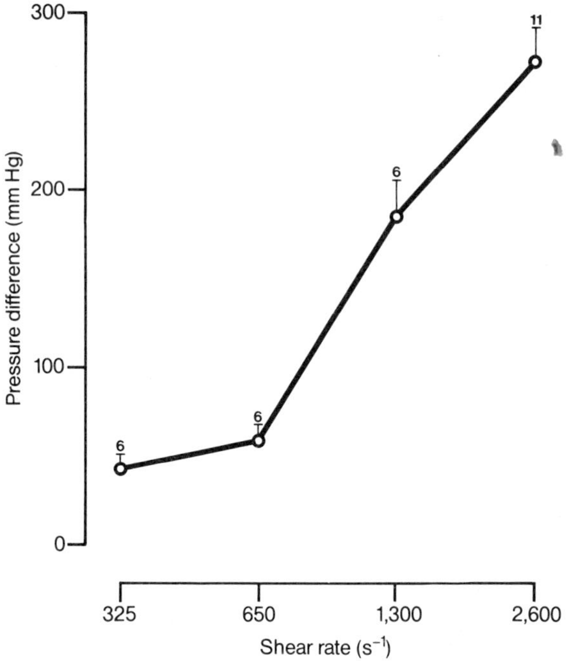

FIGURE 8. Shear rate dependence of chamber occlusion. Native rabbit blood was perfused through the small annular chamber at 5, 10, 20, and 40 ml/min flow rate producing the shear rates indicated. The blood pressure at the entrance and the exit of the chamber was monitored. The difference between these two pressures after 15 min perfusion time is shown.

Perfusion of blood of patients with hemophilia shows that platelet thrombus formation is significantly reduced in the absence of antihemophilic factor at 650 s^{-1} shear rate.[7] Interestingly, this effect is less pronounced at higher shear rates,[8] indicating again that mechanisms probably not related to coagulation are important for thrombus stability at high shear. Perfusion studies with blood of heparinized rabbits show that initial thrombus growth was similar to control perfusions at 650 s^{-1}

TABLE 2. Effect of Heparin on Platelet Thrombus Growth Induced by Subendothelium in Native Blood at 650 s^{-1} Shear Rate[a]

Perfusion Time (min)	n		Max. Thrombus Height (μm)		Thrombus Area ($\mu m^2/\mu m$)	
	Control	Heparin	Control	Heparin	Control	Heparin
3	12	4	53 ± 7	51 ± 7	2.1 ± 0.5	1.4 ± 0.4
5	12	4	155 ± 20	90 ± 15	19.2 ± 4.7	5.3 ± 1.5
10	8	5	311 ± 31	105 ± 39	74.4 ± 11.8	13.8 ± 6.1
20	7	5	382 ± 40	44 ± 29	113.0 ± 32.0	8.2 ± 7.6

[a]Heparin (500 U/kg) was given intravenously to rabbits 5–10 min prior to a perfusion experiment. Blood was recirculated from a carotid artery through the small chamber at 10 ml/min into a jugular vein. Mean ± SE are given.

shear rate. At perfusion times >3 min, platelet thrombi in blood of heparinized rabbits grew at a lower rate than those of controls, and at 20 min, their average maximum heights were below the one at 3 min (TABLE 2). The fact that the thrombus area decreased less than the height indicates that the majority of thrombi did not break off, but bent down to the surface. Whereas the thrombi at 3 min perfusion time were tall and slim, those in heparinized blood at 20 min were large and flat. These observations indicate that the main effect of heparin is not on the initial growth of platelet thrombi, but on their stability. Since patients with hemophilia have only been studied after 5 and 10 min perfusion time at 650 s^{-1} shear rate, additional time points are needed for a more general conclusion regarding the role of thrombin for thrombus stability.

Recent studies with native blood of patients at flow conditions in which little or no defect of platelet adhesion was observed in von Willebrand's disease (1300 s^{-1}) showed that platelet thrombus height and volume in this disorder were significantly reduced compared to normal controls or patients with hemophilia.[8] Thus, von Willebrand factor may mediate not only the adhesion of platelets to subendothelium, but also platelet-platelet cohesion necessary for normal thrombus development.

Interestingly, thrombus growth and stability was normal or even increased in patients with severe fibrinogen deficiency[7,8] (Straub *et al.*, unpublished). This was true for a number of flow conditions. Fibrin was never observed. These observations indicate that the formation of fibrin from plasma fibrinogen was not crucial for early platelet thrombus stability. Other adhesive proteins (TABLE 1) may substitute for fibrinogen as "glue" between platelets in these patients.[25]

CONCLUSION

Perfusion systems for the exposure of vascular surfaces to flowing blood *in vitro* were originally set up to mimic the sequence of events which were observed on vascular subendothelium *in vivo*,[1] and to bridge the gap between sophisticated test-tube experiments *in vitro* and the much more complex situation *in vivo*. We believe that the latter goal is still one of the major purposes for the use of such systems. However, their use has also led to a number of discoveries and has helped to elucidate the role of some adhesive proteins and platelet membrane glycoproteins in thrombogenesis. The most important contribution made, probably relates to the full recognition of the role of blood flow and red cells in thrombogenesis. Our results show that the wall shear rate in a vessel is very important in determining the extent of platelet versus fibrin involvement in thrombogenesis, as well as in determining the growth rate and stability of platelet thrombi. They implicate that the approaches to be taken for therapy and prevention of thrombosis must differ for different parts of the vascular tree since they depend on the shear rate which prevails.

ACKNOWLEDGMENTS

We thank Christine Michael and Käthi Schietinger for their skillful technical assistance.

REFERENCES

1. BAUMGARTNER, H. R. 1973. The role of blood flow in platelet adhesion, fibrin deposition, and formation of mural thrombi. Microvasc. Res. **5:** 167–179.

2. BAUMGARTNER, H. R. & R. MUGGLI. 1976. Adhesion and aggregation: morphological demonstration and quantitation *in vivo* and *in vitro*. *In* Platelets in Biology and Pathology. J.L. Gordon, Ed.: 23–60. Elsevier/North Holland. Biomedical Press. New York.
3. TURITTO, V. T. & H. R. BAUMGARTNER. 1982. Platelet-surface interactions. *In* Hemostasis and Thrombosis, basic principles and clinical practice. R.W. Colman, V.J. Marder & E.W. Salzman, Eds.: 364–379. J.B. Lippincott Company. Philadelphia.
4. SAKARIASSEN, K. S., P. A. M. M. AARTS, P. G. DE GROOT, W. P. M. HOUDIJK & J. J. SIXMA. 1983. A perfusion chamber developed to investigate platelet interaction in flowing blood with human vessel wall cells, their extracellular matrix, and purified components. J. Lab. Clin. Med. **102:** 522–535.
5. BAUMGARTNER, H. R. 1976. Effects of anticoagulation on the interaction of human platelets with subendothelium in flowing blood. Schweiz. Med. Wochenschr. **106:** 1367–1368.
6. BAUMGARTNER, H. R. 1979. Effect of acetylsalicylic acid, sulfinpyrazone, and dipyridamole on platelet adhesion and aggregation in flowing native and anticoagulated blood. Haemostasis **8:** 340–352.
7. WEISS, H. J., V. T. TURITTO, W. J. VICIC & H. R. BAUMGARTNER. 1984. Fibrin formation, fibrinopeptide A release, and platelet thrombus dimensions on subendothelium exposed to flowing native blood: Greater in factor XII and XI than in factor VIII and IX deficiency. Blood **63:** 1004–1014.
8. TURITTO, V. T., H. J. WEISS & H. R. BAUMGARTNER. 1984. Platelet interaction with rabbit subendothelium in von Willebrand's disease: altered thrombus formation distinct from defective platelet adhesion. J. Clin. Invest. **74:** 1730–1741.
9. SAKARIASSEN, K. S., P. A. BOLHUIS & J. J. SIXMA. 1979. Human blood platelet adhesion to artery subendothelium is mediated by factor VIII-von Willebrand factor bound to the subendothelium. Nature **279:** 636–638.
10. GRABOWSKI, E. F., K. K. HERTHER & P. DIDISHEIM. 1976. Human versus dog platelet adhesion to cuprophane under controlled conditions of whole blood flow. J. Lab. Clin. Med. **88:** 368–374.
11. MUGGLI, R., H. R. BAUMGARTNER, T. B. TSCHOPP & H. J. KELLER. 1980. Automated microdensitometry and protein assays as a measure for platelet adhesion and aggregation on collagen-coated slides under controlled flow conditions. J. Lab. Clin. Med. **95:** 195–207.
12. BAUMGARTNER, H. R., V. T. TURITTO & H. J. WEISS. 1980. Effect of shear rate on platelet interaction with subendothelium in citrated and native blood. II. Relationships among platelet adhesion, thrombus dimensions, and fibrin formation. J. Lab. Clin. Med. **95:** 208–221.
13. HARKER, L. A. & S. R. HANSON. 1979. Experimental arterial thromboembolism in baboons. Mechanism, quantitation, and pharmacologic prevention. J. Clin. Invest. **64:** 559–569.
14. BAUMGARTNER, H. R., H. KUHN & T. B. TSCHOPP. 1983. Factors influencing the growth, stability, and fate of arterial thrombi. *In* Atherosclerosis, vol. VI. G. Schettler, A. M. Gotto, G. Middelhoff, A. J. R. Habenicht & K. R. Jurutka, Eds.: 649–658. Springer-Verlag. Berlin.
15. GOLDSMITH, H. L. 1972. The flow of model particles and blood cells and its relation to thrombogenesis. *In* Progress in Hemostasis and Thrombosis, vol. 1. T. H. Spaet, Ed.: 97–139. Grune & Stratton. New York.
16. TURITTO, V. T., H. J. WEISS & H. R. BAUMGARTNER. 1980. The effect of shear rate on platelet interaction with subendothelium exposed to citrated human blood. Microvasc. Res. **19:** 352–365.
17. TSCHOPP, T. B., H. J. WEISS & H. R. BAUMGARTNER. 1974. Decreased adhesion of platelets to subendothelium in von Willebrand's disease. J. Lab. Clin. Med. **83:** 296–300.
18. WEISS, H. J., T. B. TSCHOPP, H. R. BAUMGARTNER, I. I. SUSSMAN, M. M. JOHNSON & J. J. EGAN. 1974. Decreased adhesion of giant (Bernard-Soulier) platelets to subendothelium—Further implications on the role of the von Willebrand factor in hemostasis. Am. J. Med. **57:** 920–925.
19. NIEUWENHUIS H. K., K. S. SAKARIASSEN, W. P. M. HOUDIJK, P. F. E. M. NIEVELSTEN &

J. J. SIXMA. 1984. Deficiency of platelet membrane glycoprotein Ia associated with a decreased platelet adhesion to subendothelium: a defect in platelet spreading. Submitted.

20. CAEN, J. P., H. MICHEL, G. TOBELEM, E. BODEVIN & S. LEVY-TOLEDANO. 1977. Adhesion and aggregation of human platelets to rabbit subendothelium. A new approach for investigation: Specific antibodies. Experientia **33:** 91–93.
21. BAUMGARTNER, H. R., T. B. TSCHOPP & D. MEYER. 1980. Shear rate dependent inhibition of platelet adhesion and aggregation on collagenous surfaces by antibodies to human factor VIII/von Willebrand factor. Br. J. Haematol. **44:** 127–139.
22. STEL, H. V., K. S. SAKARIASSEN, B. J. SCHOLTE, E. C. I. VEERMAN, T. H. VAN DER KWAST, P. G. DE GROOT, J. J. SIXMA & J. A. VAN MOURIK. 1984. Characterization of 25 monoclonal antibodies to factor VIII-von Willebrand factor: relationship between ristocetin-induced platelet aggregation and platelet adherence to subendothelium. Blood **63:** 1408–1415.
23. HOUDIJK, W. P. M., K. S. SAKARIASSEN & J. J. SIXMA. 1984. Role of factor VIII-von Willebrand factor and fibronectin in the interaction of platelets in flowing blood with human collagen types I and III. J. Clin. Invest. **75:** 531–540.
24. WEISS, H. J., V. T. TURITTO & H. R. BAUMGARTNER. 1978. Effect of shear rate on platelet interaction with subendothelium in citrated and native blood. I. Shear-dependent decrease in adhesion in von Willebrand's disease and the Bernard-Soulier syndrome. J. Lab. Clin. Med. **92:** 750–764.
25. PLOW, E. F., A. H. SROUJI, D. MEYER, G. MARGUERIE & M. H. GINSBERG. 1984. Evidence that three adhesive proteins interact with a common recognition site on activated platelets. J. Biol. Chem. **259:** 5388–5391.
26. TURITTO, V. T. & H. R. BAUMGARTNER. 1975. Platelet deposition on subendothelium exposed to flowing blood: Mathematical analysis of physical parameters. Trans. Am. Soc. Artif. Intern. Organs **XXI:** 593–600.
27. BAUMGARTNER, H. R., R. MUGGLI, T. B. TSCHOPP & V. T. TURITTO. 1976. Platelet adhesion, release, and aggregation in flowing blood: effects of surface properties and platelet function. Thrombos. Haemostas. **35:** 124–138.
28. BAUMGARTNER, H. R. & C. HAUDENSCHILD. 1972. Adhesion of platelets to subendothelium. Ann. N.Y. Acad. Sci. **201:** 22–36.
29. SAKARIASSEN, K. S., M. OTTENHOF-ROVERS & J. J. SIXMA. 1984. Factor VIII-von Willebrand factor requires calcium for facilitation of platelet adherence. Blood **63:** 996–1003.

The Receptor Model for Transport of Cholesterol in Plasma[a]

MICHAEL S. BROWN AND JOSEPH L. GOLDSTEIN

Departments of Molecular Genetics and Internal Medicine
University of Texas Health Science Center at Dallas
Southwestern Medical School
Dallas, Texas 75235

In recent years, a model has emerged that attempts to explain the mechanism by which cholesterol is transported through the plasma (see refs. 1 and 2 for recent reviews). The essential feature of this model is that the bulk of cholesteryl esters are transported through plasma in a net unidirectional fashion, sequestered within the lipid cores of apoprotein B-containing lipoproteins. These esters leave the plasma only when the lipoprotein that contains them is taken up by cells and degraded through the process of receptor-mediated endocytosis.

Exogenous cholesterol, which enters plasma as a result of intestinal absorption, is transported in lipoproteins that differ from the ones that transport endogenous cholesterol, which enters plasma from liver and extrahepatic tissues (FIGURE 1). Lipoproteins that carry exogenous cholesterol contain apoprotein B–48; lipoproteins that carry endogenous cholesterol contain apoprotein B–100.[3] The apoprotein B molecules emerge from the intestine or liver as integral parts of the primodial particles in the two pathways. They emerge as chylomicrons and very low density lipoproteins (VLDL), respectively. Like the driver of a bus, these apoproteins remain with the particle as it makes intermediate stops in extrahepatic tissues, where the triglycerides exit and additional cholesteryl esters enter. Although other apoproteins jump on and off the particle as it traverses its route through the circulation, the apoprotein B molecules stay in place and are removed only when the particle is destroyed in lysosomes.[1]

Two different receptors mediate the cellular uptake of the cholesterol-containing lipoproteins.[4] One receptor, believed to exist predominantly on hepatocytes, mediates the uptake of lipoproteins that carry exogenous cholesterol (chylomicron remnants). The other receptor, which is expressed on hepatocytes and a wide variety of body cells, is the LDL receptor. Unlike the chylomicron remnant receptor, which binds only lipoproteins of the exogenous pathway, the LDL receptor binds endogenous lipoproteins (IDL and LDL) as well as exogenous lipoproteins.[1,4] Interestingly, both receptors recognize apoprotein E, a constituent of the lipoproteins in the exogenous and endogenous pathways.[4,5] The chylomicron remnant receptor recognizes apo E when it is present on a chylomicron remnant or when it is complexed with phospholipids, but not when it is on a particle that contains apoprotein B–100. The LDL receptor recognizes apoprotein E when it is present together with apo B–100, apo B–48, or simply in phospholipid vesicles. The LDL receptor also recognizes apo B–100 in the absence of apo E. Thus, under normal physiological circumstances, exogenous lipoproteins (chylomicron remnants) exit from plasma primarily by binding to

[a]This work was supported by research grants from the National Institutes of Health (HL–20948) and from the Moss Heart Fund.

chylomicron remnant receptors on the liver, while the bulk of the endogenous lipoproteins (IDL and LDL) exit plasma by binding to LDL receptors on liver and extrahepatic tissues.

Although the model in FIGURE 1 describes the fate of the cholesteryl esters in chylomicrons, IDL, and LDL, it may not hold true for the cholesteryl esters that circulate in high density lipoproteins (HDL). Evidence suggests that the cholesteryl esters of HDL may be able to enter tissues in some fashion that does not involve receptor-mediated endocytosis.[6,7] So far, the studies of this uptake mechanism are

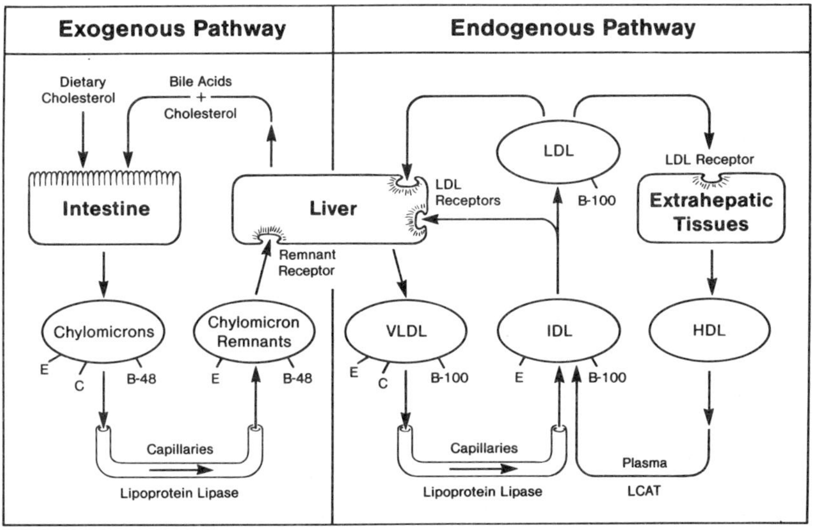

FIGURE 1. Separate pathways for receptor-mediated metabolism of lipoproteins carrying endogeneous and exogenous cholesterol. HDL denotes high density lipoprotein; LCAT, lecithin:cholesterol acyltransferase; LDL, low density lipoprotein; IDL, intermediate density lipoproteins; and VLDL, very low density lipoproteins. The distinction between exogenous and endogenous cholesterol applies to the immediate source of the cholesterol in plasma lipoproteins. After the exogenous cholesterol has been delivered to the liver and has been secreted in VLDL, it is considered endogenous cholesterol. The role of chylomicrons, VLDL, IDL, and LDL is discussed in the text. HDL is shown as the lipoprotein that removes cholesterol from extrahepatic cells. The cholesterol on HDL is delivered to IDL through the action of plasma LCAT and a cholesteryl ester-transport protein. This process is reviewed elsewhere.[20] (Reprinted from ref. 2., with permission from the *N. Engl. J. Med.*).

indirect, and the mechanism or quantitative importance of this apparent non-endocytic delivery process are not well understood.

The receptor-mediated endocytosis model allows us to understand familial hypercholesterolemia (FH), a disease in which LDL receptors are genetically defective.[2] It also suggests a mechanism to explain how high fat diets, aging, and a deficiency of thyroid hormone raise plasma cholesterol levels. These three factors appear to act by causing a partial suppression of LDL receptors in the liver, thus producing an acquired receptor deficiency state.[2,8]

The explanatory power of the receptor model stems from its ability to account for the observed metabolic abnormalities in patients with FH and in Watanabe-Heritable Hyperlipidemia (WHHL) rabbits. Both of these hypercholesterolemic states are caused by mutations in the gene for the LDL receptor.[2] Humans or rabbits that are homozygous for these defects produce few or no LDL receptors. As a result, LDL cannot be removed from plasma with normal efficiency, and the particles circulate for 3–5 times longer than normal. Eventually, the LDL particles are removed by poorly understood alternate pathways that operate with low efficiency. As a result of the sluggish catabolism, LDL accumulates to high levels in plasma, and atherosclerosis ensues. Inasmuch as chylomicron remnants are removed by a separate receptor, their metabolism is unimpaired in FH subjects and in WHHL rabbits.[2,9]

An important finding to emerge from the studies of the WHHL rabbit was the observation that the LDL receptor is required to remove intermediate density lipoproteins (IDL) from plasma.[2,10] IDL are formed from VLDL by the action of lipoprotein lipase in extrahepatic tissues. In normal rabbits, most of the IDL are immediately taken up by the liver and catabolized. However, in WHHL rabbits, which lack the LDL receptor, the vast bulk of IDL particles are not taken up by the liver, but rather, they remain in the plasma where they undergo further lipolysis and become LDL.

Because of its role in removing IDL from plasma, the LDL receptor helps to determine the rate of production of LDL, as well as its removal.[2,8,10] When the LDL receptor is absent, LDL overproduction occurs because IDL, which would normally leave the circulation, remains in the circulation and becomes LDL. This is the so-called "shunt" pathway for the production of LDL.

Although the shunt pathway was first appreciated in rabbits,[2,10] a review of previously published data indicates that this pathway operates, at least to some extent, in FH homozygotes as well. Thus, when ^{125}I-labeled VLDL was administered to FH homozygotes, it gave rise to IDL particles which remained for a prolonged period in the circulation and were apparently converted to LDL in increased amounts.[11] Although precise quantitative conclusions cannot be drawn from these human data, the observations raise the possibility that the apparent overproduction of LDL seen in FH homozygotes might all be attributable to increased shunting from VLDL. Consistent with this notion are the observations in perfused WHHL rabbit livers, which show that these livers do not overproduce LDL directly.[12]

Because of the central role of the LDL receptor in body cholesterol metabolism, it is important that its properties become understood. For this reason, we have carried out an intensive study of this receptor during the past few years. The LDL receptor was purified from bovine adrenal cortex by Schneider *et al.*[13] A partial amino acid sequence was obtained,[14] and antibodies were prepared.[15] These tools were used by Russell *et al.*,[16,17] and Yamamoto *et al.*[18] to isolate a full-length complementary DNA (cDNA) for the human LDL receptor.

The nucleotide sequence of the cDNA revealed that the human LDL receptor is a protein of 839 amino acids. It contains five domains: (1) an NH_2-terminal sequence of 292 amino acids that is extremely rich in disulfide-bonded cysteine residues (42 of 292 residues) and appears to constitute the lipoprotein binding site; (2) a sequence of 400 amino acids that bears a strong homology to the polyprotein precursor of epidermal growth factor, a protein hormone; (3) a stretch of 48 amino acids that includes 18 serine and threonine residues, each of which appears to contain a carbohydrate chain attached in O-linkage; (4) a single membrane-spanning region of 22 amino acids; and, (5) a COOH-terminal domain of 50 amino acids that extends into the cytoplasm of the cell.

Studies are currently under way to determine which parts of the receptor's structure permit it to cluster in coated pits, the sites on the cell surface where receptor-mediated endocytosis takes place.[19] Through analysis of the genes from patients with FH, we also hope to learn how the mutations in this disease affect the structure of the protein so as to disrupt its function.

REFERENCES

1. Brown, M. S., P. T. Kovanen & J. L. Goldstein. 1981. Regulation of plasma cholesterol by lipoprotein receptors. Science **212:** 628–635.
2. Goldstein, J. L., T. Kita & M. S. Brown. 1983. Defective lipoprotein receptors and atherosclerosis: Lesions from an animal counterpart of familial hypercholesterolemia. N. Engl. J. Med. **309:** 288–295.
3. Kane, J. P. 1983. Apolipoprotein B: Structural and metabolic heterogeneity. Ann. Rev. Physiol. **45:** 637–650.
4. Brown, M. S. & J. L. Goldstein. 1983. Lipoprotein receptors in the liver: Control signals for plasma cholesterol traffic. J. Clin. Invest. **72:** 743–747.
5. Mahley, R. W. & T. L. Innerarity. 1983. Lipoprotein receptors and cholesterol homeostasis. Biochim. Biophys. Acta **737:** 197–222.
6. Gwynne, J. T. & J. F. Strauss III. 1982. The role of lipoproteins in steroidogenesis and cholesterol metabolism in steroidogenic glands. Endocrine Reviews **3:** 299–329.
7. Glass, C., R. C. Pittman, D. B. Weinstein & D. Steinberg. 1983. Dissociation of tissue uptake of cholesterol ester from that of apoprotein A-I of rat plasma high density lipoprotein: Selective delivery of cholesterol ester to liver, adrenal, and gonad. Proc. Natl. Acad. Sci. USA **80:** 5435–5439.
8. Goldstein, J. L. & M. S. Brown. 1984. Progress in understanding the LDL receptor and HMG CoA reductase, two membrane proteins that regulate the plasma cholesterol. J. Lipid Res. **25:** 1450–1461.
9. Kita, T., J. L. Goldstein, M. S. Brown, Y. Watanabe, C. A. Hornick & R. J. Havel. 1982. Hepatic uptake of chylomicron remnants in WHHL rabbits: A mechanism genetically distinct from the low density lipoprotein receptor. Proc. Natl. Acad. Sci. USA **79:** 3623–3627.
10. Kita, T., M. S. Brown, D. W. Bilheimer & J. L. Goldstein. 1982. Delayed clearance of very low density and intermediate density lipoproteins with enhanced conversion to low density lipoprotein in WHHL rabbits. Proc. Natl. Acad. Sci. USA **79:** 5693–5697.
11. Soutar, A. K., N. B. Myant & G. R. Thompson. 1982. The metabolism of very low density and intermediate density lipoproteins in patients with familial hypercholesterolaemia. Atherosclerosis **43:** 217–231.
12. Hornick, C. A., T. Kita, R. L. Hamilton, J. P. Kane & R. J. Havel. 1983. Secretion of lipoproteins from the liver of normal and Watanabe heritable hyperlipidemic rabbits. Proc. Natl. Acad. Sci. USA **80:** 6096–6100.
13. Schneider, W. J., U. Beisiegel, J. L. Goldstein & M. S. Brown. 1982. Purification of the low density lipoprotein receptor, and acidic glycoprotein of 164,000 molecular weight. J. Biol. Chem. **257:** 2664–2673.
14. Schneider, W. J., C. J. Slaughter, J. L. Goldstein, R. G. W. Anderson, D. J. Capra & M. S. Brown. 1983. Use of anti-peptide antibodies to demonstrate external orientation of NH_2-terminus of the LDL receptor in the plasma membrane of fibroblasts. J. Cell Biol. **97:** 1635–1640.
15. Beisiegel, U., W. J. Schneider, J. L. Goldstein, R. G. W. Anderson & M. S. Brown. 1981. Monoclonal antibodies to the low density lipoprotein receptor as probes for study of receptor-mediated endocytosis and the genetics of familial hypercholesterolemia. J. Biol. Chem. **256:** 11923–11931.
16. Russell, D. W., T. Yamamoto, W. J. Schneider, C. J. Slaughter, M. S. Brown & J. L. Goldstein. 1983. cDNA cloning of the bovine low density lipoprotein receptor: Feedback regulation of a receptor mRNA. Proc. Natl. Acad. Sci. USA **80:** 7501–7505.
17. Russell, D. W., W. J. Schneider, T. Yamamoto, K. L. Luskey, M. S. Brown & J. L. Goldstein. 1984. Domain map of the LDL receptor: Sequence homology with the epidermal growth factor precursor. Cell **37:** 577–585.

18. YAMAMOTO, T., C. G. DAVIS, M. S. BROWN, M. L. CASEY, J. L. GOLDSTEIN & D. W. RUSSELL. 1984. The human LDL receptor: A cysteine-rich protein with multiple Alu sequences in its mRNA. Cell **39:** 27–38.
19. GOLDSTEIN, J. L., R. G. W. ANDERSON & M. S. BROWN. 1979. Coated pits, coated vesicles, and receptor-mediated endocytosis. Nature **279:** 679–685.
20. HAVEL, R. J., J. L. GOLDSTEIN & M. S. BROWN. 1980. Lipoproteins and lipid transport. Chapter 7. *In* Metabolic Control and Disease, 8th edition. P. K. Bondy & L. E. Rosenberg, Eds.: 393–494. W. B. Saunders Co. Philadelphia.

Lipoproteins Containing Apo B Extracted from Human Aortas

Structure and Function[a]

HENRY F. HOFF AND RICHARD E. MORTON

Atherosclerosis Section, Research Division
The Cleveland Clinic Foundation
Cleveland, Ohio 44106

INTRODUCTION

The earliest atherosclerotic lesion is considered by many to be the fatty streak.[1] It is characterized by the presence of numerous lipid-laden cells called foam cells,[1-3] most of which resemble tissue macrophages.[3,4] Although it has been demonstrated that such foam cells are filled with cholesteryl esters,[2] the mechanisms leading to such accumulation *in vivo* are still unknown. It is thought that such accumulation may be the result of uptake by macrophages of modified or abnormal plasma (P-) lipoproteins.[5-7] This is based on *in vitro* observations that mouse peritoneal macrophages (MPM) take up P-LDL only after the lipoprotein has been chemically modified to become more electronegative,[5] or if P-LDL is complexed to large carbohydrates such as dextran sulfate. In addition, certain lipoproteins, such as β-VLDL, which are elevated during hypercholesterolemia in some animal models, are also taken up by MPM.[6] In each of these cases, uptake is mediated by high affinity binding of the lipoprotein to a receptor on the surface of MPM which is unregulated[5] or poorly regulated (β-VLDL).[6] The internalized lipoprotein is degraded in lysosomes, and the liberated free cholesterol is subsequently re-esterified preferentially with oleate.[5,6]

Lipoproteins containing apo B and resembling plasma LDL have been demonstrated immunochemically in the grossly normal intima and in fatty-fibrous plaques of human aortas.[9-13] These lipoproteins have been shown to complex with aortic glycosaminoglycans, suggesting that their accumulation in the intima is the result of specific interactions.[14] We have isolated and purified such lipoproteins from human aortas and have demonstrated that, although similar to P-LDL, they possess some distinct characteristics.[15,16] Of most interest is the fact that these particles, in contrast to P-LDL, can induce stimulation of cholesterol esterification in MPM *in vitro*.[7,17] The purpose of this brief review is to summarize the structural and functional characteristics of lipoproteins extracted from human aortas in order to better understand the sequence of events leading to the formation of foam cells.

Procedures for Isolating Lipoproteins Containing Apo B (A-LP) from Human Aortas

Minces of aortic intima were subjected to homogenization in buffer-containing antioxidants and protease inhibitors,[17] followed by high speed centrifugation. Subse-

[a]This work was supported in part by the National Institute of Health grant no. HL-29582 and by the Bleeksma Fund.

quently, one of two procedures was utilized to isolate the aortic lipoproteins (A-LP) from such supernatants (FIGURE 1). In the first, differential ultracentrifugation was employed to isolate a d 1.006—1.063 density fraction.[15] Although possessing over 90% of the immunoreactive apo B in the supernatant, this fraction was dissimilar to plasma (P-LDL) in that it was more heterogeneous in size, and showed a different lipid composition (relative increase in free cholesterol) and protein composition (presence of excessive amounts of albumin).[15] Upon gel filtration, approximately 10% of the d

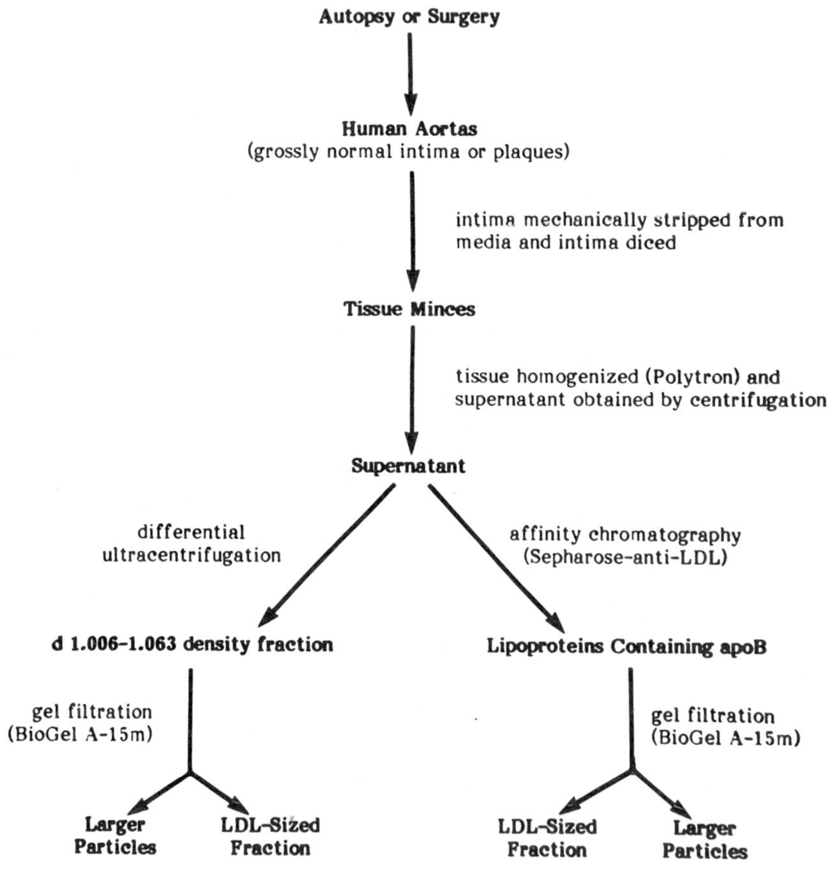

FIGURE 1. Flow diagram of isolation procedures used to obtain A-LP.

1.006–1.063 fraction co-eluted with plasma LDL.[16] This fraction was similar to P-LDL with respect to size and relative lipid composition, but possessed an increased negative charge relative to P-LDL, showed some proteolytic degradation of apo B, and demonstrated an aberrant fatty acid composition in its cholesteryl esters (enrichment in stearate and oleate; depletion in linoleate).[16] Hollander *et al.*[18] obtained similar data on the composition of an LDL-like lipoprotein isolated from human aortic plaques. In the second procedure, affinity chromatography (i.e., anti-LDL-Sepharose-4B) was

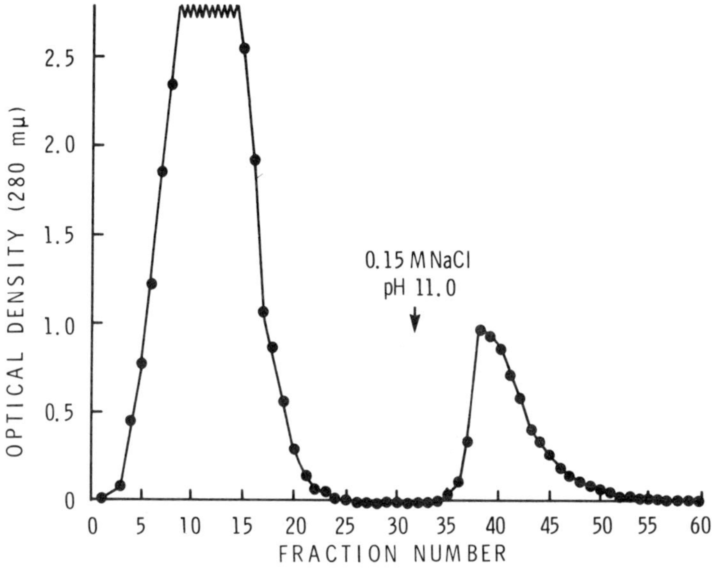

FIGURE 2. Affinity chromatography of a supernatant fraction of aortic plaque homogenate on a Sepharose anti-LDL column separating the sample into an unretained fraction (fraction numbers 2 to 25) and a retained fraction eluted with 0.15M NaCl-NH_4OH, pH 11. The latter fraction (A-LP) contained all immunoreactive apo B as measured by electroimmunoassay.

utilized to separate lipoproteins containing apo B from other material in supernatants of arterial homogenates.[16] This procedure has several advantages over ultracentrifugation. It requires less time, it avoids the possible removal of surface proteins by the high "g" forces during ultracentrifugation, and it also isolates lipoproteins containing apo B that are not in the d 1.006–1.063 density range. After application of the arterial homogenates to the affinity column, followed by extensive washing, the retained material, which contained all the immunoreactive apo B in the original fraction, was eluted with pH 11 buffer (FIGURE 2). The retained fraction represented 3.5% of the total protein applied (TABLE 1). When the fraction isolated by the affinity column was

TABLE 1. Isolation of Lipoproteins Containing Apo B from Plaque Homogenates by Affinity Chromatography[a]

Sample	mg Protein in Supernatant of Homogenate[b]
Amount Loaded onto Column	98.0 ± 27.0
Unretained Fraction	66.2 ± 10.8
Retained Fraction	3.5 ± 1.0
Total Material Recovered	69.6 ± 5.8

[a]A low-speed supernatant of homogenates of aortic plaques (four cases) was chromatographed on a Sepharose-anti-LDL affinity column. The retained fraction was eluted with 0.15 M NaCl-NH_4OH, pH 11.

[b]Values represent the mean weight of four samples ± S.E.M.

TABLE 2. Lipid Composition of Aortic Fractions after Anti-LDL-Sepharose Affinity Chromatography[a]

Sample Description	Number Samples	% of Total Wt. as Lipid	Relative Percent of Total Lipid: Phospholipid	Free Cholesterol	Cholesteryl Ester	Triglyceride
Affinity Column Unretained Fraction	3	58.0 ± 5.3	26.8 ± 1.8	16.4 ± 0.9	53.6 ± 3.0	3.2 ± 0.9
Affinity Column Retained Fraction	3	84.9 ± 0.9	25.6 ± 3.2	12.3 ± 1.2	54.1 ± 3.8	8.0 ± 1.9
Plasma LDL (d 1.006–1.063)	1	77.3	30.3	9.2	53.9	6.6

[a]Low-speed supernatants of plaque homogenates were chromatographed on a Sepharose-anti-LDL affinity column and separated into a retained fraction containing all the apo B, and an unretained fraction. The retained fraction was eluted from the column with saline-NH_4OH, pH 11. All values represent the mean weight percent ± S.E.M.

subjected to ultracentrifugation, 87% of the protein was found in the d > 1.006 fraction and 13% in the d < 1.006 fraction.

To assess whether lipoproteins in the arterial wall may have been altered by the homogenization procedure or by the subsequent affinity chromatography, we added double-labeled P-LDL [^{125}I in protein, ^{14}C in cholesteryl esters) to minces of aortic plaques prior to homogenization.[17] Over 90% of both labels were retained on the affinity column, and essentially all of both labels co-eluted with plasma LDL when the retained fraction was eluted and chromatographed on a gel filtration column (BioGel A-15m).[17] We also subjected the double-labeled LDL, which was co-isolated with the endogenous lipoproteins from plaques, to SDS-PAGE following delipidation. Over 90% of the label could be found in the B–100 band characteristic of apo B in P-LDL.[17] Thus, it is unlikely that endogenous lipoproteins containing apo B, such as A-LP, were

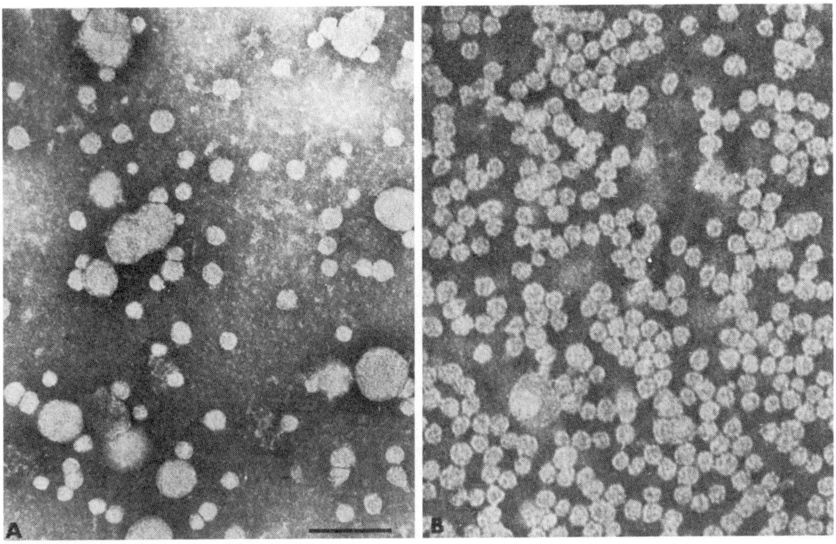

FIGURE 3. Electron micrographs of negatively stained lipoproteins in A-LP (A) and in P-LDL (B). Note the smaller particles in (A) are the same size as P-LDL. Marker indicates 1000 Å.

modified by these procedures. The lipoproteins containing apo B (A-LP) isolated by affinity chromatography were used for the studies covered in this review.

Structural Characteristics of Lipoproteins Containing Apo B (A-LP)

The retained fraction (A-LP) from the affinity column (<5% of the applied total protein) differed from the unretained fraction primarily by a higher percent triglyceide and a lower percent protein content (TABLE 2). The relative lipid composition of A-LP was quite similar to that of P-LDL, but the protein content was somewhat lower (TABLE 2). A-LP also differed from P-LDL with respect to size distribution. Although P-LDL demonstrated particles with diameters around 200 Å by negative staining and electron microscopy, A-LP contained particles both of the size of P-LDL as well as larger particles of >400 Å diameter (FIGURE 3). However, when measured over several fields, only ≃8% of particles were appreciably greater than 220Å. Using two-dimensional immunoelectrophoresis, A-LP was more electronegative than P-LDL (FIGURE 4). The broadness of the peak also suggested greater heterogeneity in surface charge for A-LP relative to P-LDL. In addition, a second peak was consistently found for A-LP at the origin of the first dimension. This probably represented the large A-LP particles. When A-LP was separated into d > or d < 1.006 fractions by ultracentrifugation, all of the d < 1.006 fraction gave a rocket close to the origin, whereas the d > 1.006 fraction gave primarily the faster migrating peak, although a small peak at the origin was still present. The small peak which was occasionally found at the origin in P–LDL (FIGURE 4) could be removed by a brief ultracentrifugation step (d 1.006, 30 min).

When A-LP was subjected to SDS-PAGE, numerous bands were discerned below the B–100 band (FIGURE 5) which were at least as intense (silver staining) as the B–100 band.[17] No band was seen in A-LP comigrating with the B–48 band present in the VLDL fraction of a non-fasting volunteer (FIGURE 5). By immunoblot, most of these bands stained positively for apo B, suggesting that they were degradation products of B–100.[17] No difference in banding pattern was found for aortic samples obtained at autopsy (within twelve hours of death) or at surgery (within five minutes of

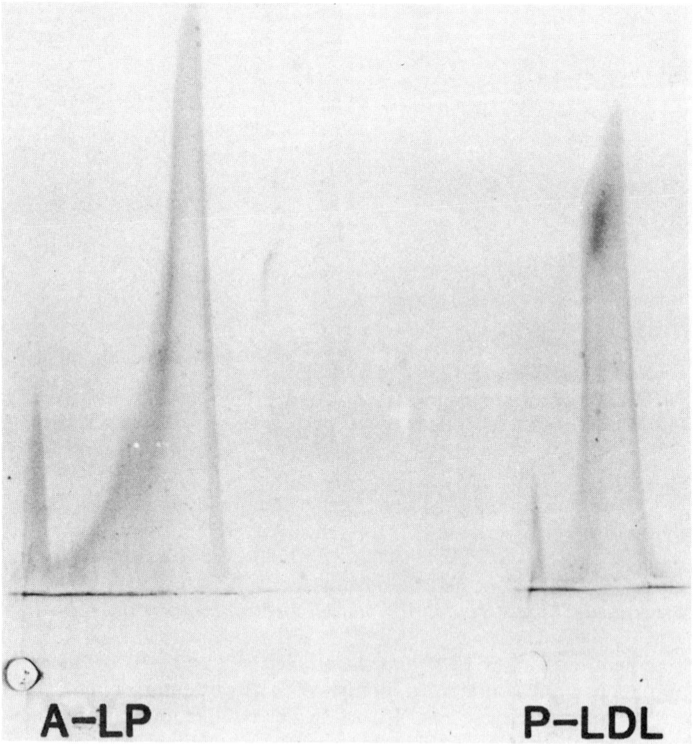

FIGURE 4. Two-dimensional immunoelectrophoresis of A-LP and of P-LDL. Anti-LDL is uniformly distributed in the upper gel. Note that the major peak in A-LP migrates further than that in P-LDL.

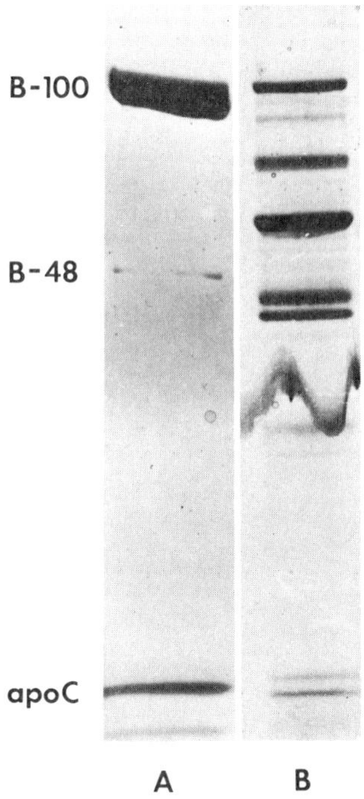

FIGURE 5. Sodium dodecyl sulfate polyacrylamide gel electrophoresis (SDS-PAGE) of P-VLDL and A-LP on gradient gels (3–12%). Gels were stained with ammoniacal silver. Note the numerous bands below the one comigrating with B–100. VLDL from a non-fasting volunteer was used so that a B–48 band would also be visible. (From ref. 17, with permission of the American Heart Association).

excision), thus suggesting that degradation of apo B had not occurred during the postmortem time interval.[17] The fragments of apo B appeared to be present within the intact lipoprotein, since gel filtration of A-LP, which would have separated any released fragments from the intact particle, did not change the SDS-PAGE pattern.

Interaction of A-LP with Mouse Peritoneal Macrophages (MPM)

In light of the increased negative charge on A-LP, we surmised that A-LP might be recognized by a receptor on MPM similar to that recognizing acetyl-LDL.[5] Using the incorporation of ^{14}C-oleate into cholesteryl oleate as a measure of lipoprotein internalization and subsequent cholesterol esterification,[5] we determined the relationship between lipoprotein concentration and stimulation of esterification. A-LP isolated from plaques caused a dose-dependent increase in cholesterol esterification[7,17] which appeared to approach saturation at about 150 μg/ml lipoprotein cholesterol (FIGURE 6). These results are consistent with the uptake of A-LP by MPM, in part, by a high affinity receptor and, in part, by a nonspecific component which was evident at higher concentrations of A-LP. Preliminary studies suggest that when A-LP is further purified by gel filtration (FIGURE 1), most of the nonspecific component was found to reside with the larger particles.

It does not appear that the isolation procedure itself caused significant recognition of A-LP by MPM. For example, compared with A-LP isolated from homogenates of aortic tissue, A-LP isolated from the supernatants of arterial minces incubated in phosphate buffer[17] was equally capable of stimulating cholesterol esterification in

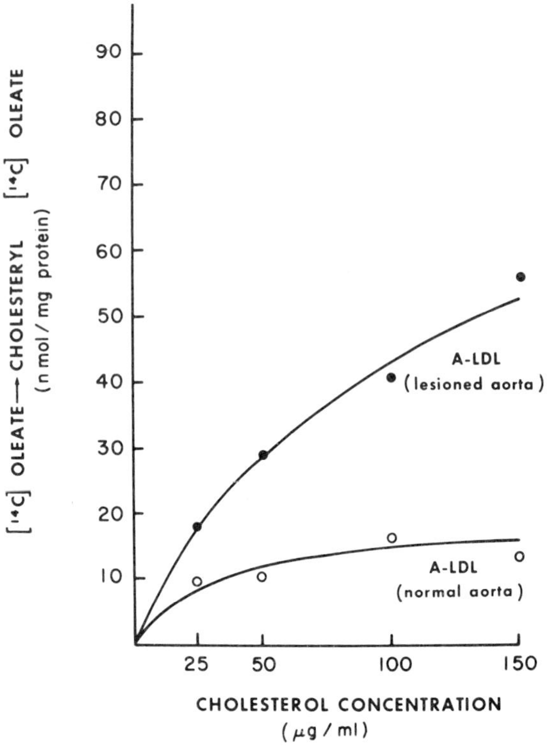

FIGURE 6. Stimulation of cholesterol esterification in mouse peritoneal macrophages (MPM) incubated with a sample of A-LP isolated from aortic plaques, and with a sample of A-LP isolated from grossly normal intima. Each monolayer of cells was incubated with lipoproteins at the indicated concentration or medium alone at 37°C for 16 hr with DMEM containing ^{14}C-oleate-albumin. Following incubation, the cellular content of cholesteryl ^{14}C-oleate was determined. Each value represents the average of duplicate determinations.

MPM. Additionally, when ^{125}I-P-LDL was added to minces of plaque and co-isolated with A-LP by affinity chromatography, the ^{125}I-P-LDL was not significantly degraded by MPM.

A preparation of A-LP isolated from a homogenate of pools of grossly normal aortic intima also stimulated cholesterol esterification in MPM, but with an apparent V_{max} appreciably less than that found for A-LP from atherosclerotic plaques (FIGURE 6). The sharp plateauing of the curve for A-LP from normal intima indicates the absence of a nonspecific component, and is consistent with the absence of larger particles in A-LP from normal intima.[15] The lower V_{max} for A-LP from normal intima, as compared to that for A-LP from plaques, suggests cellular recognition by different receptors on the MPM. This hypothesis is presently being investigated.

A-LP may be recognized, in part, by the acetyl-LDL or scavenger receptor on MPM, since fucoidin, a competitive inhibitor of this receptor,[5,7] demonstrated a dose-related inhibition of stimulation of cholesterol esterification in MPM by partially purified A-LP (affinity purified) isolated from plaques.[17] However, recent preliminary studies have demonstrated that a 30-fold excess of A-LP did not inhibit the degradation of ^{125}I-acetyl-LDL by MPM, suggesting that A-LP was not recognized by the scavenger receptor. Further studies using labeled A-LP and unlabeled acetyl-LDL are currently being undertaken to confirm this result. If A-LP is not recognized by the scavenger receptor, this result would indicate that A-LP is not identical to endothelial- or smooth muscle cell-modified P-LDL, which is recognized by the scavenger receptor on macrophages.[19]

Studies using the lysosomotropic agent, chloroquine, have indicated that uptake and internalization of A-LP by macrophages is followed by degradation in lysosomes subsequent to re-esterification of the liberated cholesterol.[17] Chloroquine was shown to inhibit stimulation of cholesterol esterification in macrophages by A-LP in a concentration-dependent manner. Moreover, when chloroquine was removed and the cells were "chased" with medium containing only the labeled oleate and albumin, cholesterol esterification commenced, presumably due to liberation of cholesterol from degraded A-LP that had accumulated in lysosomes during the "pulse" phase of the experiment.[17]

When MPM were incubated for periods of up to 48 hrs with A-LP, a linear increase in cholesterol esterification was found.[17] By contrast, P-LDL showed a negligible increase. This increase in esterification was confirmed by a significant increase in cholesteryl ester mass in MPM after 48 hrs of incubation with A-LP, as compared to the accumulation found after incubation with P-LDL for the same time (TABLE 3). When MPM were stained with oil red O and viewed by light microscopy, we found a time-dependent increase in intracellular oil red O-positive droplets (FIGURE 7). P-LDL caused few droplets to be formed after 48 hrs.[17] These results suggest that the uptake mechanism for A-LP is not down-regulated.

It is still unclear what modification, previously documented or still to be determined, is responsible for the enhanced interaction of A-LP with macrophages. It is also not clear that this recognition is related to the increased negative charge on A-LP, particularly since it is not definite that A-LP is recognized by the scavenger receptor. One possibility that needs further explanation is that the degraded apo B component of A-LP results in conformational changes on the surface of A-LP and causes its recognition by some receptors on MPM. It seems unlikely that the A-LP receptor on MPM is equivalent to the β-VLDL receptor, since the latter is down-regulated within 24 hrs,[6] whereas the receptor recognizing A-LP is unregulated over a 48 hr interval.[17] Studies are currently in progress to further characterize the structure of A-LP to discern what changes are present relative to P-LDL that might be responsible for its recognition by MPM.

TABLE 3. Accumulation of Unesterified Cholesterol and Cholesteryl Esters in Mouse Peritoneal Macrophages

Addition	Unesterified Cholesterol (μg/mg protein)	Cholesteryl Esters (μg/mg protein)
none	28.6[a]	0.4[a]
P-LDL	32.9	1.0
A-LP	50.0	169.4
Acetyl-LDL	55.8	305.7

[a]Average of duplicate determinations on duplicate wells of macrophages incubated with 100 μg/ml lipoprotein cholesterol for 48 hrs.

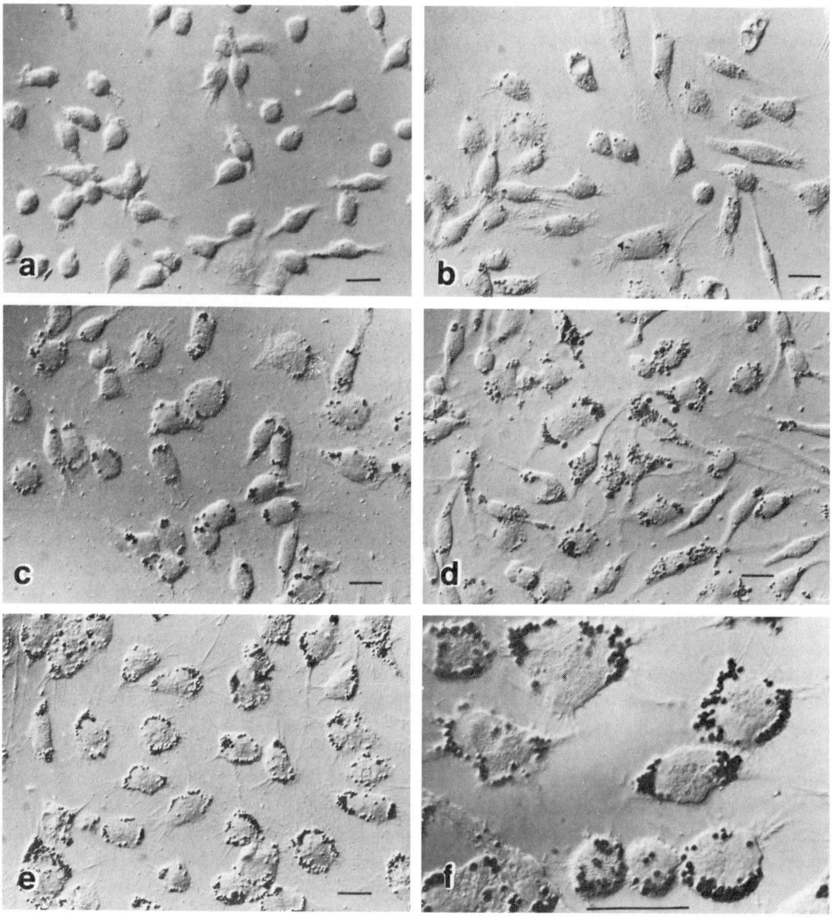

FIGURE 7. Light micrographs of oil red O-stained MPM. Cells plated on coverslips were incubated with A-LP and P-LDL at a concentration of 100 μg cholesterol/ml in 0.5 ml DMEM for time periods ranging from 6 to 48 hrs. After a 24 hr incubation period, the medium was removed, cells were washed with saline, and fresh medium containing the appropriate lipoprotein at the same concentration was added. At the end of each incubation period, cells on each coverslip were washed with saline, fixed with 5% paraformaldehyde in phosphate buffer pH 7.4, stained with oil red O, and viewed by differential interference contrast microscopy. FIGURE 7(a): 48 hr incubation with P-LDL; FIGURE 7(b): 6 hr incubation with A-LP; FIGURE 7(c): 12 hr incubation with A-LP; FIGURE 7(d): 24 hr incubation with A-LP; FIGURE 7(e): 48 hr incubation with A-LP; FIGURE 7(f): Same as FIGURE 7(e), but at higher magnification. Bar = 20 microns. (From ref. 17, with permission of the American Heart Association).

SUMMARY

We have isolated, by anti-LDL affinity chromatography, apo B-containing lipoproteins from homogenates of atherosclerotic plaques excised from the human aorta. This fraction, called A-LP, has similarities with plasma LDL, such as having similar size and relative lipid composition, along with containing apo B. However, the fraction also contains some particles larger than LDL, it is more electronegative than LDL, the relative protein content is less than in LDL, and its apo B is highly degraded. A-LP is recognized by a high affinity binding site on mouse peritoneal macrophages (MPM), as suggested by dose-response curves of stimulation of cholesterol esterification. The interaction is inhibited by negatively-charged carbohydrates such as fucoidin, but excess A-LP did not inhibit the degradation of labeled acetyl-LDL by MPM, suggesting that the binding site recognizing A-LP may not be the scavenger receptor. Finally, stimulation of cholesterol esterification by A-LP in MPM is unregulated over a 48 hr time interval, leading to massive accumulations of cholesteryl esters and a transition of these MPM to a morphology characteristic of foam cells. It is possible that when monocytes enter the arterial intima at specific sites[3,4] and become tissue macrophages, they internalize A-LP in an unregulated fashion. This, in turn, would make the monocyte-macrophage lipid-laden, and could explain the etiology of foam cells in fatty streak lesions. The modification in A-LP relative to P-LDL responsible for the enhanced recognition still needs to be elucidated.

ACKNOWLEDGMENTS

The authors acknowledge the excellent technical assistance of Ms. Gail West and the secretarial support of Ms. Muriel Daly.

REFERENCES

1. McGill, H. C., Jr. 1968. Fatty streaks in the coronary arteries and aorta. Lab. Invest. **18:** 560.
2. Lang, P. D. & W. Insull, Jr. 1970. Lipid droplets in atherosclerotic fatty streaks of human aorta. J. Clin. Invest. **49:** 1479.
3. Gerrity, R. G. 1981. The role of the monocyte in atherogenesis. I. Transition of blood-borne monocytes into foam cells in fatty lesions. Am. J. Pathol. **103:** 181.
4. Joris, I., T. Zand, J. J. Nunnar, F. J. Krolinkowski & G. Majno. 1983. Studies on the pathogenesis of atherosclerosis. 1. Adhesion and emigration of mononuclear cells in the aorta of hypercholesterolemic rats. Am. J. Pathol. **113:** 341.
5. Goldstein, J. L., Y. K. Ho, S. K. Basu & M. S. Brown. 1979. Binding site on macrophages that mediates uptake and degradation of acetylated low density lipoprotein, producing massive cholesterol deposition. Proc. Natl. Acad. Sci. USA **76:** 333.
6. Mahley, R. W., T. L. Innerarity, M. S. Brown, Y. K. Ho & J. L. Goldstein. 1980. Cholesteryl ester synthesis in macrophages: Stimulation by β-very low density lipoproteins from cholesterol-fed animals of several species. J. Lipid Res. **21:** 970.
7. Goldstein, J. L., H. F. Hoff, Y. K. Ho, S. K. Basu & M. S. Brown. 1981. Stimulation of cholesteryl ester synthesis in macrophages by extracts of atherosclerotic human aortas and complexes of albumin/cholesterol esters. Arteriosclerosis **1:** 210.
8. Basu, S. K., M. S. Brown, Y. K. Ho, J. L. Goldstein. 1979. Degradation of low density lipoprotein dextran sulfate complexes associated with deposition of cholesteryl esters in mouse macrophages. J. Biol. Chem. **254:** 7141.
9. Hoff, H. F., C. L. Heideman, J. W. Gaubatz & A. M. Gotto, Jr. 1977. Apolipoprotein B retention in the grossly normal and atherosclerotic human aorta. Circ. Res. **41:** 684.

10. HOFF, H. F., C. L. HEIDEMAN, J. W. GAUBATZ, D. W. SCOTT, J. L. TITUS & A. M. GOTTO, JR. 1978. Correlation of apolipoprotein B retention with the structure of atherosclerotic plaques from human aortas. Lab. Invest. **38:** 560.
11. HOFF, H. F., J. W. GAUBATZ & A. M. GOTTO. 1979. Apo B concentration in the normal human aorta. Biochem. Biophys. Res. Commun. **85:** 1424.
12. SMITH, E. B., I. B. MASSIE & K. M. ALEXANDER. 1976. The release of an immobilized lipoprotein fraction from atherosclerotic lesions by incubation with plasmin. Atherosclerosis **25:** 71.
13. SMITH, E. B. & E. M. STAPLES. 1980. Distribution of plasma proteins across the human aortic wall: barrier functions of endothelium and internal elastic lamina. Atherosclerosis **37:** 579.
14. SRINIVASAN, S. R., B. RADHAKRISHNAMURTHY, E. R. DALFERES & G. S. BERENSON. 1975. Lipoprotein-acid mucopolysaccharide complexes of human atherosclerotic lesions. Biochim. Biophys. Acta **338:** 58.
15. HOFF, H. F., W. A. BRADLEY, C. L. HEIDEMAN, J. W. GAUBATZ, M. D. KARAGAS & A. M. GOTTO. 1979. Characterization of a low density lipoprotein-like particle in the human aorta from grossly normal and atherosclerotic regions. Biochim. Biophys. Acta **573:** 361.
16. HOFF, H. F. & J. W. GAUBATZ. 1982. Isolation, purification, and characterization of a lipoprotein containing apo B from the human aorta. Atherosclerosis **42:** 273.
17. CLEVIDENCE, B. A., R. E. MORTON, G. WEST, D. M. DUSEK & H. F. HOFF. 1984. Cholesterol esterification in macrophages. Stimulation by lipoproteins containing apo B isolated from human aortas. Atherosclerosis **4:** 196.
18. HOLLANDER, W. 1976. Unified concept of the role of acid mucopolysaccharides and connective tissue proteins in the accumulation of lipids, lipoproteins, and calcium in the atherosclerotic phase. Exp. Mol. Pathol. **25:** 106.
19. HENRICKSEN, T., E. M. MAHONEY & D. STEINBERG. 1983. Enhanced macrophage degradation of biologically modified low density lipoprotein. Arteriosclerosis **3:** 149.

Mechanisms Involved in the Uptake and Degradation of Low Density Lipoprotein by the Artery Wall *in Vivo*[a]

DANIEL STEINBERG, RAY C. PITTMAN,
AND THOMAS E. CAREW

Department of Medicine
University of California, San Diego
La Jolla, California 92093

THE RELATIONSHIP BETWEEN ELEVATED LOW DENSITY LIPOPROTEIN (LDL) LEVELS AND ATHEROGENESIS

The causative linkage between hyperbetalipoproteinemia and atherosclerosis is firmly established by a long chain of evidence. The most recent link added to that chain is the evidence from the landmark Lipid Research Clinic intervention trial,[1] which clearly demonstrated that lowering LDL levels in hypercholesterolemic men significantly reduced their risk of death from coronary artery disease. Since the cholesterol in atherosclerotic lesions derives primarily from the cholesterol in circulating lipoproteins, it is reasonable to conclude that hyperbetalipoproteinemia is causative by virtue of its delivery of that cholesterol to the artery at a high rate. Thus: (1) High LDL levels cause high rates of LDL entry into the artery wall; (2) This leads to high rates of uptake by cells in the artery wall (and/or trapping by extracellular matrix materials); (3) This overloads whatever unloading mechanisms normally operate to prevent accumulation of cholesterol; and, (4) The end result is accelerated atherogenesis. What we have done is simply to restate the lipid infiltration hypothesis of Virchow in slightly modified, contemporary form!

However, the causative linkage could be quite different. High plasma concentrations of LDL have been, with varying degrees of certainty, implicated as contributing to several other processes that may be involved in atherogenesis (TABLE 1), as discussed in detail elsewhere,[2] and there may be still others not yet appreciated. One or more of such factors might be equally relevant or even more relevant to lesion development than the rate of delivery of cholesterol to the tissue. A crucial question is whether the delivery of lipoprotein to and the accumulation of cholesterol in the artery wall is *sine qua non* for atherogenesis. Certainly cholesterol accumulation is the hallmark of the human lesion and most experimental lesions. Yet, not all experimental lesions are lipid rich.[3] Moreover, even if the chain of causative events were triggered by mechanisms like those listed in TABLE 1, the fact that LDL levels were high during lesion development would probably lead to concurrent lipid accumulation even if it were not an essential factor in the progression of the lesion. Until this issue is completely resolved, we must keep an open mind and explore all possibilities. In the remainder of this paper, however, we confine ourselves to the mechanisms involved in penetration of LDL into the artery wall and its metabolic fate.

[a]This work was supported by a SCOR on Arteriosclerosis grant from the National Heart, Lung, and Blood Institute (HL-14197), and a grant from the Council for Tobacco Research.

TRANSENDOTHELIAL TRANSPORT OF LDL

Nonspecific Transendothelial Transport

The classical work on transendothelial transport surely must include the early studies of Palade and coworkers (reviewed in ref. 4). Using horseradish peroxidase and a series of other low molecular weight markers, they set out to find the morphologic equivalents of the "small pores" suggested by physiologic studies of capillary permeability. What they found was that molecules as large as peroxidase, or larger (e.g., ferritin), could not penetrate the tight junctions between endothelial cells. However, the peroxidase was taken up, by endocytosis, and moved across the endothelial cells at a high rate (transit time as little as one minute). Occasionally, a vesicle originating from the luminal surface would fuse with an internal vesicle, which had, in turn, fused with a vesicle opening to the transluminal surface. In this way, a temporary through and through channel was formed, suggesting that this might be a mechanism for facilitating movement of macromolecules through the endothelium. It is still uncertain how frequently channels of this kind form or how long they persist, and so one cannot be sure to what extent they correspond to the physiologists' pores. The gaps provided could allow passage of LDL molecules, as discussed by Stein and Stein,[5] and nonspecific transport by such a mechanism remains a possibility. Whether or not such channels play an important role, nonspecific fluid endocytosis and rapid movement of endocytic vesicles across the very narrow cytoplasmic band of the capillary endothelium could, in theory, account for much or all of LDL transport. However, we should note here an important caveat before generalizing. These studies were carried out mainly on capillary endothelial cells; whether or not the conclusions apply equally to endothelial cells of the large arteries remains to be established.

Horseradish peroxidase does not bind to mammalian cell membranes, and its uptake is thus largely or entirely via fluid or bulk endocytosis. Any molecules that do bind to the surface of the endothelial cell will be taken up at a higher rate, i.e., by adsorptive endocytosis as well as by fluid endocytosis. In the case of LDL, we know from the work of Reckless *et al.*[6] and others[7–9] that aortic endothelial cells express the high-affinity LDL receptor. Thus, the uptake and degradation of LDL by cultured endothelial cells demonstrated saturability, competition, and specificity. Reckless *et al.* also measured the uptake of ^{14}C-sucrose as a measure of fluid endocytosis, and found that the uptake of LDL was considerably greater than that which could be accounted for by nonspecific fluid endocytosis.[6]

However, studies in cell culture cannot by their nature tell us a great deal about transport phenomena *in vivo*. Thus, the uptake of ^{14}C-sucrose only measures that component of fluid endocytosis that delivers the contents of the endocytotic vesicle to a lysosome so that the labeled sucrose becomes irreversibly trapped within the cell (FIGURE 1: degradation pathway); any sucrose taken up at one cell surface and then

TABLE 1. Mechanisms by Which LDL Might Initiate or Promote Atherogenesis Other Than via Delivery of Lipids to Cells of the Artery Wall

1. By damaging endothelial cells.
2. By stimulating growth of smooth muscle cells.
3. By favoring platelet aggregation.
4. By serving as a source of free fatty acids or lysophosphatides due to action of extracellular lipases.
5. By affecting the migration and/or metabolism of monocyte/macrophages.

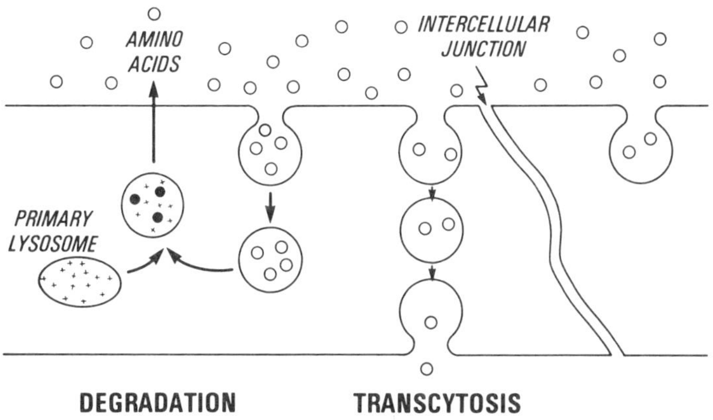

FIGURE 1. Schematic representation of vesicular transport of LDL across the endothelial cell (*transcytosis pathway*), and for irreversible transport of LDL to lysosomes (*degradation pathway*).

"retro-endocytosed" at another cell surface (as in the trancytosis pathway in FIGURE 1) would of course go unregistered in such an experiment. In fibroblasts and many other cell types it appears that LDL taken up via the specific LDL receptor is targeted predominantly or exclusively for delivery to the lysosomal compartment. If that were true in the endothelial cell, receptor-mediated uptake could not play an important role in transendothelial transport. It could only apply in endothelial cell degradation. On the other hand, since the endothelial cell exhibits specialized functions relating to transport, it, unlike other cells, could in theory utilize the receptor-mediated uptake pathway as a means to enhance LDL transport. Recently Wiklund, Carew, and Steinberg[10] have studied this matter of the role of the receptor in transport into the artery wall and their results, summarized below, indicate that transport via the specific receptor probably plays a minor role in transendothelial transport of LDL.

Wiklund *et al.* estimated the initial rates of entry of ^{125}I-labeled homologous LDL into the rabbit thoracic aorta *in vivo,* measuring uptake at 30 min and at 60 min (determining total trichloroacetic acid-precipitable radioiodine) and making appropriate corrections for trapped plasma.[10] Uptake departed only slightly from linearity over the 60-min interval, and it was calculated that any error due to concurrent degradation or efflux of labeled LDL would have changed the absolute values for uptake by no more than 10–20%. To assess the role of the LDL receptor in regulating influx, ^{125}I-labeled reductively methylated LDL was injected simultaneously with ^{131}I-labeled native LDL. The former is not recognized by the LDL receptor[11] and thus, its entry should reflect only the receptor-independent processes, while the entry of the native LDL should reflect the sum of receptor-dependent and receptor-independent processes. In fact, there was no significant difference between the two, as shown in TABLE 2. The mean values for the ratios observed in a series of individual studies were not significantly different from 1.0. It was concluded, therefore, that the transport of LDL across the endothelial barrier could not be to any large extent dependent on LDL receptor-mediated mechanisms.

Simionescu and coworkers have approached this same question using an entirely different approach.[12] Their studies were done by perfusing an isolated carotid artery in the rat with a medium containing LDL (after a suitable washout). At short time intervals (two to ten min), the artery was fixed and studied by transmission electron microscopy. LDL particles were identified on the basis of their characteristic appearance and classified according to whether they were considered to relate to receptor-mediated uptake or nonreceptor-mediated uptake pathways. For example, LDL particles on the luminal surface bound to coated pits were, of course, assigned to the "receptor pathway", while particles bound to smooth membrane were assigned to the nonspecific pathway. Similarly, LDL molecules inside coated vesicles or in lysosomes were considered in the receptor-mediated category, while particles in smooth vesicles were not. The number of LDL particles in each category was simply counted and expressed as a percentage of the total. For example, if 10% of the LDL was found in association with cellular structures assigned to the receptor pathway, it would be concluded that 10% of the uptake was receptor-mediated.

As recognized by the authors, simply calculating a proportion like this would not take into account the rate of movement of LDL particles along any particular pathway. For example, consider this pathway: coated pit to coated vesicle to lysosome. At steady state, there might be, say, 100 LDL molecules along this pathway at all times, and that is the number of particles that would be counted in the electron microscopic pictures. However, the rate at which these particles are moving along through the pathway could be 1000 per minute or 10,000 per minute, or *any* number! From a snapshot at steady state, one simply cannot evaluate rates of movement. Recognizing this problem, the authors used an initial washout period during which any LDL molecules "in the pipeline" had a chance to complete their transit. In theory, then, this should yield the fraction of particles initially entering the two defined pathways and give a valid measurement. However, the rate of entry is so fast that observations might have to be confined to the first minute or so. Palade and coworkers[4] estimated the transit time across the endothelial cell as about one minute, and in the present Simionescu studies some LDL was in fact, seen on the abluminal surface as early as two minutes. Another difficulty arises because the coated vesicle appears to lose its characteristic fuzzy coat soon after internalization. Thus, some transport via the receptor pathway may be misassigned to the nonspecific pathway. Therefore, there are some uncertainties about the quantitative interpretation of the results of Simionescu *et al.* Nevertheless, their conclusion that much or most of the transport is *not* receptor-dependent is qualitatively concordant with the results of Wiklund *et al.*[10] using a quite different approach.

RATES OF DEGRADATION IN THE ARTERY WALL *IN VIVO*

Principle of the "Trapped Ligand" Method for Determining Rates of Plasma Protein Degradation in Vivo

At first glance the problem of measuring the rates at which a given plasma protein is being degraded by particular tissues *in vivo* would seem fairly straightforward. Many have attempted to do so by simply measuring the amount of radioactive plasma protein trapped during the first few minutes after injection of a tracer dose. While disarmingly simple, this cannot be accepted as a measure of the true rate of irreversible degradation. If all the labeled protein entering the tissue were destined ineluctably for irreversible degradation, then the value would be meaningful. However, in actuality, we know that some fraction of the labeled protein entering the extracellular space of the tissue will return to the plasma compartment (or to the lymph) without undergoing cellular degradation. One simply cannot equate the amount of material entering initially with the amount undergoing degradation per unit time at steady state; that will yield an overestimate of true degradation. On the other hand, if the interval between injection of the labeled protein and measurement of tissue uptake is prolonged, then degradation and loss of degradation products from the tissue may become significant and the amount of radioactive material remaining will underestimate the true rate of degradation.

In order to circumvent these problems, Pittman and coworkers developed and validated the "trapped ligand" method.[13-15] Briefly, the method rests in principle on the fact that certain classes of molecules (sucrose being the prototype) cross membranes at only a very low rate. Thus, when ^{14}C-sucrose is taken up by cultured cells, it is delivered to the lysosome by vesicular transport and then remains trapped there, leaking at a rate less than 5% per day in most cells. If ^{14}C-sucrose is covalently linked to LDL apoprotein B, it is carried into the cell in "piggyback" fashion. After the LDL is delivered to the lysosome, the several components of the LDL are degraded by the lysosomal enzymes. The apoprotein is degraded almost completely to free amino acids, which escape rapidly back to the medium (or, *in vivo,* back to the plasma). The ^{14}C-sucrose, however, remains effectively trapped in the lysosome. In several rat tissues, the leakage rate was shown to be less than 5% per day.[16] This method allowed us to assess the uptake of LDL into various tissues, and it established that the liver is the major site of LDL degradation in several species (pig, rat, and rabbit).[14,16,17] Because uptake into the artery is extremely slow and because the specific radioactivity obtainable with ^{14}C is limited, precise measurement of arterial uptake was difficult. By shifting to a trapped ligand that could be labeled with radioiodine (tyramine cellobiose), the sensitivity of the method was increased by more than two orders of magnitude.[18] This now makes possible the quantitative assessment of arterial uptake in even very small arterial tissue samples with accuracy. It is even possible now to assess uptake *in vivo* at the cellular level by using autoradiography, as described below.

TABLE 2. Comparison of Initial Flux of Native LDL and of Reductively Methylated LDL into Normal Rabbit Aorta *in Vivo* (n = 10)[a]

Clearance of Native LDL (nl serum/g/h)	Clearance of Methyl LDL / Clearance of Native LDL
1787 ± 69[b]	1.09 ± 0.13 (NS)

[a]Uptake determined at 30 min in three rabbits, and at 60 min in seven rabbits.
[b]Mean ± S.D.

LDL Degradation in the Normal Rabbit Aorta in Vivo

Overall Rates of Irreversible Degradation

Radioiodinated tyramine cellobiose-labeled LDL (^{125}I-TC-LDL) was prepared using homologous LDL and reinjected into normal recipient rabbits. After 24 to 48 hours, the animals were sacrificed and the total accumulated radioactive TC in degradation products was determined.[19] In order to correct for undegraded LDL trapped in the tissue, the rabbits were given LDL labeled both conventionally with ^{131}I and by conjugation with ^{125}I-TC. The degradation products from the former escape the tissue rapidly, so that the radioactivity remaining after 24 hours or longer should

TABLE 3. Rates of LDL Degradation in Normal Rabbit Aorta

	Clearance (nl/g/h)	Amount of Cholesterol Delivered by the LDL Being Degraded (μg/g/h)
Intima	221	0.05
Media-adventitia	328	0.07
Total aortic wall	549	0.12

represent predominantly, if not exclusively, undegraded LDL molecules. After appropriate correction, the rate of LDL-degradation was expressed, as shown in TABLE 3, in terms of clearance of serum per gram of aorta per hour. It should be emphasized that these values represent LDL entering the artery and undergoing irreversible degradation, as opposed to values for total initial rates of entry of LDL, which were discussed above and presented in TABLE 2.

From the cholesterol concentration in LDL and the observed clearances, one can calculate the absolute rates of LDL cholesterol delivery to the normal rabbit aorta. This value, approximately 0.12 micrograms cholesterol/g/h (2.9 micrograms cholesterol/g/d), tells us, at once, that the normal rabbit aorta must be able to get rid of some of the LDL cholesterol delivered to it. Otherwise it would show progressive accumulation and would reach values much higher than those actually observed in the normal rabbit aorta. In other words, "reverse cholesterol transport" must operate in the aorta as well as in other peripheral tissues.

Relative Role of Intima and Media-Adventitia in LDL Degradation

In some studies, using basically the same protocol as described in the previous section, the intima was removed by gentle swabbing and was counted separately from the media-adventitia. The degradation products in these two fractions were determined by the methods just described. Approximately 40% of all the degradation taking place in the aortic wall was occurring within the very thin intimal layer (40.3 ± 10.8%, n = 6). That layer accounts for only a very small fraction of the total mass of the aorta. Thus, the "specific activity" in degradation, i.e., degradation per unit wet weight, was almost forty times as great in the intima as in the media-adventitia. To what extent this is a reflection of the exposure of the intimal cells to a higher concentration of LDL and to what extent due to intrinsic metabolic behavior of the cells is difficult to say. From the work of Bratzler *et al.*,[20] it is clear that there is a gradient of LDL concentration across the aortic wall, and that the concentration is, of course, higher at the intimal surface.

The conclusion that the intima plays this major role in LDL degradation was borne out by autoradiographic studies. The aorta was perfusion-fixed 24 hours after injection of ^{125}I-TC-LDL and sections were coated with liquid emulsion. Inspection showed a much higher density of grains at the intimal surface, and direct grain counts confirmed that about 40% of the total grains were in the layer just above the internal elastic membrane, confirming the biochemical studies described above.

Role of the LDL Receptor in Aortic LDL Degradation

It was of interest to assess the role of the receptor in LDL degradation *in vivo.* To do this, the rate of degradation of native LDL was compared with that of reductively methylated LDL.[11] Degradation of the latter would reflect only nonreceptor-mediated degradation, while the degradation of the native LDL would represent the sum of receptor-mediated and nonreceptor-mediated degradation. The difference between the two, then, corresponds to the receptor-mediated component. Using this approach, it was shown that between 40 and 50% of the LDL degradation occurring in the normal rabbit aorta occurs by way of the receptor. This value is somewhat less, but only slightly less, than the value of 60% found for receptor-mediated degradation in the whole body. Thus it appears that the receptor does play a role *in vivo* in arterial degradation of LDL. However, it should be noted in passing that receptor-mediated uptake is clearly not a requisite for the development of atherosclerosis. The patient with homozygous familial hypercholesterolemia and the receptor-deficient WHHL rabbit develop severe premature atherosclerosis even in the virtual absence of receptor activity. Presumably the uptake by nonreceptor pathways when plasma LDL levels are sufficiently high insures a very high rate of LDL uptake and a rapid development of lesions.

It has been reported that highly confluent endothelial cells in culture express little or no LDL receptor activity.[7] Thus, one might have expected that the totally confluent monolayer of endothelial cells in the intact artery might not express receptors. These *in vivo* studies, however, clearly show that the receptors are expressed and are playing a significant role in endothelial LDL degradation under normal *in vivo* conditions in the rabbit. The data also show that the LDL receptor is functional and plays a significant role in smooth muscle cell degradation of LDL as well.

RELATIONSHIP BETWEEN FLUX AND DEGRADATION OF LDL IN THE NORMAL AORTA

Having data on both the total flux rates of LDL into the aorta (TABLE 2), and, in separate studies, for rates of LDL degradation (TABLE 3), we can begin to construct a picture of the dynamics of LDL metabolism by the aorta *in vivo*. As schematized in FIGURE 2, an amount of LDL contained in 1787 nl of serum penetrates the aortic wall (per g wet weight) every hour. The present studies cannot differentiate between entry

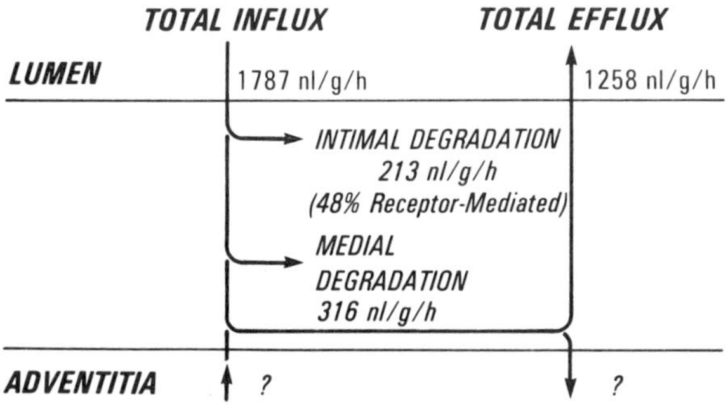

FIGURE 2. Overview of LDL metabolism in the artery wall with values entered for the normal rabbit aorta *in vivo*, as derived from the work of Carew *et al.*[19] and Wiklund *et al.*[10] In the latter paper, only the total entry of LDL across the luminal and adventitial surfaces was determined.[10] The schema shows the value for total entry at the luminal surface only for convenience. Bratzler *et al.*[20] have estimated that about one-third of LDL penetration is by way of the adventitial surface.

from the lumen and from the adventitial surface, but Bratzler *et al.*[20] have estimated that about one-third enters via the latter route. Of the total flux of LDL into the wall, about 12% (213 nl/g/h) undergoes irreversible degradation in the intima. Another 18% is degraded in the media-adventitia. The remaining 70% must be exiting the artery directly back to the plasma compartment and/or by way of capillaries and lymphatics on the adventitial surface. Thus, there appears to be a very dynamic flux of LDL into and out of the normal aortic wall. If even a small percentage of that flux were to be trapped (e.g., by binding to extracellular matrix materials), it could eventually lead to significant accumulation of extracellular lipid.

The overall entry of LDL into the artery wall does not appear to be receptor-dependent, and yet a significant fraction of the intimal degradation is receptor-dependent. This apparent paradox is understandable when we consider that only 12% of the total entry flux is degraded in the intima and thus only about 5% of the flux is degraded via the receptor. Clearly, the experimental methods employed are not sufficiently sensitive to detect a 5% difference between uptake of labeled native and methylated LDL molecules.

SITES OF LDL DEGRADATION IN THE ATHEROSCLEROTIC RABBIT AORTA *IN VIVO*

The greatly increased sensitivity of the ^{125}I-TC labeling method now makes it possible to compare rates of LDL degradation in different segments of the arterial tree at the gross anatomic level and even at the microscopic level. We can now compare the contributions of different cell types in the artery wall to overall degradation. As discussed above, the use of the trapped ligand approach allows us to measure degradation, as opposed to initial entry rate or some mixture of uptake and irreversible degradation. Stender and Zilversmit[21] have made measurements of initial rates of entry of various lipoprotein fractions into the aorta of cholesterol-fed rabbits, but if lipoprotein efflux is as significant in the atherosclerotic rabbit at it appears to be in the normal rabbit (FIGURE 2), then the entry rates need not correlate with the relative or absolute rates of catabolism of these lipoproteins. The use of the ^{125}I-TC labeling method to study lipoprotein metabolism by atherosclerotic arteries should, in principle, measure catabolism specifically and thus add a new dimension to our understanding of arterial metabolism.

Examples of application of this method are illustrated in FIGURES 3 and 4. The photograph and gross autoradiogram shown in FIGURE 3 are preliminary results from a study patterned on the model described by Minick *et al.*,[22] where a balloon catheter injury is produced in the rabbit aorta. Sixteen weeks after injury, the endothelium (light areas in photograph) has regrown from adjacent uninjured branch arteries or from uninjured areas to cover a portion of the ballooned segment. The dark areas in the photograph, delineated by injecting Evan's blue dye into the rabbit ten minutes before sacrifice, correspond to areas of smooth muscle proliferation that are not covered by true endothelium. Minick *et al.*[22] noted that rabbits undergoing this procedure, while being maintained on a cholesterol-rich diet, had the greatest cholesterol accumulations not in the non-endothelialized areas, but under the leading edge of the regrowing endothelium. Lees *et al.*[23] demonstrated the accumulation of conventionally iodinated (presumably undegraded) LDL also beneath the leading edge of endothelial regrowth. The autoradiogram in FIGURE 3 obtained 24 h after injection of ^{125}I-TC-LDL demonstrates a similar pattern: the heaviest density in the autoradiogram occurs just inside the leading edge of endothelial regrowth. The difference between this result and that of Lees *et al.* is that the trapped label approach offers presumptive evidence for increased LDL degradation under the leading edge of endothelium in addition to increased accumulation of intact LDL. However, a quantitative interpretation is not possible at this time. Preliminary studies have shown that in cholesterol-fed rabbits studied in the same way only about 50% of the activity in lesioned areas represented degraded LDL while the remainder represented intact LDL (unpublished studies). An increased accumulation of LDL under the endothelium would itself presumably lead to enhanced LDL degradation by the cells normally present, but increased cellularity in these regions may also play a role.

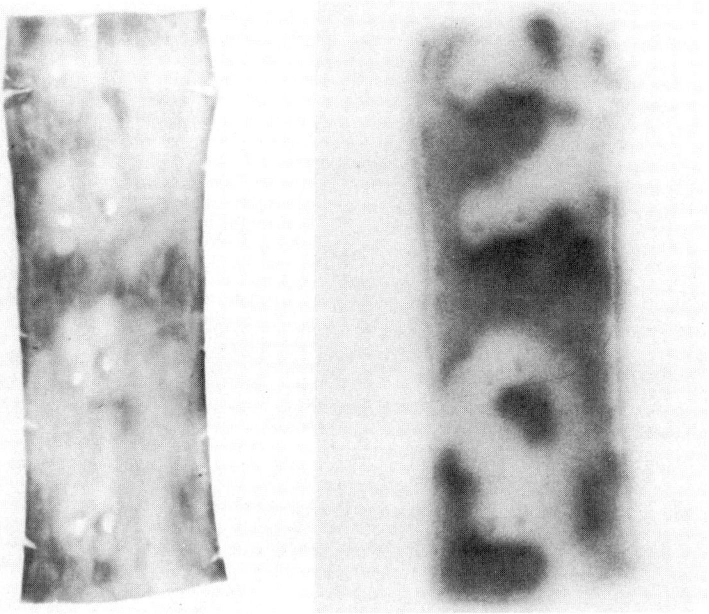

FIGURE 3. Composite photograph and autoradiogram of partially reendothelialized aortic segment sixteen weeks after injury with balloon catheter in a rabbit maintained on 2% cholesterol diet. The photograph (left) shows the areas of reendothelialization (white areas) surrounding pairs of orifices of intercostal vesicles. Dark areas (stained by Evan's blue dye injected ten minutes prior to sacrifice) reveal areas not covered by endothelium. The autoradiogram (right) demonstrates the localization of ^{125}I-TC-LDL injected prior to sacrifice of the animal.

FIGURE 4 shows that the degradation of ^{125}I-TC-LDL can be studied by autoradiography at the cellular level. ^{125}I-TC-LDL was injected into a two year-old LDL receptor-deficient (WHHL) rabbit 48 hours before sacrifice. Virtually the entire aortic surface was involved and stained strongly with Sudan IV. The figure demonstrates a marked accumulation of autoradiographic photographic grains over subendothelial foam cells from an advanced aortic lesion. The grain density over the foam cells is clearly greater than that over intercellular spaces or over adjacent endothelial cells. This section is fully representative, that is, most of the foam cells just beneath the endothelium were highly active in LDL uptake and degradation. This was true, as

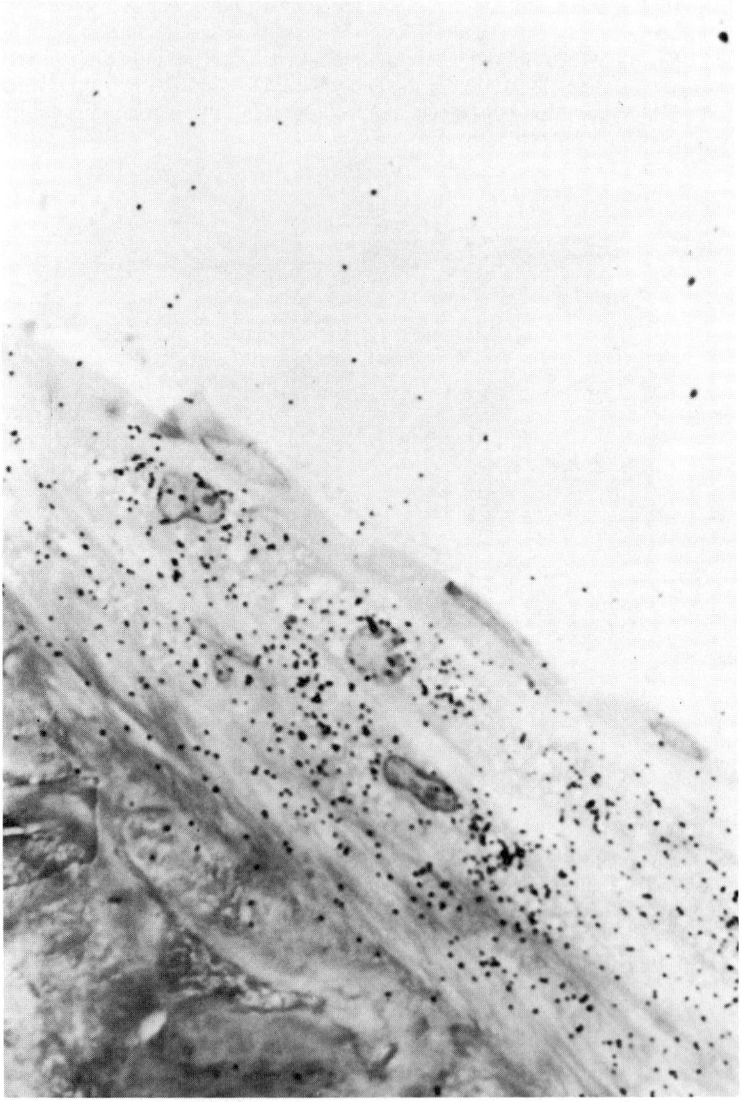

FIGURE 4. Autoradiographic localization of ^{125}I-TC-LDL in a section of an aortic atherosclerotic lesion from a two year-old WHHL rabbit. Araldite section, one micron thickness, stained with toluidine blue.

shown in FIGURE 4, even for cells already heavily loaded with lipid droplets. This finding indicates that these cells are still in a highly dynamic state, taking up and degrading LDL and its lipids. Presumably they must also be discharging lipids at some rate, and intervention to favor the latter process might be helpful. Furthermore, the fact that virtually all of the foam cells became heavily labeled during the 24 hours between injection of the labeled TC-LDL and sacrifice tends to rule against the "lipophage" hypothesis of Leary.[24] He proposed that macrophages acquired their load of lipid in the liver, or in the circulation, and only then entered the artery wall, carrying their lipid in with them. It seems most unlikely that all, or nearly all, of the foam cells we see in the artery wall could have become labeled and then entered the wall within the 48 hours available under this protocol.

An unanticipated finding from these preliminary studies is the marked gradient (see FIGURE 4) of LDL degradation within the thicker lesions. Foam cells near the luminal surface demonstrate much higher activity than those deeper in the lesions. This suggests either that foam cells just under the endothelium, for some reason, are inherently very active; that LDL in the subendothelial space may be enzymatically or chemically modified in such a way that its uptake by adjacent foam cells is enhanced; or that LDL diffusion within the lesion is very restricted. In any case, the high activity of the cells near the surface obviously reflects degradation by pathways other than the LDL receptor pathway in these receptor-deficient animals.

ACKNOWLEDGMENTS

The authors acknowledge the invaluable contributions of the following collaborators on various aspects of the studies presented: Drs. E. Roger Marchand, Eberhard von Hodenberg, and Olov Wiklund. Dr. Donald B. Zilversmit is thanked for helpful suggestions and discussions.

REFERENCES

1. LIPID RESEARCH CLINICS PROGRAM. 1984. The Lipid Research Clinics Coronary Primary Prevention Trial Results. JAMA **251:** 351–364.
2. STEINBERG, D. 1983. Arteriosclerosis **3:** 283–301.
3. SMITH, E. B. & R. H. SMITH. 1976. Atheroscler. Res. **1:** 119–136.
4. PALADE, G. E., M. SIMIONESCU & N. SIMIONESCU. 1979. Acta Physiol. Scand. Suppl. **463:** 11–32.
5. STEIN, Y. & O. STEIN. 1973. Ciba Found. Symp. **12:** 165–183.
6. RECKLESS, J. P. D., D. B. WEINSTEIN & D. STEINBERG. 1978. Biochim. Biophys. Acta **75:** 356–360.
7. VLODAVSKY, I., P. E. FIELDING, C. J. FIELDING & D. GOSPADOAROWICZ. 1978. Proc. Natl. Acad. Sci. USA **529:** 475–487.
8. COETZZ, G. A., O. STEIN & Y. STEIN. 1979. Atherosclerosis **33:** 425–431.
9. VAN HINSBERGH, V. W. M., L. HAVEKES, J. J. EMEIS, E. VAN CORVEN & M. SCHEFFER. 1983. Arteriosclerosis **3:** 547–559.
10. WILKUND, O., T. E. CAREW & D. STEINBERG. 1984. Arteriosclerosis. In press.
11. WEISGRABER, K. H., T. L. INNERARITY & R. W. MAHLEY. 1978. J. Biol. Chem. **253:** 9053–9062.
12. VASILE, E., M. SIMIONESCU & N. SIMIONESCU. 1983. J. Cell Biol. **96:** 1677–1689.
13. PITTMAN, R. C., S. R. GREEN, A. D. ATTIE & D. STEINBERG. 1979. J. Biol. Chem. **254:** 6876–6879.
14. PITTMAN, R. C., A. D. ATTIE, T. E. CAREW & D. STEINBERG. 1979. Proc. Natl. Acad. Sci. USA **76:** 5345–5349.

15. CAREW, T. E. & W. F. BELTZ. 1983. *In* Lipoprotein Kinetics and Modeling. M. Berman, S. M. Grundy & B. V. Howard, Eds.: 169–179. Academic Press. New York.
16. PITTMAN, R. C., A. D. ATTIE, T. E. CAREW & D. STEINBERG. 1982. Biochim. Biophys. Acta **710:** 7–14.
17. PITTMAN, R. C., T. E. CAREW, A. D. ATTIE, J. L. WITZTUM, Y. WATANABE & D. STEINBERG. 1982. J. Biol. Chem. **257:** 7994–8000.
18. PITTMAN, R. C., T. E. CAREW, C. K. GLASS, S. R. GREEN, C. A. TAYLOR, JR. & A. D. ATTIE. 1983. Biochem. J. **212:** 791–800.
19. CAREW, T. E., R. C. PITTMAN, R. E. MARCHAND & D. STEINBERG. 1984. Arteriosclerosis **4:** 214–224.
20. BRATZLER, R. L., G. M. CHISHOLM, C. K. COLTON, D. A. SMITH & R. D. LEES. 1977. Atherosclerosis **28:** 289–307.
21. STENDER, S. & D. B. ZILVERSMIT. Arteriosclerosis **1:**38–49.
22. MINICK, C. R., M. B. STEMERMAN & W. INSULL, JR. 1977. Proc. Natl. Acad. Sci. USA **74:** 1724–1728.
23. ROBERTS, A. B., A. M. LEES, R. S. LEES, H. W. STRAUSS, J. T. FALLON, J. TAVERAS & S. KOPRIVODA. 1983. J. Lipid Res. **24:** 1160–1167.
24. LEARY, T. 1941. Arch. Pathol. **32:** 507.

Some Speculations on the Deposition of Cholesterol in Aortic Lesions of Familial Hypercholesterolemia

DONALD M. SMALL

Biophysics Institute
Departments of Medicine and Biochemistry
Boston University School of Medicine
Boston, Massachusetts 02118

Familial homozygous hypercholesterolemia is a disease in which the plasma concentration of LDL cholesterol increases five to tenfold, even in the fetus.[1] This high level of LDL persists throughout life and results in severe premature atherosclerosis.[2] The histologic findings in familial homozygous hypercholesterolemia have recently been described by Buja *et al.*[3] In their findings, a twenty month-old fetus was found to have one minute focus of intimal lipid accumulation. However, they noted intimal involvement by a typical atherosclerotic plaque in a surgical specimen from a nine year-old. We recently had the chance to study some aortic plaques from a nine year-old boy.[4] He was known to have hypercholesterolemia and xanthomata by age one and a half years.[5] He was followed over the next several years at Rockefeller University Hospital, where cholesterol pool size and synthesis rate were measured both before and after a portacaval anastomosis.[5]

Following portacaval anastomosis, both cholesterol synthesis and total body pools of cholesterol decreased, and the serum cholesterol fell from the 700 range to about 466.[5] At age nine years, he died prematurely of his disease. Physicochemical, histologic, and autoradiographic studies were performed on the aorta,[4] using a technique in which hot stage polarizing microscopy, standard histologic staining, and autoradiography are carried out on the same or contiguous 8μ histologic sections.[6] The aorta had many large plaques. These plaques had large cholesterol clefts, some collagen, many foam cells in the upper regions, but little calcium. The bases of the plaques contained large cholesterol monohydrate crystals and extracellular cholesterol esters. Virtually, no cells were present in this region. Overlying this necrotic crystal-laden region were large numbers of foam cells filled with low melting (mean melting temperature ~30°C) cholesterol esters. The mean melting temperature of the extracellular cholesterol esters in the base of the lesion was about 15°C higher. The plaques contained up to 40% dry weight lipid and had compositions which were high in free cholesterol, similar to those reported previously for human atherosclerotic plaques (see refs. 7 and 8).

Since the patient had been given high doses of radioactive cholesterol four and a half years, two years and four months prior to death, thin frozen sections were examined by autoradiography to see if radioactive cholesterol had deposited in the lesion.[4] These sections showed many silver grains over those foam cells near the lumen. However, the base of the plaques, which were rich in cholesterol crystals and cholesterol ester, had no grains.

We concluded from this study that (i) juvenile familial homozygotes have plaques similar to those found in nonfamilial hypercholesterolemics; (ii) that cholesterol is laid down from the luminal side sequentially; (iii) that the cholesterol in the foam cells on the luminal side is not in equilibrium with the cholesterol in the base of the plaque; and, (iv) that the cholesterol present in the base of the plaque must have been laid down prior to receiving radioactive cholesterol (that is, at least four and a half years prior to death). The fact that the cholesterol crystals have virtually no silver grains indicates that they contained very little radioactivity. This may explain why the isolated crystalline cholesterol monohydrate fraction, which was taken from atherosclerotic human aortic plaques of patients previously given radioactive cholesterol, contains very little radioactivity.[9] We had previously attributed the very low crystalline cholesterol specific activity to slow exchange, but probably, it is more truly related to a combination of deposition of crystals before the radioactivity was given and extremely slow exchange.

REFERENCES

1. Brown, M. S., J. L. Goldstein, K. Vandenberghe, J. P. Fryns, P. T. Kovanen, R. Eeckels, H. van den Berghe & J. J. Cassiman. 1978. The Lancet **March 11:** 526–529.
2. Goldstein, J. L. & M. S. Brown. 1983. Familial Hypercholesterolemia, Chapt. 33. *In* The Metabolic Basis of Inherited Disease, Fifth Edition. J. B. Stanbury, J. B. Wyngaarden, D. S. Fredrickson, J. L. Goldstein & M. S. Brown, Eds.: 672–712. McGraw–Hill. New York.
3. Buja, L. M., P. T. Kovanen & D. W. Bilheimer. 1979. Am. J. Pathol. **97:** 327–345.
4. Small, D. M., A. M. Tercyak, E. Fonferko, C. McCormack, L. C. Hudgins & E. H. Ahrens, Jr. 1984. Arteriosclerosis **4:** 567a.
5. McNamara, D. J., E. H. Ahrens, Jr., R. Kolb, C. D. Brown, T. S. Parker, N. O. Davidson, P. Samuel & R. M. McVie. 1983. Proc. Natl. Acad. Sci. USA **80:** 564–568.
6. Waugh, D. A. & D. M. Small. 1984. Lab. Invest. **51**(6): 702–714.
7. Small, D. M. & G. G. Shipley. 1974. Science **185:** 222–229.
8. Katz, S. S., G. G. Shipley & D. M. Small. 1976. J. Clin. Invest. **58:** 200–211.
9. Katz, S. S., D. M. Small, F. R. Smith, R. B. Dell & D-W. S. Goodman. 1982. J. Lipid Res. **23:** 733–737.

Lipoproteins of Special Significance in Atherosclerosis

Insights Provided by Studies of Type III Hyperlipoproteinemia

ROBERT W. MAHLEY, THOMAS L. INNERARITY,
STANLEY C. RALL, JR., AND KARL H. WEISGRABER

Gladstone Foundation Laboratories for Cardiovascular Disease
Cardiovascular Research Institute
Departments of Pathology and Medicine
University of California at San Francisco
P.O. Box 40608
San Francisco, California 94140

INTRODUCTION

Much has been learned about normal metabolism by studying patients with genetic abnormalities. This is especially true of type III hyperlipoproteinemia, which has provided insights into the functional role of apolipoprotein E (apo E) in lipoprotein metabolism and of specific lipoproteins in atherogenesis. In type III hyperlipoproteinemia, the primary genetic defect is the presence of an abnormal form of the E apolipoprotein which is defective in its ability to bind to lipoprotein receptors on cells (for review, see refs. 1–4). Those patients with type III hyperlipoproteinemia have elevated plasma triglyceride and cholesterol levels, and develop accelerated atherosclerotic vascular disease involving both coronary and peripheral arteries. The hyperlipoproteinemia is characterized by an accumulation of beta-very low density lipoproteins (β-VLDL), which are of both intestinal and hepatic origin. However, not all individuals with this genetic abnormality, i.e., the primary genetic defect (defective apo E), develop type III hyperlipoproteinemia. This is one of the curious and interesting aspects of this disease. It appears that in many instances, a second event is necessary to cause expression of the abnormality. This second event may be an additional genetic defect or an environmental factor (e.g., diet, sex, body weight, age, hormonal balance, etc.), which tips the balance in favor of expression of the disease. It is this event that accentuates the effects of the presence of the abnormal form of apo E and that results in the changes in the lipoproteins that appear to predispose type III subjects to accelerated vascular disease. Other human disorders requiring a second event to induce the expression of the primary genetic defect have been described.[5] Initially, the abnormal form of apo E that occurs in these subjects will be defined, and then the alterations in the lipoproteins in type III hyperlipoproteinemia will be discussed.

APOLIPOPROTEIN E: STRUCTURE AND FUNCTION

Human apo E displays a complex isoform pattern on isoelectric focusing gels that is due to the presence of multiple alleles at a single locus and to the presence of posttranslational glycosylation of the gene product.[6–9] The major isoforms, referred to as apo E2, E3, and E4, differ by a single unit of charge on focusing gels. There are three common homozygous phenotypes (E2/2, E3/3, and E4/4) and three heterozygous phenotypes (E3/2, E4/2, and E4/3). The most common phenotype in humans is E3/3, which occurs in approximately 60% of the population, as reported in various studies (for review, see ref. 1). Type III hyperlipoproteinemia and dysbetalipoproteinemia are associated with the E2/2 phenotype. Rarely, this disorder may also occur in individuals who are heterozygous for apo E2, e.g., E3/2 and E4/2.[10,11]

Apolipoprotein E is a single polypeptide chain of 299 amino acids and has a molecular weight of 34,200. Amino acid sequence analyses have defined the structural differences among the major isoforms,[9] which are described on the basis of a comparison with the apo E3 structure. Apolipoprotein E4 differs from apo E3 at a single site, possessing arginine at residue 112 rather than cysteine, i.e., E4(Cys_{112}→Arg). Apolipoprotein E2 is genotypically heterogeneous, and three variant forms of apo E2 have been described, each differing from apo E3 at a single site. The most commonly observed apo E2 variant possesses cysteine substituted for the normally occurring arginine at residue 158, i.e., E2(Arg_{158}→Cys). Other substitutions involve the interchange of a neutral amino acid for either arginine or lysine in the apo E3 structure and are denoted E2(Arg_{145}→Cys)[12] and E2(Lys_{146}→Gln).[10] These three apo E2 variants are all found in type III hyperlipoproteinemic patients. An additional variant form of apo E is also associated with type III hyperlipoproteinemia, but it migrates in the E3 rather than the E2 position on isoelectric focusing gels.[13] Sequence analysis indicates that this apo E3 probably represents a variant form of apo E4 that has a substitution involving the loss of a positive charge and thus, migrates in the E3 position (S. C. Rall, Jr., K. H. Weisgraber, and R. W. Mahley, unpublished data). This variant is designated E3(Cys_{112}→Arg, Arg_{142}→Cys). A variant form of apo E that focuses in the E1 position has been identified with the structure E1(Gly_{127}→Asp, Arg_{158}→Cys).[14] This variant, also associated with hyperlipoproteinemia, probably arises as a result of a mutation in the gene for E2(Arg_{158}→Cys). An additional variant of apo E, an apo E3 identified by cDNA cloning procedures, has a predicted amino acid sequence that differs at two sites compared to the sequence previously reported for apo E3.[15] These substitutions involve residues 99 (threonine for alanine) and 152 (proline for alanine). In addition to the variants described above, it has been shown that there are other genetically determined variants of apo E migrating on isoelectric focusing gels in the E1,[16] E5,[17] and E7[18] positions.

An important function of apo E in lipoprotein metabolism is to serve as the protein determinant that mediates binding of lipoproteins to apo B,E(LDL) and apo E receptors (for review, see refs. 2 and 19). The apo B,E(LDL) receptors, initially described by Goldstein and Brown (for review, see refs. 20 and 21), are present in the liver and in most extrahepatic tissues. This receptor not only binds and internalizes apo B-containing lipoproteins (e.g., low density lipoproteins (LDL)), but also apo E-containing lipoproteins (e.g., specific high density lipoproteins (HDL), referred to as HDL-with apo E), chylomicron remnants, and β-VLDL. A second lipoprotein receptor, the apo E receptor, is present only on liver membranes and presumably represents the chylomicron remnant receptor.[22,23] This receptor interacts with apo E-containing lipoproteins, but not with LDL.

Apolipoprotein E3 actively and efficiently binds to both the apo B,E(LDL) and apo E receptors.[12,24] However, all variant forms of apo E that are associated with type III hyperlipoproteinemia display abnormal cell surface receptor binding activity in *in vitro* binding assays.[10,12,24–26] To both receptors, these variants possess binding activities ranging from <2% to ~45% of normal. The most severely defective mutant (<2% of normal binding) is the E2(Arg_{158}→Cys). Apolipoproteins E2(Arg_{145}→Cys) and E2(Lys_{146}→Gln) display binding activities of 45 and 40%, respectively, compared to the binding of apo E3. Likewise, β-VLDL from type III patients also display defective binding activity that parallels the activities seen with the apo E2.[24] Despite the fact that β-VLDL from type III subjects possess both apo B and apo E, the only protein determinant responsible for their binding has been demonstrated to be apo E, even though the binding activity is low.[24,27] These studies suggest a mechanism whereby the primary genetic defect in type III hyperlipoproteinemia, which is the presence of a structurally abnormal form of apo E, may cause the accumulation of remnant lipoproteins in the plasma (i.e., impaired binding of these lipoproteins to both apo B,E(LDL) and apo E receptors). This will be considered in detail later.

Identification of the variants of apo E that are defective in receptor binding activity has helped to determine the region of the apo E molecule responsible for binding to the receptors (for review, see refs. 2, 19, and 28). It is significant that the defective mutants involve substitutions of a neutral amino acid for the basic residues arginine or lysine. Previously, it has been shown that selective chemical modification of either

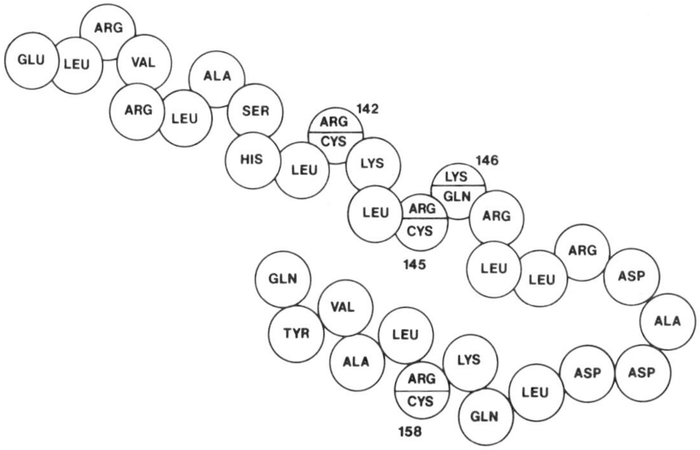

FIGURE 1. The portion of the apo E molecule postulated to represent the vicinity of the receptor binding domain. The sites of amino acid substitution known to affect binding are residues 142, 145, 146, and 158.

arginine or lysine residues within apo E (and apo B) abolishes receptor binding activity.[29,30] In addition, it is significant that the receptor-defective mutants have substitutions in a region of the apo E molecule that is uniquely enriched in both arginine and lysine residues. As described above, the defective mutants involve cysteine substitutions for arginine at residues 142, 145, and 158, or glutamine substituted for lysine at residue 146. It remains to be determined whether the substitution of a proline for alanine at residue 152, the site of a predicted β-turn, has an effect on receptor binding activity.[15] These data suggest that the region of the apo E molecule in the vicinity of residues 140 to 160 is involved in the binding domain (FIGURE 1).

Further data implicating this region as the receptor binding domain come from studies of fragments of apo E.[31] Apolipoprotein E3 was cleaved into fragments of various lengths, which were then tested for receptor binding activity. Thrombolytic cleavage produced two major fragments: the amino terminal two-thirds of the molecule (residues 1 through 191, $M_r = 22,000$), and the carboxyl terminal region (residues 216 through 299, $M_r = 10,000$). The $M_r = 22,000$ fragment possessed full receptor binding activity, whereas the $M_r = 10,000$ fragment was totally inactive. Cyanogen bromide digestion produced eight fragments. Only the largest fragment, spanning residues 126–218, possessed receptor binding activity. As shown schematically in FIGURE 2, the region of overlap for the receptor-active thrombolytic and cyanogen bromide fragments encompasses residues 126–191, the region that also encompasses the receptor-defective mutants.

An additional approach to define the receptor binding domain of apo E was the use of monoclonal antibodies to apo E to map the various regions of the molecule.[32] Of particular interest was the epitope of an apo E monoclonal antibody (1D7) that blocked receptor binding activity. Using the various mutants of apo E (substitutions at 142, 145, 146, and 158) plus a series of synthetic peptides, it was possible to localize the epitope to the vicinity of residues 140 to 150. Thus, the three lines of evidence (genetic variants, biochemical fragments, and monoclonal antibodies) all focus attention on this midportion of the apo E molecule as being the receptor binding domain of apo E.

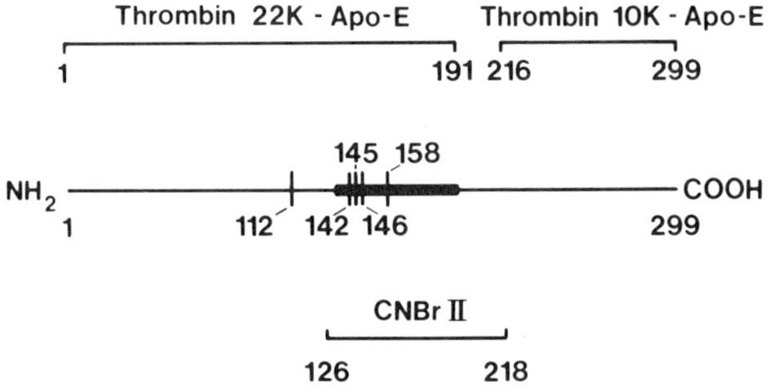

FIGURE 2. Schematic representation of the apo E molecule. Receptor binding activity resides with the $M_r = 22,000$ thrombolytic fragment and the CNBr II fragment generated by cyanogen bromide digestion.

It is now envisioned that the region of the apo E molecule responsible for the direct interaction with receptors does not involve residue 158, and it is likely that E2($Arg_{158} \rightarrow Cys$) exerts its effect on receptor binding activity by altering the conformation of the binding domain.[33] It was found that full receptor binding activity could be restored to apo E2($Arg_{158} \rightarrow Cys$) by a combination of two procedures. The treatment of apo E2 with the reagent cysteamine, which converts cysteine to a positively charged analogue of lysine via a disulfide linkage, increased the receptor binding activity by ten- to twentyfold. However, this was still only ~10% of normal apo E3 binding activity. Likewise, it was found that removal of the carboxyl terminal one-third of the apo E2 by thrombolytic cleavage activated the binding of the $M_r = 22,000$ amino terminal region of the apo E2 molecule to ~10% of normal. Furthermore, it was possible to restore fully the binding activity to the $M_r = 22,000$ fragment of apo E2 by treating it with cysteamine. An additional key observation was that the reversal of the cysteamine modification (removal of the positive charge by β-mercaptoethanol treatment) did not cause an immediate loss of receptor binding activity. This demonstrated that the positive charge at residue 158 was not required for normal receptor binding activity of the M_r = 22,000 fragment of E2(Arg_{158}→Cys). Thus, it appears that the arginine normally present at residue 158 does not directly interact with the receptor, but that its role is to stabilize the conformation of the binding domain (residues in the vicinity of 140 to 150). Apparently, the removal of the carboxyl terminal one-third of the molecule removes a conformational restraint from the E2(Arg_{158}→Cys) molecule, and this allows the positive charge at 158 (produced by cysteamine treatment) to alter the conformation of the binding domain such that it attains full receptor binding capability. When the treated M_r = 22,000 fragment achieves the proper conformation, the cysteamine modification (and the associated positive charge) can be reversed, and the molecule displays normal binding activity, which is only slowly lost with time.[33]

TYPE III HYPERLIPOPROTEINEMIA

The study of the mutant forms of apo E associated with type III hyperlipoproteinemia has provided important insights into the role of apo E in lipoprotein metabolism (for review, see refs. 1, 2, 19, and 28), and in the following discussion, the effects of the presence of receptor-defective apo E will be considered. As mentioned earlier, an additional factor (a second event) is required in many cases to induce the expression of the disease with hyperlipoproteinemia.[5] Thus, consideration will be given to the types of lipoprotein changes that occur in the plasma and to the factors that modify the expression of the disease. In addition, possible mechanisms responsible for the accelerated atherosclerosis associated with type III hyperlipoproteinemia will be identified.

The hypertriglyceridemia and hypercholesterolemia observed in type III patients are characterized by the accumulation of lipoproteins of d < 1.006 g/ml. This fraction contains pre-β-migrating VLDL, as well as β-migrating lipoproteins (β-VLDL). The β-VLDL actually represent two distinctly different lipoproteins, which can be separated by agarose chromatography.[34,35] These include (a) intestinal β-VLDL or chylomicron remnants, which are large particles (70 to 80 nm in diameter) containing apo B48 and apo E as major protein constituents, and (b) hepatic β-VLDL (cholesterol-rich VLDL or VLDL remnants), which are ~40 nm in diameter, containing apo B100 and apo E as their major apolipoproteins.

Intestinal β-VLDL (chylomicron remnants) appear to accumulate in the plasma as a result of the defective clearance of these lipoproteins secondarily to the presence of the receptor-defective apo E (for review, see refs. 1 and 2) (FIGURE 3). Normally, chylomicron remnants are cleared rapidly and efficiently by the liver, presumably by the apo E receptors (remnant receptors) or by the apo B,E(LDL) receptors (for review, see refs. 19 and 20). Apolipoprotein E appears to be the primary determinant for the recognition of these lipoproteins.[24,27] Therefore, the presence of receptor-defective apo E could contribute to the accumulation of the intestinal β-VLDL in the plasma. However, how can the observation be explained that not every individual with the receptor-defective apo E develops marked β-VLDL accumulation and hyperlipidemia?[36] (It should be pointed out that even those E2/2 subjects with normal or low lipid values have dysbetalipoproteinemia, i.e., have in their plasma detectable levels of the abnormal remnant β-VLDL.) It is reasonable to speculate that the level of expression of the hepatic lipoprotein receptors could regulate the level of these lipoproteins in the plasma and the degree of hyperlipidemia (for review, see ref. 1) (FIGURE 3). Despite the fact that all of the apo E variants associated with type III hyperlipoproteinemia are defective in their ability to bind to the apo B,E(LDL) and apo E receptors, they do possess some binding activity. Therefore, if higher levels of the receptors could be induced, it may be possible to clear the β-VLDL with the defective apo E from the plasma. It has been shown that the expression of the hepatic apo B,E(LDL) receptors can be modulated by diet, drugs, hormones, and the plasma concentrations of certain lipoproteins and bile acids.[22,23,37] By contrast, the hepatic apo E receptors are not sensitive to these factors and remain expressed at a relatively constant level.[22,23,37]

Two examples serve to emphasize the potential role of various factors that modulate the level of apo B,E(LDL) receptors, and therefore, contribute to the expression, or lack of expression, of type III hyperlipoproteinemia. Estrogen and thyroid hormones have been shown to affect the level of the apo B,E(LDL) receptors.[38–40] In experimental animals, estrogen treatment has been shown to induce the

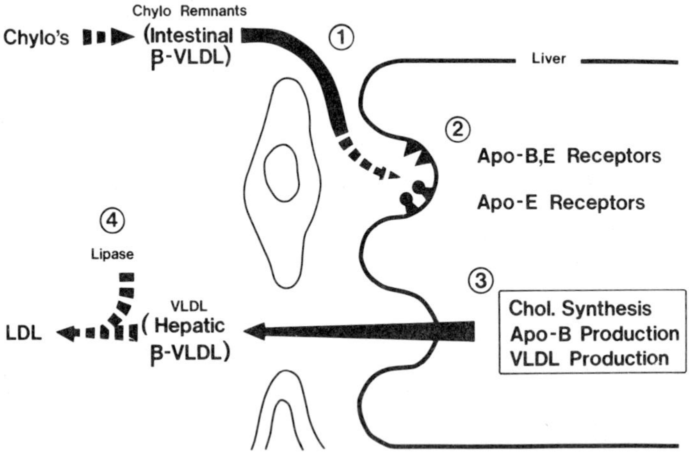

FIGURE 3. Sites in the scheme of lipoprotein metabolism where the expression of type III hyperlipoproteinemia may be modulated: (1) The presence of receptor-defective apo E could disrupt the uptake of chylomicron and VLDL remnants by the liver. (2) The level of expression of the hepatic lipoprotein receptors could regulate the level of remnants that accumulate in plasma. (3) Increased synthesis of hepatic cholesterol and/or VLDL could account for the presence of hepatic β-VLDL. (4) Impaired conversion of β-VLDL to LDL could result in elevated levels of β-VLDL and low levels of plasma LDL. (From Angelin and Mahley;[1] reproduced with permission.)

expression of high levels of apo B,E(LDL) receptors.[38,39] Consistent with this observation, type III hyperlipoproteinemia seldom occurs in women prior to menopause, and the hyperlipidemia can usually be controlled by replacement therapy.[4] Similarly, hypothyroidism predisposes an apo E2/2 subject to type III hyperlipoproteinemia, and correction of the deficiency tends to normalize the plasma lipids and lipoproteins.[4] A second example suggesting that the level of receptors affects expression of the disease may be illustrated by the fact that type III hyperlipoproteinemia does not usually occur until adulthood. The age of onset may correlate with the observation that hepatic apo B,E(LDL) receptors appear to decrease in number with age.[22,23] In summary, the appearance of high levels of intestinal β-VLDL (chylomicron remnants) in the plasma of E2/2 subjects is related to the presence of receptor-defective apo E, and the level of β-VLDL could be modulated by the level of expression of the hepatic lipoprotein receptors.

Hepatic β-VLDL (cholesterol-rich VLDL or VLDL remnants) may also occur in the plasma at high levels as a result of impaired clearance by the liver (for review, see ref. 1) (FIGURE 3). It has now become apparent that a fraction of the VLDL is cleared from the plasma, presumably by the liver, without being converted to LDL. In addition, it is possible that these lipoproteins may accumulate secondarily to hepatic overproduction of cholesterol and/or VLDL. A deficiency in the delivery of cholesterol to the liver that is secondary to the impaired clearance of chylomicron remnants may stimulate an increase in hepatic cholesterol biosynthesis and the overproduction of cholesterol-rich VLDL. Furthermore, several of the secondary factors known to exacerbate type III hyperlipoproteinemia (e.g., obesity, obesity with hypothyroidism, diabetes, and increasing age) are known to stimulate hepatic synthesis of cholesterol and/or VLDL.[41] In addition, Utermann *et al.*[42] and Hazzard *et al.*[43] have presented compelling evidence from kindred studies indicating that type III hyperlipoproteinemia occurs in association with a second heritable hyperlipidemia, such as familial combined hyperlipidemia (which is a defect that may well be associated with hepatic overproduction of VLDL and cholesterol).

Accumulation of the hepatic β-VLDL in certain E2/2 subjects may reflect a defect in the lipolytic processing of these lipoproteins to LDL (FIGURE 3). Ehnholm *et al.*[44] have demonstrated *in vitro* that hepatic β-VLDL are not converted to "LDL" by the addition of lipoprotein lipase, apo C-II, and $d > 1.21$ lipoprotein-deficient plasma, but are converted to "intermediate density lipoproteins" ("IDL") ($d = 1.006$–1.02). ("LDL" and "IDL" are shorthand notations for particles of these densities and are not meant to imply metabolic identity with *in vivo* IDL and LDL.) By comparison, normal VLDL are readily converted to LDL ($d = 1.03$–1.06). However, when apo E3 was added to the incubation mixture, it was possible to convert the hepatic β-VLDL to "LDL." In contrast, addition of apo E2 was ineffective in stimulating the lipolytic processing of these lipoproteins. It has been postulated that apo E3 (but not apo E2) can interact with a factor in the $d > 1.21$ lipoprotein-deficient plasma (probably a lipid transfer or exchange protein) that modifies the chemical composition of the hepatic β-VLDL (possibly a reduction in cholesterol content) and allows lipolytic processing to occur.[44] Therefore, apo E may possess an additional role in lipid metabolism, i.e., interaction with lipid transfer or exchange proteins. However, the mechanism whereby the addition of apo E3 facilitates the processing remains to be defined. The inability of the apo E2-containing β-VLDL to be converted to LDL may be consistent with the *in vivo* observation that type III hyperlipoproteinemic subjects have low levels of plasma LDL.

TYPE III LIPOPROTEINS AND ATHEROGENESIS

The accumulation of intestinal and hepatic β-VLDL in the plasma of patients with type III hyperlipoproteinemia correlates with the occurrence of accelerated atherosclerosis involving both peripheral and coronary arteries. The association of β-VLDL with atherogenesis may represent the best example of how a specific lipoprotein may cause lipid accumulation within specific cells of the arterial wall. It has been shown that β-VLDL from type III subjects can cause massive cholesteryl ester accumulation within macrophages in *in vitro* studies.[34,45] Furthermore, it is now established that macrophages are a major source of foam cells within atherosclerotic lesions (for review, see refs. 46 and 47). The uptake of β-VLDL by macrophages is mediated by a specific receptor, referred to as the β-VLDL receptor. The protein determinant responsible for mediating the uptake of the β-VLDL by macrophages appears to be apo E, with either apo E3 or E2 capable of mediating this interaction (T. L. Innerarity and R. W. Mahley, unpublished data). It is also of interest that in certain animals fed diets high in fat and cholesterol, one of the major changes in the lipoproteins is the induction of intestinal and hepatic β-VLDL.[46,47] The diet-induced β-VLDL resemble in many ways the β-VLDL from type III subjects, and they possess the ability to cause marked cholesteryl ester accumulation in macrophages.[48,49] This form of hyperlipoproteinemia is associated with accelerated atherogenesis, which in certain species, such as the dog,[50,51] tends to cause the most severe lipid deposits within peripheral and coronary arteries.

An additional change in the lipoproteins of subjects with type III hyperlipoproteinemia, which may be important in understanding the role of specific lipoproteins in atherogenesis, is a reduction of the total HDL in the plasma of some patients (for review, see refs. 1, 3, and 4) and an apparent increase in the HDL-with apo E (K. H. Weisgraber and R. W. Mahley, unpublished data). The potential importance of these changes relates to the role of HDL in reverse cholesterol transport and in the redistribution of cholesterol to various cells of the body. It has been postulated that HDL serves as an acceptor of cholesterol from cells, presumably including foam cells of the atherosclerotic lesion, and participates in the transport of the cholesterol to the liver for elimination from the body or to other cells that may require a source of cholesterol for membrane biosynthesis or hormone production (for review, see refs. 2, 46, and 47). Also, in animals fed high levels of fat and cholesterol, there is a decrease in HDL-without apo E and an increase in the HDL-with apo E (HDL_c). The HDL_c represent cholesterol-enriched HDL that have become progressively larger in size and are progressively enriched in apo E.[2,46,47] The apo E HDL_c (those HDL_c possessing only the E apolipoprotein) are rapidly and efficiently cleared by the liver, presumably by the apo E receptors of hepatocytes.[52] Other HDL-with apo E that also possess apo A-I may be cleared both by the liver and various cells with apo B,E(LDL) receptors. It is envisioned that these HDL-with apo E may represent anti-atherogenic lipoproteins.

The HDL-with apo E (HDL_c) accumulate in highest concentrations in those animal species that lack (or have low concentrations of) the cholesteryl ester transfer protein, e.g., dogs, rats, and swine.[53] In contrast, in those animal species with the cholesteryl ester transfer protein, some of the cholesteryl esters may be transferred out of the HDL into lower density lipoproteins, which then could transport the cholesterol to the liver and other cells. The increased concentration of HDL-with apo E in type III subjects may reflect an increase in the formation of cholesterol-enriched HDL that may participate in the reverse cholesterol transport. Their accumulation in the plasma may result (a) from the fact that the HDL-with apo E of type III subjects possess the apo E2 that is defective in receptor binding activity or (b) from a defect in the transfer of cholesteryl esters (mediated by the cholesteryl ester transfer protein) out of the HDL into the lower density lipoproteins. This latter speculation is based on an observation obtained from studies of the lipolytic processing of hepatic β-VLDL.[44] As discussed earlier, it appears that apo E3 (but not apo E2) participates with a factor present in the $d > 1.21$ lipoprotein-deficient plasma to modify the lipid composition of these particles, allowing lipolysis to proceed. Furthermore, it has been suggested that apo E is associated with the cholesteryl ester transfer process.[54]

Recently, it has been demonstrated that the HDL_3 (HDL-without apo E) are the precursors for the formation of cholesterol-enriched HDL (HDL-with apo E or

HDL_c).[55] These studies show that cholesterol can be acquired from cholesterol-loaded macrophages or from an inert support by HDL that lack apo E. The reduced levels of HDL-without apo E in type III subjects and in animals fed fat and cholesterol may reflect the use of these lipoproteins as precursors for the HDL-with apo E. When a source of lecithin:cholesterol acyltransferase is provided, the small HDL-without apo E (~10 nm in diameter) are increased in size in parallel with an increase in the cholesteryl ester and apo E content of the particles. The apo E can be acquired by redistribution from other plasma lipoproteins or by secretion from specific cells, such as macrophages[56] or other cells in various peripheral tissues of the body.[57] Three distinct sizes of HDL-with apo E are formed, including small HDL_1 (~15 nm in diameter), large HDL_1 (~20 nm), and HDL_c (~25 nm).[55] These sizes correspond to particles possessing one, two, or three layers of cholesteryl ester within the core.[55] A source of apo E is required for the formation of these large, cholesteryl ester-rich particles, and if all sources of apo E are removed in these *in vitro* systems, the large HDL will not be produced.[58] Thus, it appears that apo E may function to stabilize the surface or to allow for an increase in the core size as these large cholesteryl ester-rich HDL are formed.

SUMMARY

In summary, the study of type III hyperlipoproteinemia has provided important insights into lipoprotein metabolism that have helped to elucidate several functional roles for apo E and have provided a better understanding of the mechanisms whereby specific lipoproteins may be atherogenic or anti-atherogenic. The molecular defect in type III hyperlipoproteinemia and dysbetalipoproteinemia is the presence of a mutant form of apo E, usually apo E2, that is defective in binding to both apo B,E(LDL) and apo E receptors. The receptor-defective apo E results in an impaired clearance of remnant lipoproteins (β-VLDL). In addition, the abnormal apo E may impair the lipolytic processing of hepatic β-VLDL through its involvement in lipid transfer or exchange processes. The accumulation of β-VLDL may provide the most direct mechanism responsible for the accelerated atherosclerosis observed in type III hyperlipoproteinemia, a mechanism that involves the receptor mediated uptake of β-VLDL by macrophages, which are then converted to arterial foam cells. Alterations in the HDL of patients with type III hyperlipoproteinemia further support the concept that HDL are anti-atherogenic. The increase in HDL-with apo E provides insight into the role of these cholesterol-enriched HDL in reverse cholesterol transport and in the cellular redistribution of cholesterol, processes whereby cholesterol deposition may be reversed. It should be stressed that both the accumulation of β-VLDL and alterations in HDL (reduction in typical HDL and an increase in HDL-with apo E) are associated with accelerated atherogenesis in animals fed high levels of fat and cholesterol.

Although valuable information has been gained concerning the mechanisms involved in type III hyperlipoproteinemia by the study of the disease, the clinical expression of this disorder is variable, ranging from hypocholesterolemia to marked hypercholesterolemia in subjects with the same molecular defect (E2/2). This variability in expression is more easily understood when one considers the various factors that can promote the hyperlipoproteinemia and when one considers the mechanisms of action whereby these factors may exacerbate the effects of the presence of an abnormal apo E. In most cases, development of type III hyperlipoproteinemia requires that a second event (a predisposing environmental factor or a second genetic defect) be associated with the primary genetic defect (an abnormal form of apo E).

ACKNOWLEDGMENTS

The authors wish to thank James X. Warger for graphic assistance, Barbara Allen and Sally Gullatt Seehafer for editorial assistance, and Kerry Humphrey and Debbie Morris for manuscript preparation.

REFERENCES

1. MAHLEY, R. W. & B. ANGELIN. 1984. Type III hyperlipoproteinemia: Recent insights into the genetic defect of familial dysbetalipoproteinemia. Adv. Intern. Med. **29:** 385–411.
2. MAHLEY, R. W., T. L. INNERARITY, S. C. RALL, JR. & K. H. WEISGRABER. 1984. Plasma lipoproteins: Apolipoprotein structure and function. J. Lipid Res. **25:** 1277–1294.
3. HAVEL, R. J. 1982. Familial dysbetalipoproteinemia. New aspects of pathogenesis and diagnosis. Med. Clin. North Am. **66:** 441–454.
4. BROWN, M. S., J. L. GOLDSTEIN & D. S. FREDRICKSON. 1983. Familial type 3 hyperlipoproteinemia (dysbetalipoproteinemia). *In* The Metabolic Basis of Inherited Disease, 5th Edition. J. B. Stanbury, J. B. Wyngaarden, D. S. Fredrickson, J. L. Goldstein & M. S. Brown, Eds.: 655–671, McGraw–Hill. New York.
5. MOOLGAVKAR, S. H. & A. G. KNUDSON, JR. 1981. Mutation and cancer: A model for human carcinogenesis. J. Natl. Cancer Inst. **66:** 1037–1052.
6. ZANNIS, V. I. & J. L. BRESLOW. 1981. Human very low density lipoprotein apolipoprotein E isoprotein polymorphism is explained by genetic variation and posttranslational modification. Biochemistry **20:** 1033–1041.
7. ZANNIS, V. I., J. L. BRESLOW, G. UTERMANN, R. W. MAHLEY, K. H. WEISGRABER, R. J. HAVEL, J. L. GOLDSTEIN, M. S. BROWN, G. SCHONFELD, W. R. HAZZARD & C. BLUM. 1982. Proposed nomenclature of apoE isoproteins, apoE genotypes, and phenotypes. J. Lipid Res. **23:** 911–914.
8. UTERMANN, G., A. STEINMETZ & W. WEBER. 1982. Genetic control of human apolipoprotein E polymorphism: Comparison of one- and two-dimensional techniques of isoprotein analysis. Hum. Genet. **60:** 344–351.
9. RALL, S. C., JR., K. H. WEISGRABER & R. W. MAHLEY. 1982. Human apolipoprotein E. The complete amino acid sequence. J. Biol. Chem. **257:** 4171–4178.
10. RALL, S. C., JR., K. H. WEISGRABER, T. L. INNERARITY, T. P. BERSOT, R. W. MAHLEY & C. B. BLUM. 1983. Identification of a new structural variant of human apolipoprotein E, E2(Lys_{146}→Gln), in a type III hyperlipoproteinemic subject with the E3/2 phenotype. J. Clin. Invest. **72:** 1288–1297.
11. BRESLOW, J. L., V. I. ZANNIS, T. R. SANGIACOMA, J. L. H. C. THIRD, T. TRACY & C. J. GLUECK. 1982. Studies of familial type III hyperlipoproteinemia using as a genetic marker the apoE phenotype E2/2. J. Lipid Res. **23:** 1224–1235.
12. RALL, S. C., JR., K. H. WEISGRABER, T. L. INNERARITY & R. W. MAHLEY. 1982. Structural basis for receptor binding heterogeneity of apolipoprotein E from type III hyperlipoproteinemic subjects. Proc. Natl. Acad. Sci. USA **79:** 4696–4700.
13. HAVEL, R. J., L. KOTITE, J. P. KANE, P. TUN & T. BERSOT. 1983. Atypical familial dysbetalipoproteinemia associated with apolipoprotein phenotype E3/3. J. Clin. Invest. **72:** 379–387.
14. WEISGRABER, K. H., S. C. RALL, JR., T. L. INNERARITY, R. W. MAHLEY, T. KUUSI & C. EHNHOLM. 1984. A novel electrophoretic variant of human apolipoprotein E: Identification and characterization of apolipoprotein E1. J. Clin. Invest. **73:** 1024–1033.
15. MCLEAN, J. W., N. A. ELSHOURBAGY, D. J. CHANG, R. W. MAHLEY & J. M. TAYLOR. 1984. Human apolipoprotein E mRNA. cDNA cloning and nucleotide sequencing of a new variant. J. Biol. Chem. **259:** 6498–6504.
16. GHISELLI, G., R. E. GREGG & H. B. BREWER, JR. 1984. Apolipoprotein $E_{Bethesda}$. Isolation and partial characterization of a variant of human apolipoprotein E isolated from very low density lipoproteins. Biochim. Biophys. Acta **794:** 333–339.
17. YAMAMURA, T., A. YAMAMOTO, K. HIRAMORI & S. NAMBU. 1984. A new isoform of

apolipoprotein E—apo E-5—associated with hyperlipidemia and atherosclerosis. Atherosclerosis **50:** 159–172.

18. YAMAMURA, T., A. YAMAMOTO, S. NAMBU & K. HIRAMORI. 1984. Plasma apolipoprotein E mutants associated with atherosclerotic diseases. Arteriosclerosis **4:** 549a.
19. MAHLEY, R. W. & T. L. INNERARITY. 1983. Lipoprotein receptors and cholesterol homeostasis. Biochim. Biophys. Acta **737:** 197–222.
20. BROWN, M. S., P. T. KOVANEN & J. L. GOLDSTEIN. 1981. Regulation of plasma cholesterol by lipoprotein receptors. Science **212:** 628–635.
21. GOLDSTEIN, J. L. & M. S. BROWN. 1977. The low-density lipoprotein pathway and its relation to atherosclerosis. Annu. Rev. Biochem. **46:** 897–930.
22. HUI, D. Y., T. L. INNERARITY & R. W. MAHLEY. 1981. Lipoprotein binding to canine hepatic membranes. Metabolically distinct apo-E and apo-B,E receptors. J. Biol. Chem. **256:** 5646–5655.
23. MAHLEY, R. W., D. Y. HUI, T. L. INNERARITY & K. H. WEISGRABER. 1981. Two independent lipoprotein receptors on hepatic membranes of dog, swine, and man: Apo-B,E and apo-E receptors. J. Clin. Invest. **68:** 1197–1206.
24. HUI, D. Y., T. L. INNERARITY & R. W. MAHLEY. 1984. Defective hepatic lipoprotein receptor binding of β-very low density lipoproteins from type III hyperlipoproteinemic patients: Importance of apolipoprotein E. J. Biol. Chem. **259:** 860–869.
25. WEISGRABER, K. H., T. L. INNERARITY & R. W. MAHLEY. 1982. Abnormal lipoprotein receptor-binding activity of the human E apoprotein due to cysteine-arginine interchange at a single site. J. Biol. Chem. **257:** 2518–2521.
26. SCHNEIDER, W. J., P. T. KOVANEN, M. S. BROWN, J. L. GOLDSTEIN, G. UTERMANN, W. WEBER, R. J. HAVEL, L. KOTITE, J. P. KANE, T. L. INNERARITY & R. W. MAHLEY. 1981. Familial dysbetalipoproteinemia. Abnormal binding of mutant apoprotein E to low density lipoprotein receptors of human fibroblasts and membranes from liver and adrenal of rats, rabbits, and cows. J. Clin. Invest. **68:** 1075–1085.
27. HUI, D. Y., T. L. INNERARITY, R. W. MILNE, Y. L. MARCEL & R. W. MAHLEY. 1984. Binding of chylomicron remnants and β-very low density lipoproteins to hepatic and extrahepatic lipoprotein receptors: A process independent of apolipoprotein B48. J. Biol. Chem. **259:** 15060–15068.
28. MAHLEY, R. W. 1983. Apolipoprotein E and cholesterol metabolism. Klin. Wochenschr. **61:** 225–232.
29. MAHLEY, R. W., T. L. INNERARITY, R. E. PITAS, K. H. WEISGRABER, J. H. BROWN & E. GROSS. 1977. Inhibition of lipoprotein binding to cell surface receptors of fibroblasts following selective modification of arginyl residues in arginine-rich and B apoproteins. J. Biol. Chem. **252:** 7279–7287.
30. WEISGRABER, K. H., T. L. INNERARITY & R. W. MAHLEY. 1978. Role of lysine residues of plasma lipoproteins in high affinity binding to cell surface receptors on human fibroblasts. J. Biol. Chem. **253:** 9053–9062.
31. INNERARITY, T. L., E. J. FRIEDLANDER, S. C. RALL, JR., K. H. WEISGRABER & R. W. MAHLEY. 1983. The receptor-binding domain of human apolipoprotein E. Binding of apolipoprotein E fragments. J. Biol. Chem. **258:** 12341–12347.
32. WEISGRABER, K. H., T. L. INNERARITY, K. J. HARDER, R. W. MAHLEY, R. W. MILNE, Y. L. MARCEL & J. T. SPARROW. 1983. The receptor binding domain of human apolipoprotein E. Monoclonal antibody inhibition of binding. J. Biol. Chem. **258:** 12348–12354.
33. INNERARITY, T. L., K. H. WEISGRABER, K. S. ARNOLD, S. C. RALL, JR. & R. W. MAHLEY. 1984. Normalization of receptor binding of apolipoprotein E2. Evidence for modulation of the binding site conformation. J. Biol. Chem. **259:** 7261–7267.
34. FAINARU, M., R. W. MAHLEY, R. L. HAMILTON & T. L. INNERARITY. 1982. Structural and metabolic heterogeneity of β-very low density lipoproteins from cholesterol-fed dogs and from humans with type III hyperlipoproteinemia. J. Lipid Res. **23:** 702–714.
35. KANE, J. P., G. C. CHEN, R. L. HAMILTON, D. A. HARDMAN, M. J. MALLOY & R. J. HAVEL. 1983. Remnants of lipoproteins of intestinal and hepatic origin in familial dysbetalipoproteinemia. Arteriosclerosis **3:** 47–56.
36. RALL, S. C., JR., K. H. WEISGRABER, T. L. INNERARITY, R. W. MAHLEY & G. ASSMANN.

1983. Identical structural and receptor binding defects in apolipoprotein E2 in hypo-, normo-, and hypercholesterolemic dysbetalipoproteinemia. J. Clin. Invest. **71:** 1023–1031.

37. ANGELIN, B., C. A. RAVIOLA, T. L. INNERARITY & R. W. MAHLEY. 1983. Regulation of hepatic lipoprotein receptors in the dog. Rapid regulation of apolipoprotein B,E receptors, but not of apolipoprotein E receptors, by intestinal lipoproteins and bile acids. J. Clin. Invest. **71:** 816–831.
38. WINDLER, E. E., P. T. KOVANEN, Y-S. CHAO, M. S. BROWN, R. J. HAVEL & J. L. GOLDSTEIN. 1980. The estradiol-stimulated lipoprotein receptor of rat liver. A binding site that mediates the uptake of rat lipoproteins containing apoproteins B and E. J. Biol. Chem. **255:** 10464–10471.
39. KOVANEN, P. T., M. S. BROWN & J. L. GOLDSTEIN. 1979. Increased binding of low density lipoprotein to liver membranes from rats treated with 17 α-ethinyl estradiol. J. Biol. Chem. **254:** 11367–11373.
40. THOMPSON, G. R., A. K. SOUTAR, F. A. SPENGEL, A. JADHAV, S. J. P. GAVIGAN & N. B. MYANT. 1981. Defects of receptor-mediated low density lipoprotein catabolism in homozygous familial hypercholesterolemia and hypothyroidism *in vivo*. Proc. Natl. Acad. Sci. USA **78:** 2591–2595.
41. GRUNDY, S. M. 1982. Hypertriglyceridemia: Mechanisms, clinical significance, and treatment. Med. Clin. North Am. **66:** 519–535.
42. UTERMANN, G., N. PRUIN & A. STEINMETZ. 1979. Polymorphism of apolipoprotein E. III. Effect of a single polymorphic gene locus on plasma lipid levels in man. Clin. Genet. **15:** 63–72.
43. HAZZARD, W. R., G. R. WARNICK, G. UTERMANN & J. J. ALBERS. 1981. Genetic transmission of isoapolipoprotein E phenotypes in a large kindred: Relationship to dysbetalipoproteinemia and hyperlipidemia. Metabolism **30:** 79–88.
44. EHNHOLM, C., R. W. MAHLEY, D. A. CHAPPELL, K. H. WEISGRABER, E. LUDWIG & J. L. WITZTUM. 1984. The role of apolipoprotein E in the lipolytic conversion of β-very low density lipoproteins to low density lipoproteins in type III hyperlipoproteinemia. Proc. Natl. Acad. Sci. USA **81:** 5566–5570.
45. BERSOT, T. P., T. L. INNERARITY, R. W. MAHLEY & R. J. HAVEL. 1983. Cholesteryl ester accumulation in mouse peritoneal macrophages induced by β-migrating very low density lipoproteins from patients with atypical dysbetalipoproteinemia. J. Clin. Invest. **72:** 1024–1033.
46. MAHLEY, R. W. 1983. Development of accelerated atherosclerosis. Concepts derived from cell biology and animal model studies. Arch. Pathol. Lab. Med. **107:** 393–399.
47. MAHLEY, R. W. 1982. Atherogenic hyperlipoproteinemia. The cellular and molecular biology of plasma lipoproteins altered by dietary fat and cholesterol. Med. Clin. North Am. **66:** 375–402.
48. GOLDSTEIN, J. L., Y. K. HO, M. S. BROWN, T. L. INNERARITY & R. W. MAHLEY. 1980. Cholesteryl ester accumulation in macrophages resulting from receptor-mediated uptake and degradation of hypercholesterolemic canine β-very low density lipoproteins. J. Biol. Chem. **255:** 1839–1848.
49. MAHLEY, R. W., T. L. INNERARITY, M. S. BROWN, Y. K. HO & J. L. GOLDSTEIN. 1980. Cholesteryl ester synthesis in macrophages: Stimulation by β-very low density lipoproteins from cholesterol-fed animals of several species. J. Lipid Res. **21:** 970–980.
50. MAHLEY, R. W., T. L. INNERARITY, K. H. WEISGRABER & D. L. FRY. 1977. Canine hyperlipoproteinemia and atherosclerosis: Accumulation of lipid by aortic medial cells *in vivo* and *in vitro*. Am. J. Pathol. **87:** 205–226.
51. MAHLEY, R. W., A. W. NELSON, V. J. FERRANS & D. L. FRY. 1976. Thrombosis in association with atherosclerosis induced by dietary perturbations in dogs. Science **192:** 1139–1141.
52. FUNKE, H., J. BOYLES, K. H. WEISGRABER, E. H. LUDWIG, D. Y. HUI & R. W. MAHLEY. 1984. Uptake of apolipoprotein E-containing high density lipoproteins by hepatic parenchymal cells. Arteriosclerosis **4:** 452–461.
53. BARTER, P. J., G. J. HOPKINS & G. D. CALVERT. 1982. Transfers and exchanges of esterified cholesterol between plasma lipoproteins. Biochem. J. **208:** 1–7.

54. KLOER, H. U., G. WOLFBAUER & C. LULEY. 1983. Cholesterol ester transfer: Correlation with lipoproteins and apolipoproteins in hypertriglyceridemia. Arteriosclerosis **3:** 492a.
55. GORDON, V., T. L. INNERARITY & R. W. MAHLEY. 1983. Formation of cholesterol- and apoprotein E-enriched high density lipoproteins *in vitro*. J. Biol. Chem. **258:** 6202–6212.
56. BASU, S. K., M. S. BROWN, Y. K. HO, R. J. HAVEL & J. L. GOLDSTEIN. 1981. Mouse macrophages synthesize and secrete a protein resembling apolipoprotein E. Proc. Natl. Acad. Sci. USA **78:** 7545–7549.
57. ELSHOURBAGY, N. A., W. S. LIAO, R. W. MAHLEY & J. M. TAYLOR. 1985. Apolipoprotein E mRNA is abundant in the brain and adrenals, as well as the liver, and is present in other peripheral tissues of rats and marmosets. Proc. Natl. Acad. Sci. USA **82:** 203–207.
58. KOO, C., T. L. INNERARITY & R. W. MAHLEY. Obligatory role of cholesterol and apolipoprotein E in the formation of large cholesterol-enriched and receptor-active high density lipoproteins. J. Biol. Chem. In press.

Synthesis of Apolipoprotein E by Peripheral Tissues

Potential Functions in Reverse Cholesterol Transport and Cellular Cholesterol Metabolism[a]

DAVID L. WILLIAMS,[b] PAUL A. DAWSON,[b]
THOMAS C. NEWMAN,[b] AND LAWRENCE L. RUDEL[c]

[b]*Department of Pharmacological Sciences*
Health Sciences Center
State University of New York at Stony Brook
Stony Brook, New York 11794

[c]*Arteriosclerosis Research Center*
Bowman Gray School of Medicine
Wake Forest University
Winston-Salem, North Carolina 27103

INTRODUCTION

Apolipoprotein (apo) E is a major apolipoprotein found is plasma very low density lipoprotein (VLDL) and high density lipoprotein (HDL) subfractions. Apo E has been the subject of intensive research in recent years because of its participation in cholesterol metabolism and its potential importance for our understanding of atherosclerosis. A variety of studies indicate that apo E is intimately associated with the transport and metabolism of cholesterol. Apo E appears to play a major role in the process termed reverse cholesterol transport, which serves to move cholesterol from peripheral tissues to the liver for metabolism and elimination. Apo E appears to function in reverse cholesterol transport as a recognition signal for the hepatic removal of chylomicron remnants and cholesterol-laden HDL subfractions from the circulation.[1–4] *In vitro* studies show that apo E is responsible for the binding of cholesteryl ester enriched lipoproteins to receptors on liver membranes.[5,6] Similarly, the rapid hepatic clearance of such particles in liver perfusion experiments is mediated by apo E.[2–4] This activity of apo E may be important in preventing the accumulation of cholesterol and cholesteryl esters in the aorta and coronary arteries as occurs in atherosclerosis.

Genetic evidence also links apo E to atherosclerosis and reverse cholesterol transport. Type III hyperlipoproteinemia, a human disease associated with premature atherosclerosis,[7] is characterized by an accumulation in plasma of cholesteryl ester-enriched β-VLDL resulting from an impaired hepatic clearance of remnant particles.[8,9] Homozygosity for the ϵ 2 allele of apo E is strongly associated with type III hyperlipoproteinemia.[10] Analysis of the amino acid sequence of the major apo E alleles showed that the ϵ 2 allele codes for a polypeptide containing cysteine instead of

[a]This work was supported by American Heart Association grant no. 83–849 (DLW), and NIH grant nos. AM–18171 (DLW) and HL–14164 (LLR).

arginine at residue 158.[11] This amino acid change occurs in the receptor binding domain of apo E and is responsible for the reduced binding of β-VLDL to hepatic apo E receptors and apo B/E receptors on fibroblasts.[12,13] When apo E encoded by a normal allele was added to β-VLDL, receptor binding activity was greatly increased.[13] In addition to the effects of a mutant apo E, the absence of detectable apo E also is associated with type III hyperlipoproteinemia and elevated chylomicron remnants.[14] These findings indicate that apo E is an important factor in the removal of cholesterol-enriched lipoproteins from the circulation.

The plasma concentration of apo E appears to be under dietary and hormonal regulation. Plasma apo E is elevated in hyperlipidemic patients.[15] Studies with the rat have shown that the plasma concentration of apo E is increased in the hyperlipidemia associated with hypothyroidism.[16] Dietary cholesterol also is known to increase the apo E associated with cholesterol-rich lipoproteins in man and experimental animals.[17–21] However, little is known about the regulatory mechanisms through which these changes occur.

PERIPHERAL SYNTHESIS OF APO E

The liver and small intestine are generally thought to be the major, if not sole, sites of lipoprotein synthesis in man and experimental animals. However, we have recently shown that apo E is synthesized by human kidney and adrenal gland in addition to the liver.[21] Mouse peritoneal macrophages and human peripheral blood monocytes also synthesize and secrete apo E.[22,23] Characterization of the apo E synthesized by human kidney and adrenal tissue indicated that peripheral apo E was indistinguishable from hepatic apo E, as judged by its electrophoretic mobility in sodium dodecyl sulfate (SDS)-polyacrylamide gels and its isoform pattern upon high resolution two-dimensional gel analysis.[21] The relative rates of apo E synthesis in kidney and adrenal tissue were 0.15–1.2% of total protein synthesis, indicating that apo E is a moderately abundant protein product of these tissues. These findings raised the possibilities that apo E is made in many peripheral tissues and that peripheral apo E plays an important role in cholesterol metabolism.

Experiments have now been carried out to determine the distribution of apo E synthesis among peripheral tissues. These studies employed two species of nonhuman primate, the African green monkey (*Cercopithecus aethiops*) and the cynomolgus monkey (*Macaca fascicularis*), which are susceptible to atherosclerosis when fed an atherogenic diet.[24,25] After short-term organ culture with radiolabeled amino acids, extracts of liver and various peripheral tissues were screened with antiserum specific to apo E, and the immunoprecipitated proteins were analyzed by SDS-polyacrylamide gel electrophoresis and fluorography.[21] As shown in FIGURE 1 (lane 6), newly synthesized apo E was readily detected in the anti-apo E immunoprecipitate of liver proteins after *in vitro* incubation of liver slices with [^{35}S]methionine. The apo E band was also seen with antiserum directed against HDL proteins (lane 4), but was not detected with nonimmune goat serum (lane 5). Similar experiments showed that lung (lane 3), kidney (lane 9), and adrenal (data not shown) also synthesized apo E, while apo E synthesis was not detected in the mucosa of the small intestine. Measurement of the radioactivity in the apo E band showed that the relative rates of apo E synthesis were: liver 0.22%, kidney 0.14%, adrenal 0.10%, and lung 0.21%. In other experiments with cynomolgus monkeys (not shown), apo E synthesis also was detected in spleen, mesenteric lymph node, and testis, in addition to the above tissues. Thus, apo E is a moderately abundant product of numerous peripheral tissues.

Peripheral apo E was further characterized by high resolution two-dimensional gel analysis.[21] For this purpose, an anti-apo E immunoprecipitate of newly synthesized testis proteins of a cynomolgus monkey was mixed with purified plasma apo E prior to analysis. The staining pattern (FIGURE 2) showed plasma apo E to consist of two major isoforms with pIs of 5.97 and 5.91. The fluorogram of newly synthesized testis apo E also showed two isoforms with the same charge properties as plasma apo E, indicating apparent identity between these species . Further analysis with newly synthesized proteins from liver, lymph node, adrenal, spleen, and lung (data not shown) showed

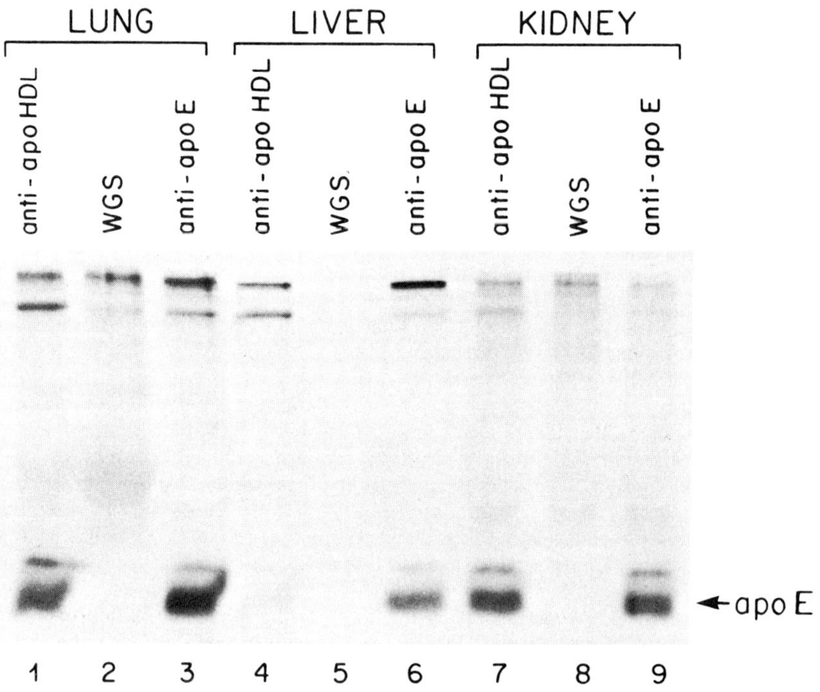

FIGURE 1. Apo E synthesis in peripheral tissues. Tissue slices from the indicated tissues of the African green monkey were incubated in short-term organ culture with [^{35}S]methionine, and tissue extracts were immunoprecipitated with anti-apo HDL (lanes 1, 4, and 7), preimmune serum (WGS) (lanes 2, 5, and 8), or anti-apo E (lanes 3, 6, and 9) as described.[21] Immunoprecipitates were analyzed by SDS–10% polyacrylamide gel electrophoresis and fluorography. The arrow indicates the mobility of plasma apo E.

that the apo E species made in the liver and peripheral tissues were indistinguishable.

Since apo E is made by numerous peripheral tissues *in vitro* at high relative rates, it seems likely that significant amounts of apo E are produced by peripheral tissues and may be quantitatively important in cholesterol transport. In order to estimate the absolute synthesis of apo E in the liver and peripheral tissues, we developed a DNA-excess solution hybridization assay to quantitate absolute amounts of apo E mRNA. This measurement should establish the potential for apo E synthesis and,

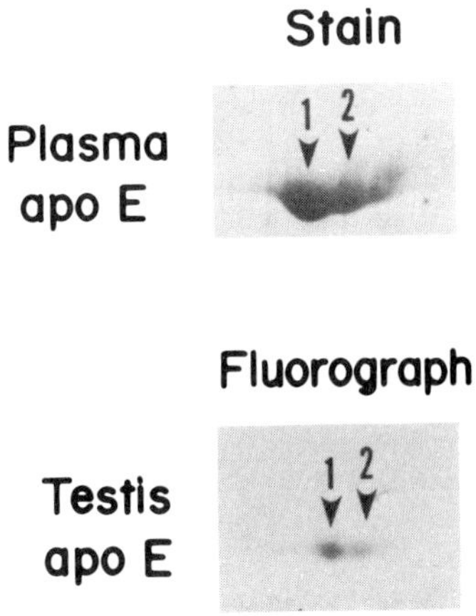

FIGURE 2. Two-dimensional gel analysis of peripheral apo E. After short-term organ culture of testis slices with [^{35}S]methionine, a tissue extract was immunoprecipitated with anti-apo E.[21] The washed immunoprecipitate was mixed with purified plasma apo E and subjected to high resolution two-dimensional gel analysis.[21] The upper panel shows the Coomassie blue staining pattern of plasma apo E. The lower panel shows the fluorogram of the newly synthesized testis apo E. Both samples show two major isoforms with pIs of 5.97 and 5.91. The isoelectricfocusing dimension was run from left to right with the basic end to the left. The SDS–10% polyacrylamide gel electrophoresis dimension was run from top to bottom.

assuming that apo E is not under regulation at the translational level, an estimate of the absolute rate of apo E synthesis in various tissues. The hybridization assay[26] employs a single stranded probe prepared from the human apo E cDNA clone isolated by Breslow *et al.*[27] TABLE 1 shows the results of measurements of apo E mRNA in various tissues of a male cynomolgus monkey. When expressed on the basis of total RNA (column A), apo E mRNA was more abundant in the adrenal than the liver. Apo E mRNA in the mesenteric lymph node was about the same as the liver, while values in thymus, spleen, kidney, testis, and brain ranged from 25–60% of the liver value. The apo E mRNA content of muscle RNA was considerably less.

By determining the contents of total RNA and DNA in these tissues, the apo E mRNA values may be expressed on the basis of mRNA molecules/cell. These data (TABLE 1, column B) show that the cellular content of apo E mRNA is the highest in liver, brain, and adrenal, while most other tissues have 10–20% as much apo E mRNA as the liver. Thus, while there are significant differences in the apo E mRNA contents

TABLE 1. Apo E mRNA in Liver and Peripheral Tissues

Tissue	A Apo E mRNA[b] pg/μg RNA	B Apo E mRNA molecules/cell	C Apo E mRNA μg/organ
Liver	20.8 ± 1.7	540	10.2
Adrenal	33.6 ± 6.3	480	0.07[a]
Testis	12.1 ± 0.6	110	0.04[a]
Brain	10.6 ± 0.5	430	1.6
Spleen	10.2 ± 0.2	42	0.45
Kidney	6.8 ± 0.3	84	0.4[a]
Thymus	5.0 ± 0.3	15	0.07
Lymph node	19.5 ± 0.3	86	—
Skeletal muscle	0.5 ± 0.1	44	1.9

[a]Value shown is for both organs.

[b]Apo E mRNA was measured in total RNA extracted from the indicated cynomolgus monkey tissues with a DNA-excess solution hybridization assay.[26] All values are from a single animal. Each value is the mean ± S.D. of 8–12 determinations.

of various tissues, the important point is that most tissues contain substantial amounts of this mRNA and would be expected to synthesize apo E at cellular rates comparable to the liver. These data are in agreement with the relative rates of apo E synthesis in human adrenal and kidney,[21] as well as those cited above for various peripheral tissues of nonhuman primates.

The total content of apo E mRNA per organ may also be determined from these data using the organ weights as measured at necropsy. As shown in TABLE 1 (Column C), most of the apo E mRNA is present in the liver. However, summation of the apo E mRNA in all tissues indicates that approximately 30% of total apo E mRNA was present in extrahepatic tissues. Since all tissues were not measured, this is likely to be a minimal estimate. Measurements made on other cynomolgus and African green monkey tissues showed that 20–40% of the apo E mRNA was extrahepatic (data not shown). These values indicate that peripheral tissues have the potential to contribute a significant fraction of plasma apo E. In addition, the magnitude of apo E synthesis and the apo E mRNA content of peripheral tissues argues strongly that apo E synthesis is a property of many cell types and is not limited to tissue macrophages. However, the identity of peripheral cell types responsible for apo E synthesis remains to be established.

POTENTIAL FUNCTIONS OF PERIPHERAL APO E

The functional significance of peripheral apo E synthesis is not yet known. Since our understanding of apo E is mainly focused on its role as a recognition signal for the hepatic uptake of cholesteryl ester-enriched lipoproteins, potential roles for peripheral apo E in reverse cholesterol transport may be suggested. FIGURE 3 illustrates a scheme in which apo E is secreted from a peripheral cell either associated or unassociated with the release of cholesterol from the cell. The latter possibility seems more likely since apo E secretion and cholesterol release do not appear to be coupled in cultured macrophages.[28] The secreted apo E within the interstitial fluid could associate with acceptor lipoproteins, which serve to remove cholesterol from cells[29] and target these

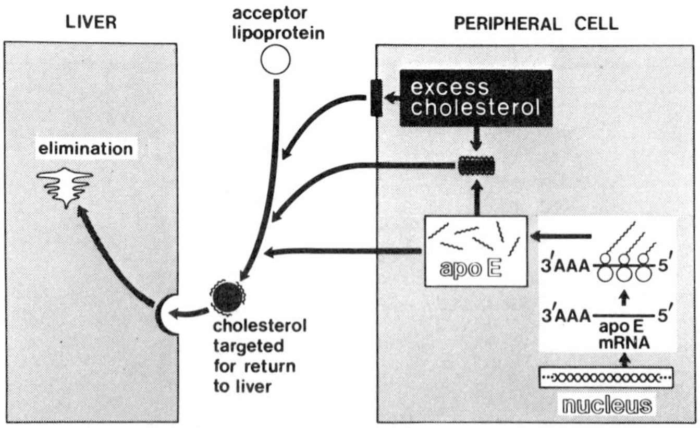

FIGURE 3. Potential role of peripheral apo E in reverse cholesterol transport. The model is described in the text.

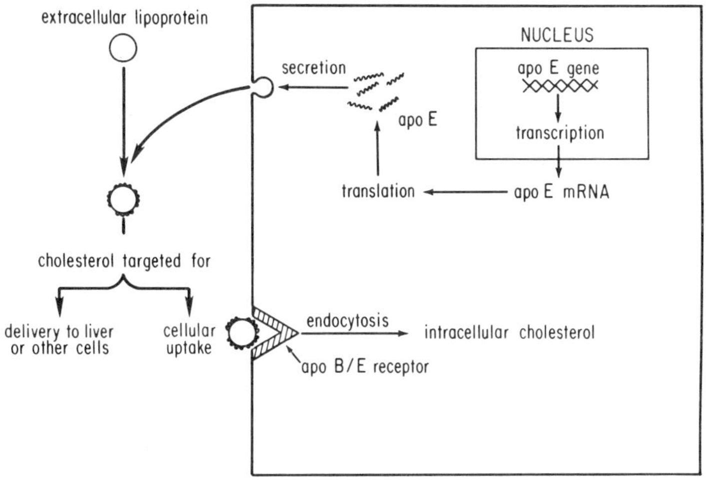

FIGURE 4. Potential role of peripheral apo E to capture lipoprotein cholesterol for peripheral cells. The model is described in the text.

particles for eventual hepatic uptake. Consistent with this possibility are the recent demonstrations that peripheral lymph contains lipoprotein particles enriched in free cholesterol and apo E as compared to their plasma counterparts.[30,31] Such particles might represent initial or early stages of the reverse cholesterol transport pathway in which the apo E has been derived from synthesis in peripheral tissues.

One difficulty with this scheme (FIGURE 3) is that apo E does not appear to be limiting in the plasma compartment. Thus, one would anticipate that an acceptor lipoprotein would acquire apo E once it reached the plasma compartment irrespective of apo E production in peripheral tissues. One may also speculate that peripheral apo E has local functions in addition to, or other than, reverse cholesterol transport. FIGURE 4 illustrates a scheme in which peripheral apo E acts to capture cholesterol for peripheral cells. In this case, secreted apo E associates with an extracellular lipoprotein to target this particle for cellular uptake by the apo B/E receptor. This mechanism could act to facilitate cholesterol uptake in tissues such as the adrenal and testis, which have a major requirement for lipoprotein cholesterol for steroid hormones production.[32] Interestingly, the adrenal gland and testis have high levels of apo E synthesis and apo E mRNA. Also shown in FIGURE 4, is the possibility of the lipoprotein being targeted for delivery to the liver or to other peripheral cells. This situation could occur if the cell did not require cholesterol and the apo B/E receptors were down regulated.[33] When formulated in this fashion (FIGURE 4), peripheral apo E serves simply as a ligand to target lipoprotein cholesterol for uptake by whichever cells are expressing apo B/E receptors.

These speculations (FIGURES 3 and 4) emphasize that we know little about the significance or regulation of apo E synthesis in peripheral tissues. The measurements of apo E synthesis and apo E mRNA suggest that peripheral apo E may play a quantitatively important role in cholesterol transport. The important task is to elucidate the functional nature of peripheral apo E synthesis at it relates to reverse cholesterol transport, cellular cholesterol metabolism, and atherosclerosis.

ACKNOWLEDGMENTS

We are grateful to Dr. Jan Breslow for providing the apo E cDNA clone. We also thank Penelope Strockbine and Ramesh Shah for excellent technical assistance. The valuable assistance given by Dr. Christopher Jerome in necropsy of the animals is gratefully acknowledged. Paul Dawson is a trainee in Pharmacological Sciences (NIH GM 07518).

REFERENCES

1. MAHLEY, R. W. & T. L. INNERARITY. 1983. Biochim. Biophys Acta **737: 197–222.**
2. SHERRILL, B. C., T. L. INNERARITY & R. W. MAHLEY. 1980. J. Biol. Chem. **255:** 1804–1807.
3. SHELBURNE, F., J. HANKS, W. MEYERS & S. QUARFORDT. 1980. J. Clin. Invest. **65:** 652–658.
4. WINDLER, E., Y-S. CHAO & R. J. HAVEL. 1980. J. Biol. Chem. **255:** 5475–5480.
5. HUI, D. Y., T. L. INNERARITY & R. W. MAHLEY. 1981. J. Biol. Chem. **256:** 5646–5655.
6. MAHLEY, R. W., D. Y. HUI, T. L. INNERARITY & K. H. WEISGRABER. J. Clin. Invest. **68:** 1197–1206.
7. MORGANROTH, J., R. I. LEVY & D. S. FREDRICKSON. 1975. Ann. Intern. Med. **82:** 158–174.
8. SCHNEIDER, W. J., P. T. KOVANEN, M. S. BROWN, J. L. GOLDSTEIN, G. UTERMANN, W. WEBER, R. J. HAVEL, L. KOTITE, J. P. KANE, T. L. INNERARITY & R. W. MAHLEY. 1981. J. Clin. Invest. **68:** 1075–1085.
9. GREGG, R. E., L. A. ZECH, E. J. SCHAEFER & H. B. BREWER, JR. 1981. Science **211:** 584–586.
10. ZANNIS, V. I. & J. L. BRESLOW. 1980. J. Biol. Chem. **255:** 1759–1762.
11. RALL, S. C., JR., K. H. WEISGRABER & R. W. MAHLEY. J. Biol. Chem. **257:** 4171–4179.
12. RALL, S. C., JR, K. H. WEISGRABER, T. L. INNERARITY & R. W. MAHLEY. 1982. Proc. Natl. Acad. Sci. USA **79:** 4696–4700.
13. HUI, D. Y., T. L. INNERARITY & R. W. MAHLEY. 1984. J. Biol. Chem. **259:** 860–869.
14. GHISELLI, G., E. J. SCHAEFER, P. GASCON & H. B. BREWER, JR. 1981. Science **214 :**1239–1241.
15. BLUM, C. B., L. ARON & R. SCIACCA. 1980. J. Clin. Invest. **66:** 1240–1250.
16. DORY, L. & P. S. ROHEIM. 1981. J. Lipid Res. **22:** 287–296.
17. MAHLEY, R. W., K. H. WEISGRABER & T. INNERARITY. 1976. Biochemistry **15:** 2979–2985.
18. MAHLEY, R. W. & K. H. WEISGRABER. 1974. Circ. Res. **35:** 722–733.
19. MAHLEY, R. W., K. H. WEISGRABER, T. INNERARITY & H. B. BREWER. 1975. Biochemistry **14:** 2817–2823.
20. MAHLEY, R. W., T. INNERARITY, T. P. BERSOT, A. LIPSON & S. MARGOLIS. 1978. Lancet **ii:** 807–809.
21. BLUE, M-L., D. L. WILLIAMS, S. ZUCKER, S. A. KHAN & C. B. BLUM. 1983. Proc. Natl. Acad. Sci. USA **80:** 283–287.
22. BASU, S. K., M. S. BROWN, Y. K. HO, R. J. HAVEL & J. L. GOLDSTEIN. 1981. Proc. Natl. Acad. Sci. USA **78:** 7545-7549.
23. BASU, S. K., Y. K. HO, M. S. BROWN, D. W. BILHEIMER, R. G. W. ANDERSON & J. L. GOLDSTEIN. 1982. J. Biol. Chem. **257:** 9788–9795.
24. ARMSTRONG, M. L. 1976. *In* Primates in Medicine, vol. 9. E. I. Goldsmith & J. Moor-Jankowski, Eds.: 16–40. S. Karger. Basel.
25. KRAMSCH, D. M. & W. HOLLANDER. 1968. Exp. Mol. Pathol. **9:** 1–22.
26. WILLIAMS, D. L., T. C. NEWMAN, G. S. SHELNESS & D. A. GORDON. 1984. Methods Enzymol. In press.
27. BRESLOW, J. L., J. MCPHERSON, A. L. NUSSBAUM, H. W. WILLIAMS, F. LOFQUIST-KAHL, S. K. KARATHANASIS & V. I. ZANNIS, 1982. J. Biol. Chem. **257:** 14639–14641.

28. Basu, S. K., J. L. Goldstein & M. S. Brown. 1983. Science **219:** 871–873.
29. Fielding, C. J. & P. E. Fieldings. 1981. Proc. Natl. Acad. Sci. USA **78:** 3911–3914.
30. Forte, T. M., C. E. Cross, R. A. Gunther & G. C. Kramer. 1983. J. Lipid Res. **24:** 1358–1367.
31. Sloop, C. H., L. Dory, R. Hamilton, B. R. Krause & P. S. Roheim. 1983. J. Lipid Res. **24:** 1429–1440.
32. Brown, M. S., P. T. Kovanen & J. L. Goldstein. 1979. Recent Prog. Horm. Res. **35:** 215–249.
33. Goldstein, J. L. & M. S. Brown. 1977. Annu. Rev. Biochem. **46:** 897–930.

The Association of Serum Lipids, Lipoproteins, and Apolipoproteins with Coronary Artery Disease Assessed by Coronary Arteriography

HERBERT K. NAITO

Section of Lipids, Nutrition, and Metabolic Diseases
The Department of Biochemistry
Division of Laboratory Medicine
The Cleveland Clinic Foundation
Cleveland, Ohio 44106

There is little doubt that serum lipids and lipoproteins are intimately involved in atherogenesis. Epidemiological, clinical, and animal experimental research have clearly demonstrated a positive association between serum total cholesterol (TC) concentrations and coronary artery disease (CAD). However, measurements of lipoprotein lipids and lipoprotein proteins (apoproteins) appear to enhance the assessment of CAD risk. For example, the measurements of low-density lipoprotein (LDL) as LDL-Cholesterol and high-density lipoprotein (HDL) as HDL-Cholesterol show a better statistical correlation with coronary atherosclerosis than either TC or triglycerides (TG) alone.[1–4] Furthermore, expression of the lipoprotein lipids as ratios (i.e., LDL-C/TC, HDL-C/TC, or LDLC/HDL-C) appears to increase the statistical relationship with the severity and extent of CAD even more.[5,6] Recent studies on serum total apoprotein and lipoprotein protein measurements are beginning to suggest that, they too, are sensitive markers for the assessment of CAD risk[1,7–12] and even for peripheral vascular disease.[13] Finally, partitioning the major lipoprotein classes into LDL_1 and LDL_2, or HDL_2 and HDL_3, increases their sensitivity, specificity, and hence, their predictive value.[14–16] To answer some of these questions, we did a double-blind study whereby we simultaneously examined the relationship of serum lipids (TC and TG), lipoprotein lipids (HDL-phospholipid, HDL-cholesterol, HDL-triglycerides), and lipoprotein proteins (HDL-apo A) with the severity of coronary atherosclerosis. Part of this data has already been published elsewhere.[6,16] The HDL subfraction data and apolipoprotein data are new.

METHODS

Two-hundred and twenty-six male subjects who had a cardiac workup performed (including cineangiography) at The Cleveland Clinic Foundation were sequentially selected for our study. Multiple fasting (>12 hours) blood samples were drawn before the day of catheterization and were immediately used for serum lipid and lipoprotein determinations in the Lipid-Lipoprotein Laboratory, which is standardized and certified by the Center for Disease Control. The procedures are described in detail elsewhere.[6] In brief, TC, TG, phospholipid (P), and agarose lipoprotein electrophoreses were done on the serum. Lipid analyses were performed on the HDL and LDL fractions according to the procedures described in the Manual of Laboratory Operations, Lipid Research Clinic Program.[17] HDL subfractions (HDL_2-cholesterol and HDL_3-cholesterol) were quantitated according to the method of Warnick *et al.*,[18] with modifications.[19] The apo B, apo A, and A–I were done by electroimmunoassay according to the Laurell method[20] with modifications.[21] Apo A–II was obtained by subtracting the difference between apo A and A–I concentrations. No serum samples were used for analyses if the collection was made within three months of a myocardial event, and no data was used if the lapse between catheterization and biochemical analyses were greater than one year.

At the time of catheterization, detailed histories were taken of each patient and stored in the Department of Cardiology's Cardiovascular Information Registry computer bank. The cinecoronary arteriography method of Sones and Shirey[22] was used. Twenty-six preselected sites of the three coronary arteries and the left main trunk were graded for degree of coronary stenosis, i.e., percent obstruction. Statistical calculations were carried out using the BCP (Biomedical Computer Programs) developed by the Health Sciences Computing Facility, Department of Biomathematics, School of Medicine, University of California (Los Angeles, CA), and run on our Burroughs 4700 computer, as well as the PROPHET (NIH funded and developed by Bolt, Beraneck, and Newman Corp., Cambridge, MA.) time-sharing computer system. The PROPHET system was primarily used for analysis of variance and covariance, for Kruskal-Wallis non-parametric analysis of variance, and for correlation analysis. The receiver operating characteristic (ROC) analyses were done using a Fortran program supplied by Dr. Charles Metz at the University of Chicago.

RESULTS

For the sake of obtaining mean values for the patients in our study, we first arbitrarily categorized the subjects into four groups, based on the degree of coronary stenosis: Group I (controls): No lesions whatsoever in any of the coronary arteries; Group II (mild): Between 1–50% obstruction; Group III (moderate-severe): 51–99% occlusion; and, Group IV (severe): 100% occlusion with any of the 26 preselected sites in the coronary arteries evaluated. TABLE 1 contains some demographic and clinical data on the subjects. Of the 226 subjects, 21 had no coronary lesions whatsoever, and were thus, included in the "control" group (Gr I). It must be emphasized that while all of the individuals in this group had no vascular lesions, some had vascular lesions or calcification. In order to minimize the complication of scoring the severity of coronary lesions, we used the most severely occluded coronary artery as the end point for classification. This data (TABLE 1) suggest that no statistically significant differences were found between the four groups, with respect to the number of individuals with a family history of premature CHD, high blood pressure (>140/90 mm Hg), smoking (number of cigarettes/day), obesity (>10% over ideal body weight), diabetes mellitus (abnormal glucose tolerance test), and thyroid dysfunction (abnormal serum T_4, T_3 levels). Only the control group (n = 21) had a lower number of individuals who were considered obese as compared to groups II, III, and IV. Thus, the four groups were virtually homogeneous.

Group II (n = 33) had an average percent occlusion of the coronary arteries of 22.3%, while groups III (n = 68) and IV (n = 104) had 89.3% and 100%, respectively.

Based on the above classification, a one-way analysis of variance for comparing group mean values showed that TC, TG, LDL-C, HDL-C, HDL-TG, LDL-C/TC, and LDL-C/HDLC-C were not statistically significant at the 95% confidence level (see

TABLE 1. Demographic and Clinical Data ($\overline{X} \pm 1$ S.D.)

	Degree of Coronary Stenosis				
Parameters	0%	1–50%	51–99%	100%	
Group	I	II	III	IV	Statistics[a]
Degree of obstruction (%)	0 ± 14.2	22.3 ± 9.6	89.3 ± 0.0	100.0	
Age at cath. (years)	50.6 ± 8.5	51.6 ± 9.1	52.7 ± 7.3	53.1 ± 8.9	$p > 0.50$
Family history for CHD (%)	59	35	59	58	$p = 0.40$
Blood pressure					
Systolic (mm Hg)	128.1 ± 15.9	131.3 ± 22.8	135.3 ± 16.5	133.1 ± 19.3	$p > 0.3$
Diastolic (mm Hg)	82.2 ± 9.9	85.1 ± 13.5	84.1 ± 8.5	84.3 ± 10.4	$p > 0.5$
Hypertensive (%)	29	45	40	41	$p = 0.66$
Cigarette smoking (%)	57	31	55	55	$p = 0.40$
Obese (%)	5[b]	9	12	17	$p = 0.81$
Thyroid dysfunction (%)	0	0	3	1	$p = 0.90$

[a]Overall chi-square.

[b]$p < 0.05$ using simultaneous testing for equality of class proportions between multinomial populations.[26]

TABLE 2). While the HDL-P/TC ratio was highly significant ($p < 0.002$), HDL-C/TC ($p < 0.01$), LDL-C/HDL-P ($p < 0.02$), and HDL-P ($p < 0.02$) were also statistically significant, but to a lesser degree than HDL-P/TC. Since the majority of the phospholipid is generally carried in HDL, it is likely that HDL-P measurements more accurately reflect HDL as a whole, which appears to be a better biochemical marker for CAD risk assessment.

Since the publication of the original data,[6,16] we went back and randomly selected ten frozen samples (−80°C) from each of the four groups, and analyzed the serum HDL_2-cholesterol, HDL_3-cholesterol, apo A, apo A–I, apo A–II, and apo B concentrations, which are shown in TABLE 3. The new data, while only preliminary, suggest that HDL_2-cholesterol, apo A–I, and apo B, but not HDL_3-cholesterol or apo A–II, are highly correlated ($p = 0.001$) with the degree of coronary artery stenosis. TABLE 4 clearly illustrates that the correlation coefficient data suggest that the best associations with coronary artery stenosis are found with the HDL subfractions or apoproteins A–I or B, and this is particularly emphasized when the biochemical parameters are expressed as ratios. The association of HDL_2-Cholesterol/HDL_3-Cholesterol or HDL_2-Cholesterol/HDL-Cholesterol ratios with CAD correlates better with the degree of coronary stenosis by a factor of fivefold when compared to HDL-cholesterol, or threefold when compared to the HDL-Cholesterol/Total Cholesterol ratio, which was once believed to be one of the best lipoprotein lipid biochemical markers for the assessment of CHD risk.[1,16] The best correlation was found with HDL_2-C/HDL-C ($r = -0.67$, $p < 0.001$) and Apo A–I/Apo B ($r = 0.62$, $p < 0.0001$). The ROC curves suggest that statistically the two ratios were not different from each other. No correlation was found with VLDL-cholesterol ($r = 0.02, p = 0.86$), HDL_3-C ($r = 0.02$, $p = 80$), Apo A–II ($r = 0.03$, $p = 0.50$), HDL-triglycerides ($r = 0.09$, $p = 0.18$), triglycerides ($r = 0.11$, $p = 0.21$), or surprisingly, LDL-C/TC (where $r = 0.09$, $p = 0.17$), with the severity of coronary stenosis.

Our data is in agreement with other investigators who found that patients with myocardial infarction (MI) had comparatively low levels of Apo A–I or HDL_2, and/or had high apo B levels. Avogaro *et al.*[2,37,11,12] have reported that Apo A–I and B, and in particular their ratio, is more powerful than lipid measurements by themselves or lipoprotein lipids in discriminating ischemic heart disease (IHD) cases from non-cases. Desager *et al.*,[10] like other investigators,[4,8] found that LDL-C and apo B values were highly correlated with the severity of coronary vascular disease (CVD). In addition, they, as well as others, stated that HDL-C is more closely correlated to the severity of CVD, and that HDL-C alone[23] or in combination with LDL-C[4,8,24] maintained a highly predictive value for CVD. While, Avogaro[25] reported that 91% of MI survivors have been correctly classified by the calculation of the Apo A–I/Apo B ratio, Dresager *et al.*[10] found it particularly difficult to predict the one-vessel CVD using this ratio. They concluded from their study of 317 patients that apo A–I and B, as measured in the plasma of patients undergoing coronary angiography, contributed to a better discrimination of the CVD, but did not allow better predictive value to the lipid fraction with regard to the CVD. Using a cutoff point of 0.545, we obtained a sensitivity of 89% and a specificity of 93% for HDL_2-C/HDL_3-C ratio. For the HDL_2-C/HDL-C ratio, we obtained a sensitivity and specificity of 90% and 93%, respectively. Using a cutoff point of 1.325, the Apo A–I/Apo B ratio had a 87% sensitivity and 80% specificity. In contrast, total cholesterol (using a cutoff point of 224 mg/dl) had a sensitivity and specificity of 63% and 67%, respectively. Using a cutoff point of 0.194, the HDL-C/TC had a sensitivity of 71% and specificity of 87%. Thus, our data suggest that the HDL-subfractions have a higher sensitivity and specificity, especially when expressed as a ratio, i.e., HDL_2-C/HDL_3-C or as HDL_2-C/HDL-C, than serum apo A–I/apo B

TABLE 2. Serum and Lipoprotein Data on the 226 Subjects Undergoing Cineangiographic Analysis ($\overline{X} \pm 1$ S.D.)

Parameters	Degree of Coronary Obstruction 0%	1–50%	50–99%	100%	Statistics[a]
Total Cholesterol (mg/dl)	252.8 ± 8.0	257.9 ± 49.1	274.9 ± 56.2	268.3 ± 49.9	$p = 0.24$
Triglycerides (mg/dl)	144.8 ± 60.4	181.6 ± 108.5	174.3 ± 78.3	186.3 ± 43.7	$p = 0.19$
LDL-Cholesterol (mg/dl)	167.2 ± 38.1	170.8 ± 38.4	187.9 ± 38.8	193.8 ± 43.7	$p = 0.08$
HDL-Cholesterol (mg/dl)	51.1 ± 18.1	49.3 ± 14.4	46.8 ± 11.7	44.9 ± 11.7	$p = 0.13$
HDL-Phospholipid (mg/dl)	111.4 ± 30.6	104.0 ± 22.0	98.2 ± 21.0	95.9 ± 22.6	$p = 0.02$
HDK-Triglycerides (mg/dl)	14.8 ± 8.2	12.2 ± 6.6	14.2 ± 7.1	14.9 ± 9.5	$p = 0.41$
$\frac{\text{LDL-C}}{\text{TC}}$	0.661 ± 0.078	0.663 ± 0.094	0.686 ± 0.070	0.682 ± 0.065	$p = 0.29$
$\frac{\text{HDL-C}}{\text{TC}}$	0.205 ± 0.061	0.198 ± 0.071	0.176 ± 0.050	0.171 ± 0.047	$p = 0.01$
$\frac{\text{HDL-P}}{\text{TC}}$	0.451 ± 0.124	0.416 ± 0.115	0.370 ± 0.102	0.367 ± 0.099	$p = 0.002$
$\frac{\text{LDL-C}}{\text{HDL-C}}$	3.61 ± 1.47	3.79 ± 1.50	4.26 ± 1.41	4.32 ± 1.42	$p = 0.08$
$\frac{\text{LDL-C}}{\text{HDL-P}}$	1.61 ± 0.62	1.73 ± 0.58	2.02 ± 0.68	2.03 ± 0.76	$p = 0.02$

[a]Analysis of variance.

ratio. The HDL subfraction values are slightly (but not statistically) better than the Apo A–I/Apo B ratio.

Studies by Miller *et al.*[14,15] suggest that the HDL_2 subfraction concentration was more markedly reduced than the HDL_3 concentration in patients with angiographically documented CHD. In our study, the HDL_3-C did not change in concentration with the increasing severity of the coronary artery stenosis. On the other hand, HDL_2-C decreased 42.8% when compared to controls. It is interesting to note that the HDL-protein (i.e., HDL-apo A) was also highly correlated ($r = 0.51, p < 0.001$) with the degree of coronary artery stenosis (See TABLE 3 and 4). This lipoprotein-protein parameter had a correlation value similar to HDL_2-C and serum apo A–I. It would have been interesting to see the comparison with LDL-apo B, which we did not do. Sniderman and Kwiterovich[26] postulated that hyperapobetalipoproteinemia is of particular importance in normolipidemic individuals prone to premature CHD. In their study, they found that the group with significant CAD (>50% stenosis of at least one major coronary artery) had a mean plasma LDL apo B level of 118 ± 22 mg/dl, which was significantly higher than that of 82 ± 15 mg/dl in the patients without CAD as determined by coronary angiography. While the mean plasma levels of total cholesterol, triglycerides, and LDL cholesterol in the group with CAD were also higher

TABLE 3. Serum High-Density Lipoprotein Subfractions and Apolipoprotein Levels of Patients Undergoing Cineangiography ($\bar{X}$ ± 1 S.D.)[a]

Parameters (mg/dl)	Group I	Group II	Group III	Group IV	Statistics[b]
HDL_2-C	21 ± 4	17 ± 6	16 ± 6	12 ± 4	$p = 0.001$
HDL_3-C	30 ± 5	32 ± 6	31 ± 5	33 ± 5	$p = 0.7$
HDL-Apo A	192 ± 31	160 ± 16	147 ± 25	145 ± 24	$p = 0.001$
Apo A–I	161 ± 30	150 ± 34	125 ± 30	118 ± 24	$p = 0.001$
Apo A–II	42 ± 7	40 ± 6	46 ± 6	43 ± 9	$p = 0.1$
Apo B	107 ± 25	116 ± 24	129 ± 20	137 ± 26	$p = 0.001$

[a]n = 10 patients per group.
[b]Analysis of variance.

than in those free of disease, results of stepwise discriminant function analyses indicted that the plasma LDL apo B separated those with disease from those without disease significantly better than the other variables. In the same study, plasma LDL apo B levels were also measured in forty patients with primary type IIa hyperlipoproteinemia, most of whom were judged to be heterozygous for FH based on the presence of tendon xanthomas or family studies. When the plasma LDL apo B level was plotted, many subjects with CAD had plasma LDL apo B concentrations as high as those with FH, but their LDL-cholesterol level (mean 134 mg/100 ml) was considerably lower than that of the FH subjects (mean 250 mg/100 ml). The average ratio of LDL-cholesterol to LDL apo B in FH was 1.8. Thus, the measurement of plasma LDL apo B in the FH group did not provide any additional information above that given by the measurement of LDL-cholesterol. Conversely, the measurement of plasma LDL apo B in the normocholesterolemic coronary group provided significant information not given by the LDL-C levels.

Miller and his associates[14,15] have postulated that plasma HDL_2 concentration is a better predictor of CHD than HDL_3 concentration. We have come to similar conclusions, but have emphasized the use of the ratios of the subfractions as a more sensitive means of assessing the relative risk for CHD. The use of apolipoproteins

TABLE 4. Correlation of the Various Biochemical Parameters with the Degree of Coronary Stenosis

Ranking	Parameters	Correlation Coefficient	r-squared	p values
1.	HDL_2-Cholesterol / HDL_3-Cholesterol	−0.67	0.45	<0.001
2.	HDL_2-Cholesterol / HDL-Cholesterol	−0.64	0.41	<0.001
3.	Apo A–I / Apo B	−0.62	0.38	<0.001
4.	HDL_2-Cholesterol	−0.58	0.34	<0.001
5.	HDL-Apo A	−0.51	0.026	<0.001
6.	Apo A–I	−0.50	0.25	<0.001
7.	Apo A	−0.47	0.22	0.001
8.	Apo B	0.42	0.18	0.001
9.	HDL-Phospholipid / Total Cholesterol	−0.24	0.06	<0.001
10.	HDL-Cholesterol / Total Cholesterol	−0.20	0.04	<0.002
11.	LDL-Cholesterol / HDL-Phospholipid	0.19	0.04	<0.004
12.	HDL-Phospholipid	−0.18	0.03	<0.008
13.	LDL-Cholesterol	0.16	0.02	<0.02
14.	LDL-Cholesterol / HDL-Cholesterol	0.16	0.03	<0.02
15.	Total Cholesterol	0.14	0.02	<0.04
16.	HDL-Cholesterol	−0.13	0.02	<0.05
17.	Triglycerides	0.11	0.01	<0.21
18.	HDL-Triglycerides	0.09	0.01	<0.18
19.	LDL-Cholesterol / Total Cholesterol	0.09	0.01	<0.17
20.	APO A–II	0.03	0.001	0.50
21.	HDL_3-Cholesterol	0.02	0.0004	0.80
22.	VLDL-Cholesterol	0.02	0.0004	0.8

(particularly as Apo A–I/Apo B ratio) is also more useful than today's current laboratory assessment techniques, i.e., total cholesterol, triglycerides, LDL-C, and HDL-C. In summary, as newer analytical markers become readily available in the clinical laboratory, the clinical ability and enhancement of the assessment of CHD risk will become more prominent. The increase in specificity and sensitivity of these newer biochemical markers will increase the emphasis on the research of these biochemical constituents to better understand their metabolism and pathophysiologic role in the vascular disease process.

REFERENCES

1. HEISS, G. & H. A. TYROLER. 1983. Are apoproteins useful for evaluating ischemic heart disease? A brief overview of the literature. *In* Proceedings of the Workshop on Apolipoprotein Quantification. K. Lippel, Ed.: 7–22. NIH Publ. No. 83–1266, MHLBI. Bethesda, Maryland.
2. AVOGARO, P., G. BITTOLO BON, G. CAZZOLATO, G. B. QUINCI & F. BELUSSI. 1978. Plasma levels of Apolipoprotein A–I and Apolipoprotein B in human atherosclerosis. Artery **4:** 385–394.
3. AVOGARO, P., G. CAZZOLATO, G. BITTOLO BON & G. B. QUINCI. 1979. Are apolipoproteins better discriminators than lipids for atherosclerosis? Lancet **I:** 901–903.
4. SNIDERMAN, A., S. SHAPIRO, D. MARPOLE, B. SKINNER, B. TENG & P. O. KWITEROVICH. 1980. Association of coronary atherosclerosis with hyperapobetalipoproteinemia increased protein but normal cholesterol levels in human plasma low density [(beta)] lipoproteins. Proc. Natl. Acad. Sci. USA **77:** 604–608.
5. KLADETZKY, R. G., G. ASSMANN, S. WALGENBACH, P. TAVCHERT & H. D. HELB. 1980. Lipoprotein and apoprotein values in coronary angiography patients. Artery **7:** 191–205.
6. NAITO, H. K., R. L. GREENSTREET, J. A. DAVID, W. L. SHELDON, E. K. SHIREY, R. C. LEWIS, W. L. PROUDFIT & R. G. GERRITY. 1980. Artery **8:** 101–112.
7. RIESEN, W. P., R. MORDASINI, C. SALZMANN, A. THELER and H. P. GURTNER. 1980. Apoproteins and lipids as discriminators of severity of coronary heart disease. Atherosclerosis **37:** 157–162.
8. WHAYNE, T. F., P. ALAUPOVIC, M. D. CURRY, E. T. LEE, P. S. ANDERSON and E. SCHECHTER. 1981. Plasma apolipoprotein B and VLDL-, LDL-, and HDL-cholesterol as risk factors in the development of coronary artery disease in male patients examined by angiography. Atherosclerosis **39:** 411–424.
9. FAGER, G., O. WIKLUND, S. O. OLOFSON, L. WILHELMSEN and G. BONDJERS. 1981. Multivariate analysis of serum apolipoproteins and risk factors in relation to acute myocardial infarction. Arteriosclerosis **1:** 273–279.
10. DESAGER, J. P., M. ROUSSEAU, W. F. RIESEN & C. HARVENGT. 1984. Limitations of the predictive value for coronary vascular disease of the plasma lipids and Apoproteins AI, AII, B levels as measured before coronarography in 317 patients. *In* Latent Dyslipoproteinemia and Atherosclerosis. J. L. deGennes, J. Polonovski & R. Paoletti, Eds.: 165–174. Raven Press. New York.
11. PARRA, H., C. FIEUET, B. BONIFACE, M. BERTRAND, P. DUTHILLEUL & F. C. FRUCHART. 1984. Lipoproteins, apolipoproteins, and coronary artery disease assessed by coronary arteriography. *In* Latent Dyslipoproteinemia and Atherosclerosis. J. L. deGennes, J. Polonovski & R. Paoletti, Eds.: 187–197. Raven Press. New York.
12. RIESEN, W. F. & R. C. MORDASINI. 1984. Abnormal Apo A and Apo B levels in patients with atherosclerotic vascular lesions. *In* Latent Dyslipoproteinemia and Atherosclerosis. J. L. deGennes, J. Polonovski & R. Paoletti, Eds.: 247–253. Raven Press. New York.
13. PILGER, E., H. PRISTAUTZ, K. P. PFEIFFER & G. KOSTNER. 1983. Risk factors for peripheral arterosclerosis. Retrospective evaluation by stepwise discriminant analysis. Atherosclerosis **3:** 64–76.
14. MILLER, N. E., F. HAMMET, S. SALTISSI, S. RAO, H. VAN ZELLER, J. COLTART & B. LEWIS.

1981. Relation of angiographically defined coronary artery disease to plasma lipoproteins subfractions and apolipoproteins. Br. Med. J. **282:** 1741–1744.
15. MILLER, N. E. 1984. High density lipoprotein, atherosclerosis, and ischemic heart disease. *In* Atherosclerosis: Mechanisms and Approaches to Therapy. N. E. Miller, Ed.: 153–168. Raven Press. New York.
16. NAITO, H. K. 1984. HDL-Cholesterol: Metabolism, clinical significance, and laboratory considerations. *In* Clinical Laboratory Annual. H. Homburger & J. G. Batsakis, Eds.: 271–336. Appleton-Century-Crofts, Norwalk, Conn.
17. MANUAL OF LABORATORY OPERATIONS. LIPID RESEARCH CLINIC PROGRAM. 1974. Lipid and lipoprotein analysis, vol. 1. DHEW Publ. No. (NIH) 75–628, U.S. Government Printing Office, Washington, D.C. pp. 9–50.
18. WARNICK, G. R., J. M. BENDERSON & J. J. ALBERS. 1982. Quantitation of high-density lipoprotein subclasses after separation by dextran sulfate and Mg^{2+} precipitation. Clin. Chem. **28:** 1574.
19. TALAMEH, Y., R. WEI & H. K. NAITO. 1983. Measurement of HDL-cholesterol (C) and its subclasses using dextran sulfate (DS)-$MgCl_2$. Clin. Chem. **29:** 1226.
20. LAURELL, C-B. 1966. Quantitative estimation of proteins by electrophoresis in agarose containing antibodies. Anal. Biochem. **15:** 45–52.
21. TALAMEH, Y. & H. K. NAITO. 1984. An optimized electroimmunoassay (EIA) technique for measuring serum apolipoproteins B, A, A–I, and A–II. Clin Chem. **30:** 993.
22. SONES, F. M. & E. K. SHIREY. 1962. Cine coronary arteriography. Mod. Concepts Cardiovasc. Dis. **31**(7): 735–738.
23. JENKINS, P. J., R. W. HARPER & P. J. NESTEL. 1978. Severity of coronary atherosclerosis related to lipoprotein concentration. Br. Med. J. **2:** 388–391.
24. MOORE, R. B., J. M. LONG, J. P. MATTS, K. AMPLATZ, R. L. VARCO, H. BUCHWALD and the POSCH GROUP. 1979. Plasma lipoproteins and coronary arteriography in subjects in the program on the surgical control of the hyperlipidemias. Atherosclerosis **32:** 101–119.
25. AVOGARO, P., G. CAZZOLATO, G. BITTOLO BON, E. RORAI & E. PONTOGLIO. 1982. Lipoprotein derangement in human atherosclerosis. *In* Lipoproteins and Coronary Atherosclerosis. G. Noseda, C. Fragiacomo, R. Fumagalli & R. Paoletti, Eds.: 123–128. Elservier Biomedical. Amsterdam.
26. GOODMAN, L. A. 1964. Simultaneous confidence intervals for contrasts among multinomial populations. Ann. Math. Stat. **35:** 716–725.

Expression of LDL Receptor Binding Determinants in Very Low Density Lipoproteins[a]

WILLIAM A. BRADLEY, ANTONIO M. GOTTO, JR., AND SANDRA H. GIANTURCO[b]

Department of Medicine
Baylor College of Medicine
and
The Methodist Hospital
Houston, Texas 77030

INTRODUCTION

The interaction of cholesterol-ladened lipoproteins with the low density lipoprotein receptor has been elegantly described by the pioneering studies of Brown and Goldstein and their colleagues.[1,2] Since up to two-thirds of low density lipoproteins are catabolized by this mechanism,[3,4] the consequences of impairment or absence of the LDL receptor are directly related to elevated levels of LDL with an increased risk for coronary heart disease. Thus, one mechanistic link between elevated plasma cholesterol levels (in the form of LDL) and the pathogenesis of atherosclerosis can be inferred in hypercholesterolemia. However, an understanding of the relationship of elevated plasma triglyceride concentration (i.e., hypertriglyceridemias) to atherogenesis has yet to be established. The initial description of the specific interaction with the LDL receptor of large triglyceride-rich very low density lipoproteins (VLDL) from patients with hypertriglyceridemia (HTG), in contrast to those from normal subjects, suggested an alternate catabolic pathway for these TG-rich lipoproteins not available to their normal counterparts.[5] This finding raised the following question: Is the abnormal ability of large TG-rich lipoproteins from hyperlipidemic subjects to interact with the LDL receptor related to atherogenesis? The observation that uptake of HTG-VLDL, but not normal VLDL, is toxic to endothelial cells *in vitro*[6] suggested one potential receptor-mediated mechanism of atherogenesis in hypertriglyceridemia. Moreover, HTG-VLDL ($S_f > 60$) specifically interact with the β-VLDL receptor of murine peritoneal macrophage, thus causing engorgement with triglyceride and foam cell formation.[7] This interaction could be atherogenic. Van Lenten *et al.*[8] have extended our initial observation to show that postprandial, but not fasting normal VLDL are taken up by the same receptor in human monocyte-macrophages.

Our recent goals have been to understand the interaction of TG-rich lipoproteins with receptors, and to establish the binding determinant differences among lipoprotein

[a]This work was supported in part by a grant in the Specialized Center of Research in Arteriosclerosis (HL–27341).

[b]This author is an established investigator of the American Heart Association.

classes as well as between VLDL from normal and hypertriglyceridemic subjects. Furthermore, we have demonstrated that processing by plasma proteases may alter the site of catabolism of the large TG-rich lipoproteins.[9]

The following discussion will review and summarize our results concerning the unique binding determinants of hypertriglyceridemic VLDL, how these determinants change in the metabolic cascade from large TG-rich VLDL to LDL, and how receptor-mediated uptake of normal VLDL differs from that of HTG-VLDL.

VERY LOW DENSITY LIPOPROTEINS

The studies of the interaction of VLDL, unlike those of LDL, have been somewhat confounded by their innate heterogeneity, by the presence of transferable peptides, and by their ability to interact with charged surfaces. The problems of carrying out studies with this family of lipoproteins have been recently reviewed[10] and will not be elaborated upon here, except to emphasize that one major step in accurately examining the metabolism of VLDL is to recognize that subfractionation is essential when comparing cell receptor properties or studying turnover *in vivo.*

We further point out that the comparisons of "d 1.006 g/ml tops" as representative VLDL can be very misleading. Within this fraction, the distribution of large triglyceride-rich versus smaller cholesterol-rich lipoproteins in normal and hyperlipidemic subjects is very different; there is also the potential of great variability within populations. In normals, this fraction is approximately one-third S_f 60–400 and two-thirds S_f 20–60; this is in stark contrast to most patients with hypertriglyceridemia, in which two-thirds of the VLDL is S_f 60–400 and one-third of S_f 20–60. The consequences of such differences in unfractionated VLDL are only apparent when these fractions are purified and compared. We have found the Lindgren method of cumulative flotation[11] an easy and consistent procedure to obtain relatively homogeneous VLDL subclasses. With this method, it was initially shown that the interaction of large HTG-VLDL ($S_f > 60$) with the LDL receptor is a high-affinity process; in the same particle (subfraction) from normal individuals, only nonspecific (low-affinity) mechanisms for uptake occur.[5,12] Comparable subclasses from normals and hypertriglyceridemic subjects are very similar in composition; subtle differences in apoproteins account for differences in receptor interaction. Not only are there differences in the ability of different subclasses to bind to lipoprotein receptors, but within the hypertriglyceridemia VLDL series there is actually a change in ligand specificity.

Ligands of the LDL Receptor

Two principal apoproteins are known to bind with high affinity to the LDL receptor. The primary ligand of physiological significance, originally described by Goldstein and Brown, is apolipoprotein B (apo B), the major protein of LDL.[1,2] Later, it was shown by Brown and Goldstein, in collaboration with Mahley and his colleagues,[13] that a diet-induced particle, an abnormal HDL containing apo E (and no apo B), also binds avidly to the LDL receptor of human skin fibroblasts. This duplicity of ligands for the LDL receptor is an intriguing observation and suggests that similar domains of the very chemically distinct apo B and apo E might exist. The nature of these domains must be somewhat similar since chemical modifications of the positively charged residues of each apoprotein cause loss of receptor recognition.[14–16] This observation also suggests that this receptor-mediated process is so physiologically important that a backup (redundant) system is necessary.

Apo E Mediates Receptor Binding of HTG-VLDL ($S_f > 60$)

Since VLDL contain both apo B and apo E, our initial attempts to understand the specific uptake of HTG-VLDL (S_f 100–400) by the LDL receptor, as opposed to the same subfraction from normal individuals, addressed the role of these apoproteins in binding. Did apo E or apo B alone mediate binding of HTG-VLDL, or were both required? How did these differ from the apo E and apo B of normal VLDL?

We demonstrated a time-dependent loss in the ability of the HTG-VLDL to interact with the receptor.[7] This loss of activity was correlated with the degradation of apo E in these particles[18] by a VLDL-associated protease. This process could be simulated by thrombin treatment of either the apo E[17] or VLDL.[18] We, therefore, used thrombin as a probe to show a specific hydrolysis of some, but not all apo E on HTG-VLDL (S_f 100–400), and to show that the thrombin-accessible apo E is responsible for the interaction with the LDL receptor.[18] The hydrolysis of apo E occurred at residues 191–192, between arginine and alanine, yielding two fragments designated E–22 and E–12, the amino- and carboxy-terminal regions, respectively. Immunologically stained Western transfers demonstrated two startling facts about this hydrolysis: (1) The hydrolysis was specific and cleaved only a portion of the apo E of HTG-VLDL (S_f 100–400); and, (2) the amino terminal, E–22, exclusively was lost from the surface of the lipoprotein upon recentrifugation, while E–12 was retained.

The loss of LDL receptor recognition of thrombin-treated HTG-VLDL (S_f 100–400) could be restored totally by the reincorporation of one mole of intact apo E into the HTG-VLDL. However, reincorporation of the E–12 fragment into the HTG-VLDL did not restore receptor recognition, and addition of the E–22 fragment yielded less than 50% of the original recognition. We concluded, therefore, that a minimum of one mole of intact apo E of the appropriate conformation (thrombin accessible) per mole of HTG-VLDL (S_f 100–400) is required for efficient receptor binding and uptake.

A crucial observation in this study concerned the fact that it was sufficient to have thrombin cleave the region 191–192 of apo E in the native particle in order to destroy receptor recognition. Before reisolation by centrifugation, which caused specific loss of the E–22 fragment, the ability to bind to the receptor was totally lost and was not regained until one mole of intact apo E was reincorporated into the VLDL surface. This is in direct contrast to a recent observation[19] incorporating apo E into small phospholipid vesicles. Using dimyristoylphosphatidylcholine (DMPC) and apo E–2 isoform, it was suggested that not only is the E–22 fragment necessary for receptor recognition, but that the E–12 region may interfere with the folding of this isoform of apo E into the appropriate conformation for binding to the receptor. Although this may be true in these small artificial vesicles, it is not the case for large native TG-rich lipoproteins,[18] for CER-VLDL (beta-VLDL), nor for apo E-HDL_c (unpublished observation). Indeed, if the E–12 domain of apo E inhibited binding to the LDL receptor, then thrombin treatment of HTG-VLDL, which was reputed to relieve the constraint on the putative binding region, should cause either no loss in binding or even an increased binding to the receptor. As stated above, just the opposite occurred. Our findings suggest that in native particles, the E–12 region is necessary for the proper anchoring of the apo E to the phospholipid surface, and that, by contrast, in small DMPC vesicles, apo E–2 is in a very different conformation that is more capable of interacting with the LDL receptor. As will be discussed below, the presence of apo E in a particle does not satisfy the condition for binding to the LDL receptor. A specific conformation is necessary. This is not necessarily dependent on the isoform of apo E. In the case of large TG-rich VLDL, this conformation is susceptible to hydrolysis by thrombin as well.

CONFORMATION OF APO E IN NATIVE VLDL

If apo E is the primary ligand of HTG-VLDL (S_f 100–400) interaction with the LDL receptor, then why is this same subclass of VLDL from normal subjects, which contains both apo B and apo E, incapable of interaction with the LDL receptor?[5,12] To answer this question, we used thrombin as a probe of VLDL structure.

Unlike our studies with HTG-VLDL (S_f 100–400), thrombin was incapable of cleaving any of the apo E of normal VLDL (S_f 100–400). Using immunochemical electrophoretic blots, we demonstrated that the apo E of normal VLDL (S_f 100–400) is inaccessible to thrombin under conditions which readily cleave isolated apo E and which cleave the portion of the apo E that inactivated the HTG-VLDL (S_f 100–400) interaction with the LDL receptor.[18] As indicated in TABLE 1, we have determined that there are at least two conformations of apo E present in large HTG-VLDL. One conformation is cleaved by thrombin with an associated loss of binding to the LDL receptor, which is absent in normal VLDL (S_f 100–400). A second conformation is thrombin inaccessible and is not recognized by the LDL receptor. This second conformation of apo E is present in both normal and hypertriglyceridemic VLDL. Although the thrombin-accessible, LDL receptor-accessible apo E is usually not present on the normal VLDL, we can generate this conformation by the direct incorporation of one mole of apo E per mole of normal VLDL (S_f 100–400).[4] This is a specific property of apo E, since incorporation of an equimolar amount of apo A–I does not generate the receptor recognition domain.[4] Furthermore, the receptor recognition domain can be generated by the specific incorporation of at least one mole of apo E into one mole of either thrombin- or trypsin-inactivated HTG-VLDL (S_f 100–400).

We used a specific apo E radioimmunoassay (RIA) which did not contain detergent[18,20] to measure a change in the amount of apo E present in HTG-VLDL ($S_f >$ 60) after thrombin treatment and reisolation. This percent change in immunoassayable apo E usually reflects a decrease of approximately 1–2 moles of apo E per mole of VLDL. After thrombin treatment and prior to removal of the E–22 fragment by reisolation, the apo E immunoreactivity measured is either the same or increased, depending upon the antisera. We interpret this to indicate a conformational shift or a change in equilibrium of the E–22 fragment on the surface of HTG-VLDL with the aqueous phase. In normal VLDL ($S_f >$ 60), however, no such change in apo E immunoreactivity is measured with thrombin treatment either before or after reisolation. Our quantitative data with RIA confirm the results of our Western blots and our receptor binding experiments which showed that apo E of normal VLDL ($S_f >$ 60)

TABLE 1. Conformations of Apo E in Normal and HTG-VLDL as Assessed by Thrombin Cleavage and LDL Receptor Binding

Lipoprotein	Thrombin Accessibility		LDL Receptor Interaction
	yes	no	
Normal VLDL (S_f 100–400)	−	+	no
Normal VLDL (S_f 60–100)	−	+	no
Normal VLDL (S_f 20–60)	−	+	yes[a]
HTG-VLDL (S_f 100–400)	+	+	yes
HTG-VLDL (S_f 60–100)	+	+	yes
HTG-VLDL (S_f 20–60)	+/−	+	yes[b]

[a]Apo B-mediated LDL receptor binding.
[b]Primarily apo B mediated.

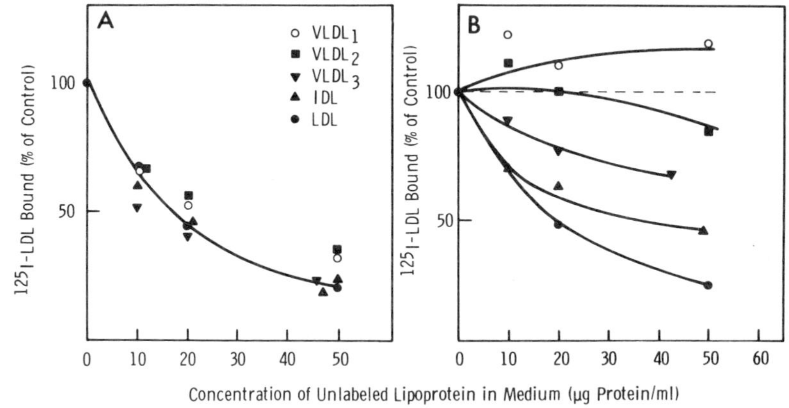

FIGURE 1. Abilities of trypsinized hypertriglyceridemic lipoproteins to compete with the binding of ^{125}I-LDL. Cells were grown to approximately 75% confluency in complete medium containing 10% fetal calf serum, and then washed and placed on 2 ml of medium containing 5% LPDS for 36 hours. The medium was then removed and replaced with fresh medium containing 5% LPDS, ^{125}I-LDL (5 µg protein/ml), and the indicated concentrations of native lipoproteins (Panel A), or trypsinized, reisolated HTG-VLDL$_1$ (S_f 100–400), HTG-VLDL$_2$ (S_f 60–100), HTG-VLDL$_3$ (S_f 20–60), IDL, or native LDL (Panel B), for comparison, for 3 hours at 37°C. Lipoproteins were isolated from a hypertriglyceridemic subject, incubated with trypsin (Worthington 3× crystallized, 1% by weight, two hours at 37°C), reisolated by the same flotation procedures used to isolate the starting materials, and tested for competition with the specific binding of ^{125}I-LDL. The cells were then washed extensively with chilled albumin-containing buffer, and total cell-associated radioactivity was determined. Each point is the average of duplicates, which varied by less than 8%. HTG-VLDL$_1$ (○); HTG-VLDL$_2$ (■); HTG-VLDL$_3$ (▼); IDL (PC8 ▲); LDL (●). Panel A illustrates competition of each lipoprotein prior to trypsinization, and Panel B, after it. LDL is shown as the control in each panel (After Bradley *et al.*[21])

is not cleaved by thrombin and is not available for LDL receptor binding. These data also indicate that there is a consistent mass difference of at least 1–2 moles of additional apo E in the surface of HTG-VLDL ($S_f > 60$) as compared to the same subclass of normal VLDL. This reflects the thrombin-accessible, LDL receptor-accessible apo E of HTG-VLDL ($S_f > 60$).

The LDL Receptor Binding Determinants Change in the Cascade from HTG-VLDL to LDL

It has long been recognized that apo B is the ligand for receptor-mediated uptake of LDL. Since we have shown that apo E and not apo B is the primary ligand for uptake of large HTG-VLDL,[17,18] it is of structural and metabolic interest to determine at what point in the metabolic cascade from HTG-VLDL (S_f 100–400) to LDL that the switch in ligand recognition occurs.

In this study, we used both thrombin and trypsin as reagents to eliminate apo E determinants of the lipoproteins for binding to the LDL receptor. Competitive binding (FIGURE 1) and HMG-CoA reductase suppression studies showed that thrombin treatment can abolish uptake of HTG-VLDL (S_f 100–400) and HTG-VLDL (S_f 60–100); it has almost no effect on HTG-VLDL (S_f 20–60), and no effect on IDL or

LDL. Trypsin, on the other hand, completely degrades the apo E of all lipoproteins, but has no effect on LDL binding (apo B mediated) to the receptor. Therefore, receptor binding after trypsinization of lipoproteins is due to residual apo B binding determinants. Trypsin abolishes the binding of HTG-VLDL (S_f 100–400) and HTG-VLDL (S_f 60–100), reduces (but does not abolish) the binding of HTG-VLDL (S_f 20–60), and has little to no effect on IDL or LDL.[21]

Immunochemical blots of SDS gels and radioimmunoassay demonstrated that while thrombin cleaves only a population of apo E into the E–22 and E–12 fragments, trypsin completely degrades all apo E in each HTG-lipoprotein class or subclass. Although the apo B immunoreactivities of VLDL subclasses are not significantly altered after treatment with thrombin, analysis by SDS disc gel electrophoresis on 3% acrylamide revealed that thrombin cleaves some of the B–100 of each VLDL subclass into four to six major large fragments. A loss of apo B epitopes (immunoreactivity) was found in both IDL and LDL after thrombin treatment (after, but not prior to, recentrifugation), even though these retained full receptor binding activity. Although the fragments produced in each of these lipoproteins were essentially identical, virtually all of the B–100 in IDL and LDL was hydrolyzed by thrombin, whereas only a portion of the B–100 of the VLDL was hydrolyzed at all. Three of these fragments had electrophoretic mobilities similar to B–74, B–26, and B–48. Trypsin, on the other hand, converted all B–100 of all lipoproteins to fragments smaller than MW 100K, yet still did not abolish binding of LDL, IDL, or HTG-VLDL (S_f 20–60). From the above observations, we concluded that both thrombin and trypsin treatment change the structure of apo B, but neither destroys apo B mediated binding to the LDL receptor. However, when apo E is hydrolyzed, apo E mediated binding is abolished. These facts, therefore, allow us to conclude that the LDL receptor binding determinants switch from apo E to apo B within HTG-VLDL (S_f 20–60), which is the precise subfraction where we observe receptor-mediated uptake in normal individuals (a primarily apo B-mediated process). This information is summarized schematically in FIGURE 2.

Several interesting conceptual points should be considered here. In large particles (i.e., VLDL $S_f > 60$), the apo B is not available for binding to the LDL receptor, and therefore, must be in a different conformation from that in smaller lipoproteins ($S_f < 60$). This conclusion is supported by recent reports using apo B polyclonal[22] and monoclonal antibodies indicating different apo B epitope expression in VLDL and LDL.[23,24] When these large particles do bind to the LDL receptor, apo E is the ligand as demonstrated in the case of HTG-VLDL ($S_f > 60$).[18] However, the presence of apo E in such lipoproteins is not sufficient for binding as we indicated for normal VLDL ($S_f > 60$). For large particles, then, it is also necessary to have the appropriate conformation of apo E to bind to the LDL receptor. It also appears that in VLDL ($S_f > 60$), not only is apo B not involved in binding, but that its presence is unnecessary for binding. Intralipid-apo E complexes, fractionated to HTG-VLDL (S_f 100–400) size, bind efficiently to the LDL receptor in the absence of apo B.[25] This indicates that apo B is not necessary to maintain the conformation of apo E for binding to the LDL receptor. From these observations, one might anticipate the possibility that a normal VLDL could bind to the LDL receptor if it acquires one mole of apo E of the proper conformation, as might occur in certain nutritional states.

SUMMARY AND CONCLUSIONS

We have used both proteolysis and reconstitution experiments to characterize the determinants for LDL receptor binding of HTG-VLDL. In these studies, we showed that the removal of approximately one mole of apo E per mole of HTG-VLDL (S_f 100–400) and HTG-VLDL (S_f 60–100) by thrombin-specific cleavage results in loss of receptor binding and concomitant loss of suppression of HMG-CoA reductase. This is in direct contrast to the lack of effect thrombin cleavage has on the receptor-mediated uptake of LDL, an apo B-mediated process. We were able to reconstitute receptor binding in thrombin-treated HTG-VLDL (S_f 100–400) by the specific reincorporation of one mole of apo E into the VLDL. The incorporation of one mole of apo E into normal non-suppressive VLDL (S_f 60–400) also enables this lipoprotein to bind to the receptor as effectively as LDL. Trypsin, which destroys apo E-mediated, but not apo B-mediated binding to the LDL receptor, abolishes binding of HTG-VLDL (S_f 100–400) and HTG-VLDL (S_f 60–100), but not that of HTG-VLDL (S_f 20–60), IDL, or LDL to the LDL receptor. Therefore, we conclude that apo E of the appropriate conformation is required for receptor-mediated uptake by the LDL receptor of large

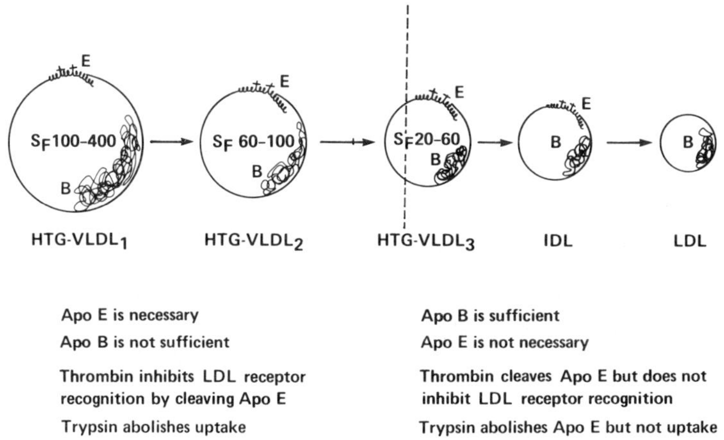

FIGURE 2. Schematic summary of protease inactivation of HTG-VLDL$_1$ and HTG-VLDL$_2$, but not HTG-VLDL$_3$, IDL, or LDL. The dashed line indicates where on this catabolic continuum the switch occurs from apo E to apo B as the primary ligand for LDL receptor binding, that is, within the HTG-VLDL$_3$ subclass. HTG-VLDL$_1$ = (S_f 100–400); HTG-VLDL$_2$ = (S_f 60–100); and HTG-VLDL$_3$ = (S_f 20–60).

TG-rich lipoproteins ($S_f > 60$). This conformation of apo E is probably related to the surface on which it is found (i.e., size of the particle) and the mode of incorporation into the phospholipid surface (i.e., transferred from plasma HDL). In large TG-rich particles, it appears that the intact apo E is necessary for the proper orientation of the molecule on the surface, with the carboxy-terminal one-third needed to anchor the apoprotein to the phospholipid surface.

We believe that the binding of apo E to the LDL receptor is a redundant system and is used as a backup system in abnormal pathological states such as hypertriglyceridemia, abetalipoproteinemia, and hypobetalipoproteinemia. In the case of hypertriglyceridemia, where the lipolysis mechanism is overloaded, the abnormal binding of HTG-VLDL ($S_f > 60$) provides an alternate catabolic route for their removal from plasma. In the cases of abeta- and hypobetalipoproteinemia, where the normal particles for cholesterol delivery are either absent or at low levels, apo E-containing particles can serve to deliver cholesterol to cells as has been recently observed *in vitro.*[26]

The initial observation that in cultured fibroblasts HTG-VLDL (S_f 100–400) interacted with high affinity with the LDL receptor, while its normal counterpart did not, led to a series of hypotheses concerning the interaction of these abnormal triglyceride-rich lipoproteins with lipoprotein receptors. Since then, we have demonstrated differences in the ligand expression in normal and hypertriglyceridemic VLDL, and have shown the ligand switch from apo E to apo B in the metabolic cascade from large HTG-VLDL to LDL. We further have shown that these receptor-mediated differences exist for several arterial cell types including macrophages and endothelial cells. In macrophages, these TG-rich lipoproteins are taken up through the β-VLDL receptor and cause triglyceride accumulation and foam cell formation; endothelial cells take up these HTG-lipoproteins through receptor-mediated processes with subsequent cell death. These observations support our hypothesis that indeed triglyceride-rich lipoproteins in hypertriglyceridemia are involved in aberrant processes leading to atherogenesis.

Our studies are far from the final answer concerning the role of triglyceride in atherosclerosis. It has yet to be shown that, as in the case of LDL, receptor-mediated processes are operable and that this is an alternate route of catabolism of HTG-VLDL *in vivo.* If this occurs *in vivo,* we need to determine the mechanism(s) by which these particles may cause atherosclerosis, and the fate of triglyceride and cholesterol delivered to arterial cells by the abnormal VLDL.

[**Note Added in Proof:** Since this manuscript was written, Krul *et al.* (J. Clin. Invest. **75:** 361–369, 1985) have also demonstrated, using monoclonal antibodies to apo B and apo E, that apo E is the primary ligand for the LDL receptor in large VLDL $S_f > 60$ from hypertriglyceridemic patients and that apo B is the primary ligand in smaller VLDL $S_f < 60$ and LDL. This elegant monoclonal antibody study confirms our original findings using thrombin as a probe.]

ACKNOWLEDGMENTS

The authors wish to thank Dr. Sarada C. Prasad for radioimmunoassays, Flora Brown for tissue culture, Alice Lin and Shiah-Lian Hwang for excellent technical assistance, and Rosetta Ray for expert manuscript preparation. In addition, we want to thank Dr. John Fenton for his generous gift of α-human thrombin, and Dr. Peter Jones for providing plasma from hypertriglyceridemic subjects.

REFERENCES

1. GOLDSTEIN, J. L. & M. S. BROWN. 1977. Ann. Rev. Biochem. **46:** 897–930.
2. BROWN, M. S. & J. L. GOLDSTEIN. 1983. Ann. Rev. Biochem. **52:** 223–261.
3. SHEPARD, J., S. BECKER, A. R. LORIMER & C. J. PACKARD. 1979. J. Lipid Res. **20:** 999–1006.
4. BROWN, M. S., P. T. KOVANEN & J. L. GOLDSTEIN. 1980. Ann. N. Y. Acad. Sci. **348:** 47–66.
5. GIANTURCO, S. H., A. M. GOTTO, JR., R. L. JACKSON, J. R. PATSCH, H. D. SYBERS, O. D. TAUNTON, D. L. YESHURUN & L. C. SMITH. 1978. J. Clin. Invest. **61:** 320–328.
6. GIANTURCO, S. H., S. G. ESKIN, L. T. NAVARRO, C. J. LAHART, L. C. SMITH & A. M. GOTTO, JR. 1980. Biochim. Biophys. Acta **618:** 143–152.

7. GIANTURCO, S. H., W. A. BRADLEY, A. M. GOTTO, JR., J. D. MORRISETT & D. L. PEAVY. 1982. J. Clin. Invest. **70:** 168–178.
8. VAN LENTEN, B. J., A. M. FOGELMAN, M. M. HOKOM, L. BENSON, M. E. HABERLAND & P. A. EDWARDS. 1983. J. Biol. Chem. **258:** 5151–5157.
9. GIANTURCO, S. H., A. M. GOTTO, JR. & W. A. BRADLEY. 1984. VIII Plenary Lecture—International Symposium on Drugs Affecting Lipid Metabolism. In press.
10. GIANTURCO, S. H. & W. A. BRADLEY. 1985. *In* Methods in Enzymology. J. P. Segrest & J. J. Albers, Eds. In press.
11. LINDGREN, F. T., L. C. JENSEN & F. T. HATCH. 1972. *In* Blood Lipids and Lipoproteins. G. J. Nelson, Ed.: 181–274. Wiley Interscience. New York.
12. GIANTURCO, S. H., F. B. BROWN, A. M. GOTTO, JR. & W. A. BRADLEY. 1982. J. Lipid Res. **23:** 984–993.
13. BERSOT, T. P., R. W. MAHLEY, M. S. BROWN & J. L. GOLDSTEIN. 1976. J. Biol. Chem. **251:** 2395–2398.
14. WEISGRABER, K. H., T. L. INNERARITY & R. W. MAHLEY. 1978. J. Biol. Chem. **253:** 9053–9062.
15. INNERARITY, T. L., R. W. MAHLEY, K. H. WEISGRABER & T. P. BERSOT. 1978. J. Biol. Chem. **253:** 6289–6295.
16. MAHLEY, R. W., T. L. INNERARITY & K. H. WEISGRABER. 1980. Ann. N. Y. Acad. Sci. **348:** 265–277.
17. BRADLEY, W. A., E. B. GILLIAM, A. M. GOTTO, JR. & S. H. GIANTURCO. 1982. Biochem. Biophys. Res. Commun. **109:** 1360–1367.
18. GIANTURCO, S. H., A. M. GOTTO, JR., S.-L. HWANG, J. B. KARLIN, A. H. Y. LIN, S. C. PRASAD & W. A. BRADLEY. 1983. J. Biol. Chem. **258:** 4526–4533.
19. INNERARITY, T. L., K. H. WEISGRABER, K. S. ARNOLD, S. C. RALL, JR. & R. W. MAHLEY. 1984. J. Biol. Chem. **259:** 7261–7267.
20. BRADLEY, W. A., J. B. KARLIN, S. C. PRASAD, A. M. GOTTO, JR. & S. H. GIANTURCO. 1983. *In* Proceedings of the Workshop on Apolipoprotein Quantification. K. Lippel, Ed.: 200–211. NIH Publication #83-1266. Bethesda, Maryland.
21. BRADLEY, W. A., S-L. C. HWANG, J. B. KARLIN, H. Y. LIN, S. C. PRASAD, A. M. GOTTO, JR. & S. H. GIANTURCO. 1984. J. Biol. Chem. **259:** 14728–14735.
22. SCHONFELD, G., W. PATSCH, B. PFLEGER, J. L. WITZTUM & S. W. WEIDMAN. 1979. J. Clin. Invest. **65:** 1288–1297.
23. CURTISS, L. K. & T. S. EDGINGTON. 1982. J. Biol. Chem. **257:** 15213–15221.
24. MARCEL, Y. L., P. DOUSTE-BLAZY & R. W. MILNE. 1983. *In* Proceedings of the Workshop on Apolipoprotein Quantification. K. Lippel, Ed.: 414–424. NIH Publication #83-1266. Bethesda, Maryland.
25. GIANTURCO, S. H. & W. A. BRADLEY. 1984. Fed. Proc. **43:** 1328.
26. INNERARITY, T. L., T. P. BEROT, K. S. ARNOLD, K. H. WEISGRABER, P. A. DAVIS, T. M. FORTE & R. W. MAHLEY. 1984. Metabolism **33:** 186–195.

LDL Heterogeneity and Atherosclerosis in Nonhuman Primates[a]

LAWRENCE L. RUDEL, M. GENE BOND,
AND BILLY C. BULLOCK

Arteriosclerosis Research Center
Wake Forest University Medical Center
Winston-Salem, North Carolina 27103

INTRODUCTION

We have studied the effects of atherogenic diets on plasma lipoproteins in several nonhuman primate species.[1-3] In each of these studies, individual animals were evaluated both for the extent of atherosclerosis and for the pattern of hyperlipoproteinemia so that atherogenic features of the plasma lipoproteins could be identified. Our first studies were carried out in two species of Asian macaques, *Macaca fascicularis* and *Macaca nemestrina.* The results indicated that the most potent lipoprotein predictor of the extent of coronary artery atherosclerosis was the degree of enlargement of the LDL,[1,2] and this enlargement in these species was marked. The LDL enlargement was due to the enrichment of the LDL particles with cholesteryl esters, primarily cholesteryl oleate and cholesteryl palmitate, i.e., esters presumably of tissue acyl CoA:cholesterol acyl transferase origin.[4]

The studies to be described in this presentation were carried out in African green monkeys, *Cercopithecus aethiops,* because the degree of LDL enlargement is much less marked, although it still occurs to a significant extent in response to an atherogenic diet.[5,6] This degree of diet responsiveness and the characteristics of the atherosclerotic lesions of this species[7] suggest that this nonhuman primate is one of the most appropriate animal models for atherosclerosis as it occurs in man.

MATERIALS AND METHODS

For 25 months, nineteen adult male African green monkeys were fed an atherogenic diet containing 0.74 mg cholesterol/kcal and 40% of kcal as saturated fat, and thirteen were fed a control diet containing 0.03 mg cholesterol/kcal. Diet compositions have been published.[8] Plasma lipoproteins were isolated by ultracentrifugation from fasting blood samples from each animal and were separated by agarose column chromatography. Then they were characterized as described before.[9,10] All animals were necropsied, and the coronary arteries, abdominal aorta, and carotid arteries were removed and evaluated for the extent and severity of atherosclerosis by a morphometric determination of intimal area performed according to described procedures.[11] Statistical analyses of variance, correlation, and regression were performed as outlined by Edwards.[12,13]

[a]This work was supported by NIH grant no. HL-14164.

TABLE 1. Effects of Atherogenic Diet on Plasma Cholesterol and Lipoproteins in African Green Monkeys[a]

Diet	N	Plasma Concentration				LDL MW (g/μmole)	LDL (μM)	CE Ratio (w/w)
		Chol	ILDL	LDL (mg/dl)	HDL			
Control	13	151 ± 5[b]	27 ± 4	159 ± 12	604 ± 30	3.11 ± 0.05	0.509 ± 0.04	0.657 ± 0.05
Test	19	394 ± 31[c]	75 ± 9[c]	724 ± 89[c]	564 ± 49	3.45 ± 0.09[c]	1.975 ± 0.22[c]	1.222 ± 0.10[c]

[a]Abbreviations: N = Number of animals; Chol = Cholesterol; ILDL = Intermediate-sized low density lipoproteins; LDL = Low density lipoproteins; HDL = High density lipoproteins; MW = Molecular weight; CE Ratio = Weight ratio of Cholesteryl oleate/Cholesteryl linoleate.

[b]All values, mean ± sem.

[c]Statistically different from control, $p < 0.05$.

TABLE 2. Effects of Atherogenic Diet on Atherosclerosis in African Green Monkeys

Diet	N	Abdominal Aorta	Coronary Arteries	Carotid Arteries
			Intimal Area (mm^2)	
Control	13	0.177 ± 0.04[a]	0.004 ± 0.001	0.001 ± 0.000
Test	19	1.041 ± 0.29[b]	0.100 ± 0.04[b]	0.168 ± 0.083[b]

[a]All values, mean ± sem.
[b]Statistically different from control, $p < 0.05$.

TABLE 3. Correlations between Measurements of Abdominal Aorta Atherosclerosis and Plasma Lipids and Lipoproteins

Abdominal Aorta Intimal Area with:	N	Correlation Coefficient	Significance
Plasma CE ratio (CO/CL)	25	0.88	$p < 0.0001$
Total plasma chol (mg/dl)	29	0.83	$p < 0.0001$
LDL size (mol. wt.)	29	0.83	$p < 0.0001$
LDL concentration (μM)	29	0.81	$p < 0.0001$
HDL concentration (mg/dl)	12	−0.73	$p < 0.006$
ILDL concentration (mg/dl)	32	0.54	$p < 0.002$

TABLE 4. Correlations between Measurements of Coronary Artery Atherosclerosis and Plasma Lipids and Lipoproteins

Coronary Artery Intimal Area with:	N	Correlation Coefficient	Significance
LDL size (mol. wt)	32	0.80	$p < 0.0001$
Plasma CE ratio (CO/CL)	27	0.72	$p < 0.0001$
LDL concentration (μM)	32	0.70	$p < 0.0001$
Total plasma chol (mg/dl)	32	0.67	$p < 0.0001$
ILDL concentration (mg/dl)	32	0.64	$p < 0.0002$
HDL concentration (mg/dl)	19	−0.51	$p < 0.03$

TABLE 5. Correlations between Measurements of Carotid Artery Atherosclerosis and Plasma Lipids and Lipoproteins

Carotid Artery Intimal Area with:	N	Correlation Coefficient	Significance
LDL concentrations (μM)	28	0.73	$p < 0.0001$
Total plasma chol (mg/dl)	29	0.64	$p < 0.0003$
HDL concentration (mg/dl)	29	−0.50	$p < 0.008$
Plasma CE ratio (CO/CL)	25	0.49	$p < 0.02$
LDL size (mol. wt.)	28	0.48	$p < 0.02$
ILDL concentration (mg/dl)	29	0.34	NS

RESULTS AND DISCUSSION

The effects of the atherogenic diet on plasma cholesterol and lipoproteins is shown in TABLE 1. The mass concentrations of total cholesterol, intermediate-sized low density lipoproteins (ILDL), and LDL were all increased, as were the average LDL molecular weight, the particle concentration of LDL (μM), and the ratio of cholesteryl oleate to cholesteryl linoleate in plasma lipoproteins. The latter measurement is for whole plasma since we were unable to demonstrate a significant difference in the cholesteryl ester composition of LDL versus HDL. Together, these two esters made up 75–85% of the cholesteryl ester mass in these samples.

TABLE 6. Multiple Regression Analysis of Abdominal Aorta, Coronary Artery, and Carotid Artery Atherosclerosis vs. Plasma Cholesterol and Lipoprotein Measurements

	R^2	Significance (of the regression)
Abdominal Aorta Intimal Area with:		
LDL particle conc. (μM)	0.83	$p < 0.0001$
LDL mw (g/μmole)	0.87	
HDL mass (mg/dl)	0.89	
Total plasma chol (mg/dl)	0.89	
CE ratio (CO/CL)	0.89	
Coronary Artery Intimal Area with:		
LDL mw (g/μmole)	0.64	$p < 0.0001$
HDL mass (mg/dl)	0.68	
Total plasma chol (mg/dl)	0.70	
LDL particle conc. (μM)	0.71	
CE ratio (CO/CL)	0.71	
Carotid Artery Intimal Area with:		
LDL particle conc. (μM)	0.65	$p < 0.0001$
Total plasma chol (mg/dl)	0.75	
CE ratio ((CO/CL)	0.77	
LDL mw (g/μmole)	0.78	
HDL mass (mg/dl)	0.78	

TABLE 2 shows the effects of the atherogenic diet on the extent of atherosclerosis as measured by the average intimal area. In each artery, the extent of atherosclerosis was significantly increased in the animals receiving the atherogenic diet. This occurred even though only about 50% of the animals fed this diet actually developed lesions during the 25 months of diet induction.

When the data were analyzed by correlation analyses to identify relationships between the lipoprotein measurements and the atherosclerosis end point, highly significant correlations were found for most measurements, seen in TABLES 3, 4, and 5. Multiple regression analyses were then carried out in an attempt to identify the order of importance of the lipoprotein measurements in predicting the atherosclerosis outcome (TABLE 6). Interestingly, LDL particle concentration was found to be the most predictive measurement for abdominal aorta and carotid artery atherosclerosis, whereas the average LDL molecular weight was the most predictive measurement for coronary artery atherosclerosis. In each of these three cases, the intercorrelations among the predictor lipid and lipoprotein measurements were sufficiently high that no further significance was contributed to the regression analysis by any one additional predictor, although the R^2 for the carotid artery intimal area did increase from 0.65 to 0.78 when all predictors were included in the regression equation.

These data show that measurements of LDL concentration and molecular weight are significantly related to the extent of diet-induced atherosclerosis that occurs in African green monkeys; measurements of HDL concentration and total plasma cholesterol concentration were of less predictive value. The predictive value of size versus concentration of LDL varied for different arteries. For coronary artery atherosclerosis in this species, the average LDL size was the most highly correlated lipoprotein measurement; this has also been found to be the case in two other nonhuman primate species, although in these cases, the degree of particle enlargement was much greater than in the African green monkeys of the present study. The particle characteristic(s) of the large molecular weight LDL fractions are not completely understood, but appear to be complex. When the LDL populations from individual animals were analyzed by density gradient ultracentrifugation and gradient gel electrophoresis, a significant degree of size and density heterogeneity of particles within the LDL fraction was identified (Marzetta and Rudel, unpublished observations). Animals with enlarged LDL are apparently those animals with a hepatic cholesteryl ester accumulation that results in increased hepatic cholesteryl ester secretion as noted during liver perfusion.[6] The hepatic cholesteryl ester contribution is evidenced by the increased content of cholesteryl oleate in the plasma lipoproteins, i.e., higher CO/CL ratio (TABLE 1). Mechanisms responsible for cholesteryl ester enrichment of LDL particles appear to result in an increased atherogenicity of the particle.

REFERENCES

1. RUDEL, L. L., C. W. LEATHERS, M. G. BOND & B. C. BULLOCK. 1981. Dietary ethanol induced modifications in hyperlipoproteinemia and atherosclerosis in nonhuman primates (*Macaca nemestrina*). Arteriosclerosis **1:** 144–155.
2. RUDEL, L. L. 1980. Plasma lipoproteins in atherogenesis in nonhuman primates. *In* Use of Nonhuman Primates in Cardiovascular Research. S. S. Kalter, Ed.: 37–57. University of Texas Press. Austin.
3. CLARKSON, T. B., R. W. PRICHARD, B. C. BULLOCK, R. W. ST. CLAIR, N. D. M. LEHNER, D. C. JONES, W. D. WAGNER & L. L. RUDEL. 1976. Pathogenesis of atherosclerosis: Some advances from using animal models. Exp. Mol. Pathol. **24:** 264–286.
4. TALL, A. R., D. M. SMALL, D. ATKINSON & L. L. RUDEL. 1978. Studies on the structure of low density lipoproteins isolated from *Macaca fascicularis* fed an atherogenic diet. J. Clin. Invest. **62:** 1354–1363.
5. RUDEL, L. L., J. S. PARKS & R. M. CARROLL. 1983. Effects of polyunsaturated versus saturated dietary fat on nonhuman primate HDL. *In* Dietary Fats and Health. E. G. Perkins & W. J. Visek, Eds: 649–666. American Oil Chemists' Society. Chicago.
6. JOHNSON, F. L., R. W. ST. CLAIR & L. L. RUDEL. 1983. Studies of the production of low density lipoproteins by perfused livers from nonhuman primates: Effect of dietary cholesterol. J. Clin. Invest. **72:** 221–236.
7. BULLOCK, B. C., N. D. M. LEHNER, T. B. CLARKSON, M. A. FELDNER, W. D. WAGNER & H. B. LOFLAND. 1975. Comparative primate atherosclerosis. I. Tissue cholesterol concentration and pathological anatomy. Exp. Mol. Pathol. **22:** 151–175.
8. RUDEL, L. L., J. A. REYNOLDS & B. C. BULLOCK. 1981. Nutritional effects of blood lipid and HDL cholesterol concentrations in two subspecies of African green monkeys (*Cercopithecus aethiops*). J. Lipid Res. **22:** 278–286.

9. RUDEL, L. L., D. G. GREENE & R. SHAH. 1977. Separation and characterization of plasma lipoproteins of rhesus monkeys (*Macaca mulatta*). J. Lipid Res. **18:** 734–744.
10. RUDEL, L. L., R. SHAH & D. GREENE. 1972. A study of the atherogenic dyslipoproteinemia induced by dietary cholesterol in rhesus monkeys (*Macaca mulatta*). J. Lipid Res. **18:** 55–65.
11. CLARKSON, T. B., M. G. BOND, B. C. BULLOCK & C. A. MARZETTA. 1981. A study of atherosclerosis regression in *Macaca mulatta.* IV. Changes in coronary arteries from animals with atherosclerosis induced for 19 months and then regressed for 24 or 48 months at plasma cholesterol concentrations of 300 or 200 mg/dl. Exp. Mol. Pathol. **34:** 345–368.
12. EDWARDS, A. L. 1976. An Introduction to Linear Regression and Correlation. W. H. Freeman and Company. San Francisco.
13. EDWARDS, A. L. 1979. Multiple Regression and the Analysis of Variance and Covariance. W. H. Freeman and Company. San Francisco.

Platelets, Macrophages, Endothelium, and Growth Factors

Their Effects upon Cells and their Possible Roles in Atherogenesis

RUSSELL ROSS, DANIEL F. BOWEN-POPE,
AND ELAINE W. RAINES

Department of Pathology
University of Washington
Seattle, Washington 98195

GROWTH FACTORS

The possibility that growth factors may represent important constituents in normal growth and development received its impetus with the discovery of epidermal growth factor (EGF) and the demonstration that EGF was responsible for premature eyelid opening and tooth eruption.[1] Subsequent to the discovery, purification, and characterization of EGF, a number of other growth factors have been discovered, many of which are in the process of purification and characterization. Two of these, platelet-derived growth factor (PDGF) and macrophage-derived growth factor (MDGF), were postulated to exist, based upon the knowledge that cells in culture required whole blood serum for continuing proliferation[2] and upon the observation that when healing wounds were deprived of activated macrophages, the process of wound fibroplasia was markedly decreased.[3] Several attempts were made to purify the growth factors present in whole blood serum by chromatographic fractionation, which yielded different molecular weight constitutents that appeared to have mitogenic activity.[2]

The discovery that one of the principal growth factors present in whole blood serum was derived from the platelet, was based upon the observation that serum prepared from cell-free plasma lacked any mitogenic activity.[4,5] This led to a series of experiments demonstrating that platelets were the only blood cells that contained significant mitogenic activity, which was released during the process of blood coagulation.[5,6] This mitogen, PDGF, has been highly purified,[7–10] and has received recent widespread attention based on its extensive homology with the product of an oncogene.[11,12]

PDGF is a highly cationic (pI $\simeq$ 10) 30,000 molecular weight glycoprotein that is composed of two subunits of approximately 17,000 and 14,000 molecular weight each, which are disulfide bonded. It is released from platelets at sites where platelet adherence or aggregation will lead to platelet shape change and to secretion of the contents of the platelet's alpha-granules.

A large series of growth factors (including fibroblast growth factor,[13] tumor growth factors,[14] and growth factors derived from varying tissues) continue to be discovered and characterized. Studies during the next decade should provide information concerning the biological importance of these factors in embryogenesis, growth and development, wound repair, tumorigenesis, atherogenesis, and possibly other disease processes as well.

PLATELET-DERIVED GROWTH FACTOR

Platelet-derived growth factor was originally felt to be solely the constituent of the platelet which, by virtue of its presence in the circulation, could be delivered to sites of injury and serve as a "wound hormone." As such, it could help to initiate proliferation of connective tissue cells such as fibroblasts or smooth muscle, and thus, participate in the initiation of wound repair and serve as an important defensive mechanism. As will be delineated below, platelet-derived growth factor is representative of a class of proteins whose genetic expression may occur in a widespread group of cells, including a large number of transformed cells, and which may play a wider role in biology than that of simple wound hormone. In fact, although it is likely that PDGF may be a wound hormone, its presence and role in the process of wound repair has yet to be demonstrated and delineated.

Because of its highly cationic character,[9,15-17] PDGF tends to adhere to many surfaces. In addition, it can be shown that at physiological pH, it contains hydrophobic regions,[16,18] and thus is capable of interacting with cell membranes. When PDGF binds to cells, it does so at specific cell-surface receptors which bind with an apparent K_D of 10^{-9} M to 10^{-11} M.[19-22] PDGF not only binds with high affinity to these receptors, but it dissociates at a relatively slow rate.[23,24] Bound ^{125}I-PDGF is not irreversibly bound since it can be dissociated by rinsing cultures of cells that have been exposed to ^{125}I-PDGF with dilute acetic acid (pH 3.7) without damaging the PDGF receptor.[24,25]

Cells that bind PDGF are principally connective tissue forming cells. PDGF appears to have been highly conserved since it is present in a broad range of species, including nonmammalian species. Furthermore, PDGF appears to be present in primitive vertebrates such as skates and lampreys, since their serum contains material able to bind to PDGF receptors on 3T3 cells.[26] The numbers of PDGF receptors vary widely among different cell types. Most cells express between 25,000 and 150,000 receptors per cell, including fibroblasts, smooth muscle cells, glial cells, and chondrocytes.[24] The cell line that contains the most PDGF receptors is a line of 3T3 cells[27] that contains approximately 600,000 receptors per cell. Cells which lack PDGF receptors include epithelial cells and A–431 cells (an epidermoid carcinoma cell line that contains large numbers of EGF receptors).[28] The other principal cell line that lacks receptors for PDGF is the arterial endothelial cell, which does not appear to express PDGF receptors, but, as detailed below, appears to be capable of synthesizing and secreting PDGF in cell culture.

When PDGF binds to its specific cell-surface, high-affinity receptor, it induces a large series of intracellular events, some of which occur virtually instantaneously and appear to be intimately related to the receptor itself. The receptor for PDGF appears to be functional since the concentrations of ^{125}I-PDGF required for binding and for mitogenic stimulation are very similar,[20-22] and there is no evidence for the presence of "spare receptors," as has been proposed for insulin and for EGF, that can account for the saturation of binding of PDGF at concentrations 10–100-fold higher than those needed for maximum biological response.[29] Furthermore, PDGF does not appear to bind to other cell surface receptors, and when ^{125}I-PDGF binds to its receptor, the receptor ligand complex is internalized or "down-regulated" if binding occurs at 37° C, a response characteristic of receptors for various mitogens.[30]

Glenn *et al.*[31] used affinity cross-linking experiments to demonstrate that the receptor for PDGF is a cell-surface glycoprotein of approximately 164,000 molecular weight. Heldin and Ronnstrand[32] have confirmed these observations using photoactivatable cross-linking reagents, and have suggested that receptor size was approximately 175,000 molecular weight. When PDGF binds to its receptor, a membrane protein of the same molecular weight as the receptor is rapidly phosphorylated. This can be demonstrated by the transfer of phosphate from ATP to tyrosine moieties present in proteins isolated from the membranes of cells that had been previously exposed to PDGF. Thus, it appears that the PDGF receptor contains a PDGF-activatable tyrosine kinase, which was discovered by incubation of membranes derived from responsive cells together with ^{32}P-ATP in the presence or absence of PDGF. Analysis of the proteins that were phosphorylated due to the presence of PDGF by autoradiography of SDS-PAGE, demonstrated increases in the phosphorylation of proteins equivalent to the molecular weight of the PDGF receptor. The proteins that were phosphorylated contained both phosphotyrosine and phosphoserine,[33-35] probably due to activation of a tyrosine phosphokinase and a serine phosphokinase which may occur as a consequence of activation of the PDGF receptor. Although it has not been conclusively demonstrated that the PDGF receptor is autophosphorylated by a tyrosine kinase, the evidence derived from the studies of Heldin and Ronnstrand[32] and Pike *et al.*[35] suggests that this is, in fact, the case. Pike *et al.*[35] demonstrated that the PDGF receptor and the substrate for PDGF-stimulated phosphorylation are similar in size; that this protein is present only in cells that express PDGF receptors; that the receptor number is proportional to the amount of phosphorylation that occurs after exposure to PDGF; and that the phosphoprotein that is formed after PDGF stimulation disappears at a rate concomitant with the disappearance of the loss of receptors from the cell surface due to down-regulation. All of these observations are consistent with autophosphorylation of the PDGF receptor due to PDGF binding. It is not clear what role PDGF receptor phosphorylation plays in relation to the biological responses that follow PDGF binding to its receptor. A number of cytosolic proteins are also phosphorylated after PDGF binds to the cells,[36] and the roles of these phosphorylation reactions, including that of the PDGF-receptor complex, remain to be defined in terms of understanding the biological activity of PDGF.

When PDGF binds to its receptor, a number of cellular events occur at varying time intervals after binding. In addition to the rapidly induced phosphorylation reactions, there is an early and rapid change in phospholipid metabolism that occurs after PDGF binds to its receptor. Within five to ten minutes after binding, there is a rapid increase in the formation of intracellular diacylglycerol, which is fairly rapidly degraded into monoglyceride and free arachidonic acid.[37] The diacylglycerol formation is apparently due to the activation of a membrane-associated phospholipase type C. The resulting diglyceride that is formed may be important in relation to the activation of a protein kinase-C, which may be associated with calcium mobilization in the cell and which could be important in induction of cell proliferation.[38] Furthermore, the free arachidonic acid that is formed can serve as a substrate for formation of prostaglandin derivatives by cells which are so activated and, in the case of smooth muscle cells, for the formation of increased amounts of prostacyclin (PGI_2). Recently, Habenicht *et al.*[56] showed that not only does PDGF stimulate the release of free arachidonic acid, but that over a longer period of time, it stimulates both an early rise in prostaglandin formation and a somewhat later (two hours) increase in both PGE and PGI_2 due to an increased synthesis of cyclooxygenase, which is stimulated by exposure of the cells to PDGF. The increased formation of PGI_2, as well as PGE, by cells such as smooth muscle that have been stimulated by PDGF, may be important *in vivo* as a measure of protecting cells after exposure to platelets has occurred.

In addition to these rapid early events, PDGF induces increased endocytosis,[39] increased binding of LDL to its high-affinity receptor,[40] increase in cholesterol synthesis,[40] and increased protein and RNA synthesis. Cochran *et al.*[41] have demonstrated that PDGF leads to the formation of several new messenger RNAs, the specificity of which remains to be determined.

Finally, PDGF is the only growth factor isolated, thus far, that is both a mitogen and a chemotactic agent. It is chemotactic for both fibroblasts and smooth muscle,[42] and possibly for leukocytes as well.[43]

MACROPHAGE-DERIVED GROWTH FACTOR

MDGF was first observed as a result of the culture of activated peritoneal macrophages.[44] The medium conditioned by these macrophages served as a source of growth for fibroblasts and smooth muscle cells, and it was therefore suggested that activated macrophages might be an important source of fibroblast proliferation in wound repair as well as in other inflammatory phenomena. Recently, monocyte/macrophages have been shown to be the principal cell associated with the development of the early lesion of atherosclerosis, the fatty streak, suggesting that, perhaps, these cells might be the source of a growth factor in the development of the lesions of atherosclerosis.[45,46]

Glenn and Ross[47] demonstrated that elutriator-purified blood monocytes can serve as an excellent source of MDGF in culture, and MDGF has also been shown to be formed by macrophages derived from the lung.[48]

The molecular weight of MDGF has been reported to range between 20,000 and 30,000[48] (Shimokado *et al.*, unpublished data). MDGF appears to be unrelated to EGF and insulin, two well-characterized growth factors. The further purification and characterization of this factor, together with the development of antibodies against MDGF, remain to be completed. However, recent experiments (Shimokado *et al.*, unpublished data) suggest that the major growth factors may consist of PDGF and possibly FGF.

ENDOTHELIAL-DERIVED GROWTH FACTOR

Gajdusek *et al.*[49] demonstrated that medium conditioned by arterial endothelial cells contains potent growth factors for cells such as fibroblasts or smooth muscle. DiCorleto and Bowen-Pope[50] were able to demonstrate that the material secreted by endothelial cells in culture contains both a PDGF-like molecule, as well as another growth factor(s) that is distinct from PDGF. Since arterial endothelial cells lack receptors for PDGF on their surface, it is difficult to know whether they are, in fact, capable of binding PDGF in an autocrine fashion since these studies must be performed at 37° C and under conditions where the numbers of PDGF receptors, if they were present on the surface of the cell, would be sufficiently small as to be difficult to detect. The PDGF-like molecule formed by arterial endothelial cells appears to be identical to PDGF in that it competes for binding to the PDGF receptor, and both its binding and mitogenic activity can be abolished by a monospecific antiserum against PDGF developed in a goat. It is not clear whether confluent quiescent endothelial cells *in vivo* form PDGF. It is possible that they do not, but when endothelial injury occurs, PDGF may then be formed. This speculation results from the suggestion that formation of PDGF in cell culture may be a manifestation of endothelial cells that are artifactually and possibly continuously activated because of the peculiar nature of the growth of endothelium on plastic tissue culture dishes.

THE ROLE OF THESE GROWTH FACTORS IN ATHEROGENESIS

In experimentally induced atherosclerosis, it has been demonstrated by numerous investigators that endothelial injury due to sources such as intra-arterial catheters, hypercholesterolemia, homocysteinemia, and perhaps immune-induced injury, all result in monocyte/macrophage and, subsequently, platelet interactions at such sites of injury. Attempts to prevent platelet interactions pharmacologically,[51] or by inducing a thrombocytopenia,[52,53] or by studying swine homozygous for von Willebrand's disease and lacking Factor VIII,[54] have all demonstrated that platelet interactions are a necessary prerequisite for the intimal smooth muscle proliferative response of advanced atherosclerosis to occur. The early presence of monocyte/macrophages in lesions of atherosclerosis, like the fatty streak, suggests that this cell type and factors derived from activated macrophages may be important in smooth muscle chemotaxis and in proliferation and development of atherosclerotic lesions.[46,55] Nevertheless, to date there is no definitive data that the growth factors derived from platelets, activated macrophages, or endothelial cells play a role in atherogenesis, so this must remain highly speculative. There is preliminary data by Sprugel *et al.* (unpublished) that balloon catheter induced de-endothelialization, which is normally followed by platelet adherence, smooth muscle cell chemotaxis, and intimal proliferation, can be markedly inhibited by using an anti-PDGF antibody *in vivo.* These studies are preliminary, and further studies must be pursued before it can be definitively demonstrated that PDGF, in fact, is one of the major culprits involved in the induction of the proliferative lesions of atherosclerosis. These approaches, however, should ultimately lead to development of new means of diagnosis, prevention, and intervention in atherosclerosis.

REFERENCES

1. Cohen, S. 1962. J. Biol. Chem. **237:** 1555–1562.
2. Temin, H. M., R. W. Pierson, Jr. & N. C. Dulak. 1972. *In* Growth, Nutrition, and Metabolism of Cells in Culture, vol. 5. G. H. Rothblat & V. J. Cristofalo, Eds.: 50–81. Academic Press. New York.
3. Leibovich, S. J. & R. Ross. 1975. Am. J. Pathol. **78:** 71.
4. Balk, S. D. 1971. Proc. Natl. Acad. Sci. USA **68:** 271–275.
5. Ross, R., J. Glomset, B. Kariya & L. Harker. 1974. Proc. Natl. Acad. Sci. USA **71:** 1207–1210.
6. Kohler, N. & A. Lipton. 1974. Exp. Cell Res. **87:** 297–301.
7. Heldin, C-H., B. Westermark & A. Wasteson. 1981. Biochem. J. **193:** 907–913.
8. Antoniades, H. N. 1981. Proc. Natl. Acad. Sci. USA **78:** 7314–7317.
9. Deuel, T. J., J. S. Huang, R. T. Proffitt, J. U. Baenziger, D. Chang & B. B. Kennedy. 1981. J. Biol. Chem. **256:** 8896–8899.
10. Raines, E. W. & R. Ross. 1982. J. Biol. Chem. **257:** 5154–5160.
11. Doolittle, R. F., M. W. Hunkapiller, L. E. Hood, S. G. Devare, K. C. Robbins, S. A. Aaronson & H. N. Antoniades. 1983. Science **221:** 275–277.
12. Waterfield, M. D., G. T. Scrace, N. Whittle, P. Stroobant, A. Johnsson, A. Wasteson, B. Westermark, C-H. Heldin, J. S. Huang & T. F. Deuel. 1983. Nature **304:** 35–39.
13. Gospodarowicz, D., H. Dialecki & G. Greenburg. 1978. J. Biol. Chem. **253:** 3736–3743.
14. Todaro, G. J., C. Fryling & J. E. Delarco. 1980. Proc. Natl. Acad. Sci. USA **77:** 5258–5262.
15. Heldin, C-H., A. Wasteson & B. Westermark. 1977. Exp. Cell Res. **109:** 429–437.
16. Ross, R., A. Vogel, P. Davies, E. Raines, B. Kariya, M. J. Rivest, C. Gustafson & J.

GLOMSET. 1979. *In* Hormones and Cell Culture, Cold Spring Harbor Conferences on Cell Proliferation, vol. 6, p. 3–16. Cold Spring Harbor, New York.

17. ANTONIADES, H. N., C. D. SCHER & C. D. STILES. 1979. Proc. Natl. Acad. Sci. USA **76:** 1809–1813.
18. HELDIN, C-H., B. WESTERMARK & A. WASTESON. 1979. Proc. Natl. Acad. Sci. USA **76:** 3722–3726.
19. HELDIN, C-H., B. WESTERMARK, and A. WASTESON. 1981. Proc. Natl. Acad. Sci. USA **78:** 3664–3668.
20. BOWEN-POPE, D. F. & R. ROSS. 1982. J. Biol. Chem. **257:** 5161–5171.
21. HUANG, J. S., S. S. HUANG, B. KENNEDY & T. F. DEUEL. 1982. J. Biol. Chem. **257:** 8130–8136.
22. WILLIAMS, L. T., P. TREMBLE & H. N. ANTONIADES. 1982. Proc. Natl. Acad. Sci. USA **79:** 5867–5870.
23. HELDIN, C-H., A. WASTESON & B. WESTERMARK. 1982. J. Biol. Chem. **257:** 4126–4221.
24. BOWEN-POPE, D. F. & R. ROSS. 1985. *In* Peptide Hormones, a Volume of Methods in Enzymology, vol. 109. L. Birnbaumer & B. W. O'Malley, Eds.: 69–100. Academic Press. New York.
25. BOWEN-POPE, D. F., P. E. DICORLETO & R. ROSS. 1983. J. Cell Biol. **96:** 679–683.
26. SINGH, J. P., M. A. CHAIKIN & C. D. STILES. 1982. J. Cell Biol. **95:** 667–671.
27. PRUSS, R. M. & H. R. HERSCHMAN. 1977. Proc. Natl. Acad. Sci. USA **74:** 3918–3921.
28. FABRICANT, R. N., J. E. DELARCO & G. J. TODARO. 1977. Proc. Natl. Acad. Sci. USA **74:** 565–569.
29. CUATRECASAS, P. & M. D. HOLLENBERG. 1976. *In* Advances in Protein Chemistry, vol. 30. L. B. Anfinsen, J. T. Edsall & F. M. Richards, Eds.: 251–451. Academic Press. New York.
30. KAPLAN, J. 1981. Science **212:** 14–20.
31. GLENN, K., D. BOWEN-POPE & R. ROSS. 1982. J. Biol. Chem. **257:** 5172–5176.
32. HELDIN, C-H. & L. RONNSTRAND. 1983. J. Biol. Chem. **258:** 10054–10061.
33. EK, B. & C-H. HELDIN. 1982. J. Biol. Chem. **257:** 10486–10492.
34. NISHIMURA, J., J. S. HUANG & T. F. DEUEL. 1982. Proc. Natl. Acad. Sci. USA **69:** 4303–4307.
35. PIKE, L. J., D. F. BOWEN-POPE, R. ROSS & E. G. KREBS. 1983. J. Biol. Chem. **258:** 9383–9390.
36. COOPER, J. A., D. F. BOWEN-POPE, E. RAINES, R. ROSS & T. HUNTER. 1982. Cell **31:** 263–273.
37. HABENICHT, A. J. R., J. A. GLOMSET, W. C. KING, C. NIST, C. D. MITCHEL & R. ROSS. 1981. J. Biol. Chem. **256:** 12329–12335.
38. NISHIZUKA, Y. 1984. Nature **308:** 693–698.
39. DAVIES, P. R. & R. ROSS. 1978. J. Cell Biol. **79:** 663–671.
40. CHAIT, A., R. ROSS, J. ALBERS & E. L. BIERMAN. 1980. Proc. Natl. Acad. Sci. USA **77:** 4084–4088.
41. COCHRAN, B. H., A. C. REFFEL & C. D. STILES. 1983. Cell **33:** 939–947.
42. GROTENDORST, G. R., T. CHANG, H. E. J. SEPPA, H. K. KLEINMAN & G. R. MARTIN. 1982. J. Cell. Physiol. **113:** 261–266.
43. DEUEL, T. F., R. M. SENIOR, J. S. HUANG & G. L. GRIFFIN. 1982. J. Clin. Invest. **69:** 1046–1049.
44. LEIBOVICH, S. J. & R. ROSS. 1976. Am. J. Pathol. **84:** 501.
45. GERRITY, R. G. 1981. Am. J. Pathol. **103:** 191–200.
46. FAGGIOTTO, A., R. ROSS & L. HARKER. 1984. Arteriosclerosis **4:** 323–340.
47. GLENN, K. & R. ROSS. 1981. Cell **25:** 603–615.
48. BITTERMAN, P. B., S. I. RENNARD, G. W. HUNNINGHAKE & R. G. CRYSTAL. 1982. J. Clin. Invest. **70:** 806–822.
49. GAJDUSEK, C., P. DICORLETO, R. ROSS & S. SCHWARTZ. 1980. J. Cell Biol. **85:** 467–472.
50. DICORLETO, P. E. & D. F. BOWEN-POPE. 1983. Proc. Natl. Acad. Sci. USA **80:** 1919–1923.
51. HARKER, L., R. ROSS, S. SLICHTER & C. SCOTT. 1976. J. Clin. Invest. **58:** 731–741.

52. MOORE, A., R. J. FRIEDMAN, D. P. SINGAL, J. GAULDIE & M. BLAJCHMAN. 1976. Thromb. Diath. Haemorrh. **35:** 70–79.
53. FRIEDMAN, R. J., M. B. STEMERMAN, B. WENZ, S. MOORE, J. GAULDIE, M. GENT, M. L. TIELL & T. H. SPAET. 1977. J. Clin. Invest. **60:** 1191–1201.
54. FUSTER, V., E. J. W. BOWIE, J. C. LEWIS, D. N. FASS, C. A. OWEN, JR. & A. BROWN. 1978. J. Clin. Invest. **61:** 722–730.
55. FAGGIOTTO, A. & R. ROSS. 1984. Arteriosclerosis **4:** 341–356.
56. HABENICHT, A. J. R., M. GOERIG, J. GRULICH, D. ROTHE, R. GRONWALD, V. LOTH, G. SCHETTLER, B. KOMMERELL & R. ROSS. 1985. J. Clin. Invest. **75:** 1381–1387.

Studies on Cell Proliferation and Mevalonic Acid Metabolism in Cultured Human Fibroblasts[a]

LARRY D. WITTE, KATHY P. FAIRBANKS, VERONIQUE BARBU, AND DEWITT S. GOODMAN

Arteriosclerosis Research Center and Department of Medicine
Columbia University College of Physicians and Surgeons
New York, New York 10032

INTRODUCTION

Focal proliferation of cells in the arterial intima is a prominent feature of atherogenesis and contributes to the production of the atherosclerotic plaque.[1] Much of what we know about the molecular mechanisms that regulate cellular proliferation has been determined by studying cells in culture. Proliferation of normal diploid cells in culture (and presumably, *in vivo*) is known to be under the control of exogenous growth factors.[1,2] These include platelet-derived growth factor (PDGF),[3,4] epidermal growth factor (EGF),[5] and the insulin-like growth factors.[6] It has become well established that these polypeptide growth factors initiate their effects on cells by binding to high-affinity, specific, cell-surface receptors. Although numerous cellular events are known to occur after the stimulation of a cell by a mitogen, the detailed molecular mechanisms whereby the interaction of a growth factor with its receptor leads to later DNA synthesis remain a mystery. A recent paper by Mroczkowski *et al.*[7] presented intriguing data suggesting that the receptor itself may function as a "second messenger." Thus, these workers reported that purified EGF receptors had endonuclease activity that could nick double-stranded circular DNA and convert it to a relaxed form. However, evidence has also been accumulating over the past several years that it may be the activation of a pathway involving polyphosphoinositide-derived "second messengers"[8–10] that are responsible for the series of events leading to DNA synthesis.

Among the cellular events which occur in response to a mitogenic stimulus are those involving cholesterol synthesis and metabolism. For example, in earlier studies from this laboratory, parallel increases in both DNA synthesis and in the number of low-density lipoprotein (LDL) receptors per cell were found following the treatment of quiescent human fibroblasts with PDGF.[11] In addition, rapidly proliferating cells and tissues have been reported to show a high rate of 3-hydroxy-3-methylglutaryl coenzyme A (HMG-CoA) reductase activity.[12] This enzyme converts HMG-CoA to mevalonic acid, which is usually the rate-limiting reaction of cholesterol biosynthesis.[13] These findings suggest that as part of a cell's response to a mitogenic stimulus, it can increase its ability to obtain cholesterol via both exogenous and endogenous means. Inhibition of a cell's ability to obtain cholesterol has been shown to prevent cell growth.[15,16]

[a]This work was supported by National Institutes of Health grant no. HL-21006 (Specialized Center of Research in Arteriosclerosis) and National Institutes of Health Training grant no. HL-07343.

Several recent studies have suggested that a product of mevalonic acid other than cholesterol may also be involved in DNA synthesis and cell growth.[17-20] These studies were made possible by the availability of two potent specific inhibitors of HMG-CoA reductase—compactin and mevinolin. In brief, the studies demonstrated that in the presence of high concentrations of these reductase inhibitors, DNA synthesis could be blocked. It was further shown that the block on DNA synthesis could not be overcome with cholesterol alone, whereas mevalonic acid could overcome the block. We recently reported that in quiescent human fibroblasts stimulated with PDGF, there is a critical time period, several hours before S phase, when the cells require mevalonate in order for DNA synthesis to proceed.[20] We will briefly review these studies here and describe studies designed to explore the fate of mevalonic acid in mitogenically stimulated cells.

EXPERIMENTAL METHODS

Cell Culture

Human fibroblasts were isolated from the foreskin of a normal newborn child and cultured as previously described.[21] Cells for experiments were thawed from stock vials frozen in liquid N_2 and plated into either 35 mm dishes at 4×10^4 cells/dish or 100 mm dishes at 3×10^5 cells/dish. Stock culture medium contained 10% calf serum (v/v) in Dulbecco's modified Eagle's (DME) medium supplemented with penicillin (100 units/ml), streptomycin (100 μg/ml), and glutamine (2 m*M*). On day 3 of each experiment, the medium was replaced with fresh medium. On day 6, the monolayer was washed once with DME medium containing 2 mg/ml of bovine serum albumin (BSA), and replaced with 5% human plasma-derived serum or 5% plasma-derived lipoprotein deficient serum, prepared as previously described.[21] After 48 hours, the cells were quiescent and the experiments were begun.

Assays

For the studies reported here, the quiescent fibroblasts were mitogenically stimulated with partially purified PDGF prepared from outdated human platelet-rich concentrate as previously described.[20] DNA synthesis was determined by measuring the incorporation of ^{3}H-thymidine into DNA during a thirty minute interval.[20] Protein synthesis was assessed by determining the incorporation of ^{3}H-labeled mixed amino acids (New England Nuclear) into cells at the times indicated, according to the method of Liberti and Miller.[22] The level of HMG-CoA reductase activity was determined according to the method of Alberts *et al.*[23]

Separation of Different Cell Components

To explore the fate of mevalonic acid in PDGF stimulated cells, we added PDGF and mevinolin (30 μM, prepared as described previously)[20] to the quiescent fibroblasts at zero time. We then labeled the culture by adding 25 μCi of ^{3}H-mevalonic acid/100 mm plate during the time intervals indicated. At the end of the pulse time period, the cells were scraped into ice-cold phosphate-buffered saline (PBS). To determine the level of mevalonate incorporation into lipids, cell pellets were extracted twice with 3 ml of cold chloroform:methanol (2:1). An internal standard of ^{14}C-cholesterol

(1000 cpm) was added prior to the extraction and greater than 90% recovery was achieved.

To determine the level of incorporation of label from ^{3}H-mevalonate into nucleic acid, these compounds were separated from cell homogenates essentially as described by Yang and Novelli.[24] In brief, the cells were harvested as described above and homogenized with a dounce homogenizer. The lipids were extracted with petroleum ether twice, after which the aqueous phase was extracted with phenol and mixed by vortexing for one hour at room temperature. Then, the phases were separated by centrifugation. To the aqueous fraction was added 0.1 volume of 20% potassium acetate. The total nucleic acids were precipitated by the addition of 2.5 volumes of cold ethanol, followed by mixing for one hour at −20°C and standing overnight at −20°C. The precipitated nucleic acids were collected by centrifugation, and the pellet was dissolved in 1 ml of 10 m*M* Tris-HCl, pH 7.4, at room temperature. An aliquot was taken for liquid scintillation counting.

To arrive at an estimate of the incorporation of label from mevalonic acid into protein, we first precipitated the protein from cell homogenates with 10% ice-cold trichloroacetic acid (TCA) (final concentration), followed by extensive extraction of the TCA pellet with chloroform:methanol (2:1) to remove the lipids. The pellet was then solubilized in 0.5 *N* NaOH and an aliquot taken for liquid scintillation counting.

In other experiments, the incorporation of label mevalonate into different subcellular organelles and fractions was explored. Cell fractionation into a nuclear pellet and a postnuclear supernatant was performed as described by Sheeler.[25] In brief, the cells were harvested into homogenization buffer (0.25 *M* sucrose, 1 m*M* NA_2–EDTA, and 3 m*M* imidazol), and homogenized twice with a dounce homogenizer. The nuclei were then isolated by centrifugation.

SDS-Polyacrylamide Gel Electrophoresis

Sodium dodecyl sulfate (SDS) polyacrylamide slab gels were prepared as described by Laemmli.[26] The gels were 1.5 mm thick with a 12.5% resolving gel and a 5% stacking gel. Cell pellets were dissolved in electrophoresis sample buffer and heated for 110 seconds at 95°C before being loaded onto the gel. Following electrophoresis, the gels were stained with Coomassie brilliant bluc and destained in 7% acetic acid/5% methanol. The gels were then sliced, solubilized, and counted by liquid scintillation.

Other Methods

Protein concentrations were determined by the method of Lowry *et al.*,[27] using a protein standard solution from Sigma. Cell numbers were determined using a Model Z_f Coulter Counter or a hemocytometer. Radioassay for ^{14}C and ^{3}H was carried out in a Packard liquid scintillation counter, model 3255.

RESULTS

Stimulation of DNA Synthesis, Protein Synthesis, and HMG-CoA Reductase Activity by PDGF

The time course of action of PDGF on DNA synthesis and on the level of protein synthesis in human fibroblasts is shown in FIGURE 1A. DNA synthesis consistently was

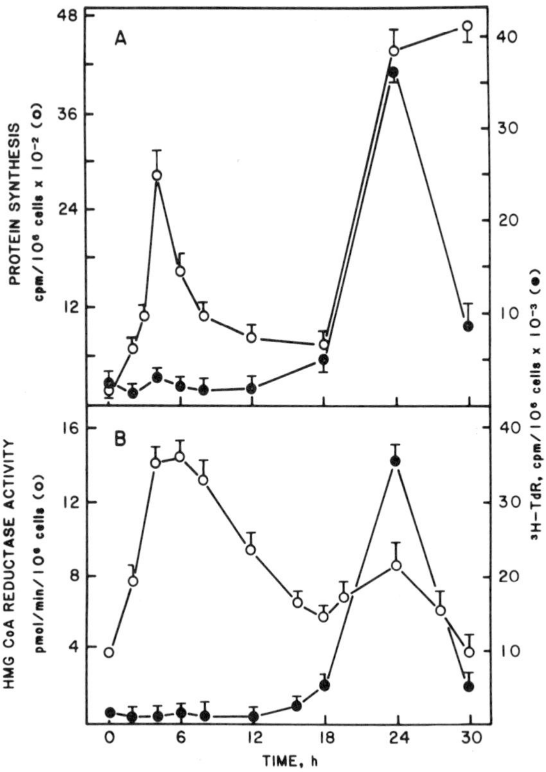

FIGURE 1. Time course of the effects of PDGF on DNA synthesis, protein synthesis, and HMG-CoA reductase activity. Quiescent cell monolayers were prepared in 35 mm plates as described under "cell culture" (see EXPERIMENTAL METHODS). PDGF (2 μg/ml) was added at zero time to two sets of plates, each in triplicate. For the studies shown in both FIGURES 1A and 1B, DNA synthesis (●) was determined with a 15 min pulse of 1 μCi ^{3}H-thymidine/well in one set of plates at the time points indicated. The second set of plates in the top panel (A) received 4 μCi/plate of ^{3}H-amino acids (NEN, specific activity = 57 mCi/mmol) for a 15 min pulse (○). The second set of plates in the bottom panel (B) were harvested at the times indicated and prepared for the assay of HMG-CoA reductase activity (○). The mean ±SD are shown for each data point.

found to peak at approximately 24 h in these cells. The incorporation of ^{3}H-amino acids into cellular proteins increased soon after PDGF addition, reaching a peak of synthesis at 4 h, subsequently dropping-off, and then rising again at the time of DNA synthesis. This experiment was repeated twice, with very similar results. In studies not shown, we found an increase in the mass of cellular protein within 12–18 h of PDGF addition, whereas an increase in cell number was not evident until approximately 30 h after PDGF treatment.

The time course of action of PDGF on DNA synthesis and HMG-CoA reductase activity is shown in FIGURE 1B. Reductase activity was determined in cell homogenates by measuring the formation of ^{14}C-mevalonate from ^{14}C-HMG-CoA. Following the addition of PDGF to quiescent fibroblasts cultured in lipoprotein deficient medium, reductase activity was found to rapidly increase, reaching a peak within 4–6 h, which was greater than threefold that found in nonstimulated cells. This level of reductase activity then slowly decreased over the next several hours, followed by a second, smaller increase at the time of DNA synthesis. Therefore, both the overall protein synthesis of the cell, as well as its HMG-CoA reductase activity, followed a biphasic pattern, with an increase occurring soon after the addition of the mitogenic stimulus (PDGF) to quiescent cells, and a second rise coinciding with DNA synthesis. In addition, if the fibroblasts were cultured in medium containing LDL (and thus having an exogenous source of cholesterol), the level of reductase stimulation was decreased; however, even at very high levels of LDL (200 μg/ml), there was still a significant biphasic increase in reductase activity (data not shown).

The Incorporation of ^{3}H-Mevalonate into Cells Following Stimulation with PDGF

As indicated above, we have recently reported[20] that there is a critical time period in the middle of the cell cycle when PDGF-stimulated cells require mevalonate in order for DNA synthesis to proceed. This critical period comprised the interval of approximately 10–20 h after PDGF addition to quiescent human fibroblasts (which was especially critical during the early part of this interval). In the studies next described, we undertook to explore the products made from labeled mevalonate and found in cells under various conditions. These studies represent the first phase of a project which has as its general objective the attempt to identify the putative product(s) of mevalonate that may be necessary to permit DNA synthesis to proceed. Our approach was to follow the incorporation of radioactivity from ^{3}H-mevalonate into cellular products when the ^{3}H-mevalonate was made available to cells during either a noncritical (0–8h)

TABLE 1. Incorporation of Radioactivity from Labeled Mevalonate into Mevinolin-treated Human Fibroblasts Following the Addition of PDGF[a]

Cell Fraction	Percent of Total Cell Associated Radioactivity 0–8h	10–18h
$CHCl_3$ MeOH (2:1)[b]	51.8	54.0
Extracted TCA pellet[c]	43.1	34.1
Phenol/ETOH precipitate[d]	<1.0	<1.0
Other water soluble compounds	<10.0	<10.0
Nuclear pellet	20.7	24.5
Postnuclear supernatant	79.3	75.5

[a]Quiescent human fibroblasts were prepared in 100 mm plates as described under "cell culture" (see EXPERIMENTAL METHODS). The monolayers were then exposed to PDGF (2 μg/ml) and mevinolin (30 μM), and divided into two sets of plates. During the time intervals indicated (0–8 h or 10–18 h), ^{3}H-mevalonate (40 μM, 25 μCi/plate) was added. The cells were harvested by scraping into cold PBS and separated into the various fractions shown above, as described in EXPERIMENTAL METHODS.

[b]Represents total cell lipid.

[c]Represents total cell protein.

[d]Represents total cell nucleic acids.

or a critical time interval (10–18h). Utilizing this protocol, we found approximately 0.01% of the ^{3}H-mevalonate added to the medium to be incorporated into the cells.

The results of one such study are presented in TABLE 1. Slightly more than half (52–54%) of the ^{3}H-mevalonate-derived counts found in the cells were recovered in the total lipid extract, with no real differences being found between the two time intervals. Thin-layer chromatography of these lipid extracts (data not shown) showed no significant differences between the two time intervals although the amount found in cholesterol was slightly higher at the 0–8 h time period as compared to the 10–18 h time interval. Cellular proteins, represented by the lipid extracted TCA pellet, showed a surprisingly high percentage of mevalonate-derived radioactivity.

In the study shown in TABLE 1, 34–43% of the cell-associated label was found in the proteins. There was not, however, a significant difference between the amount of label found in cell proteins during the two time intervals. Less than 1% of the counts in the cells could be found in the nucleic acid fraction (phenol/ETOH precipitate) at either

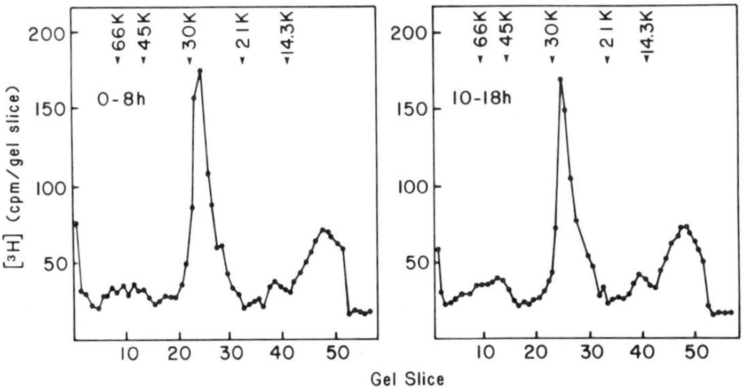

FIGURE 2. The incorporation of ^{3}H-mevalonic acid into proteins of fibroblasts treated with PDGF and mevinolin. Fibroblasts were prepared and treated as described under TABLE 1. The cell pellets were analyzed by SDS-electrophoresis, as described under EXPERIMENTAL METHODS. Molecular weight marker proteins were also run (bovine serum albumin, ovalbumin, carbonic anhydrase, soybean trypsin inhibitor, and lysozyme), with their migration points indicated by the arrows.

time period. The water soluble component comprised less than 10% of the total counts. Also shown in TABLE 1, are the percentages of mevalonate-derived radioactivity associated with the nuclear and the postnuclear supernatant. We were intrigued to find relatively large percentages of counts in the nuclear fractions (over 20% at both time intervals). The majority of these counts remained with the nuclei even after further purification, with approximately 45% of the radioactivity being extractable with chloroform:methanol (data not shown).

To explore further the cellular proteins which were labeled by the ^{3}H-mevalonate, we solubilized the pellets of cells treated in the same manner as those described under TABLE 1 in SDS sample buffer, and performed SDS-polyacrylamide gel electrophoresis on the solubilized proteins. The results of one such experiment are shown in FIGURE 2. As shown in the figure, a major labeled band was seen with a molecular weight of approximately 28–29K, along with a minor labeled band, less sharply defined, of molecular weight <14K. Other trace bands were also noted. Again, there was no apparent difference in the pattern at the two time intervals.

DISCUSSION

Mevalonic acid, or products of mevalonate metabolism, are required for cell proliferation. Several studies[17–20] have indicated that mevalonate appears to serve at least two essential roles in cell growth; one as the biosynthetic precursor for cholesterol, and another to provide a product(s) or serve some other role essential for DNA synthesis. In previous studies,[20] we demonstrated that there is a critical time period following the addition of PDGF to quiescent-cultured human fibroblasts when mevalonate (but not cholesterol) was required to allow the cells to go into DNA synthesis. This time period was from approximately 10–18 h, with DNA synthesis subsequently peaking at 24 h. In the studies reported here, we demonstrate that in the same human fibroblast system, both cellular protein synthesis and HMG-CoA reductase activity (the enzyme responsible for the generation of mevalonic acid) exhibit a biphasic pattern in response to PDGF, with an early (4–6 h) increase, followed by a decline, then a second increase at the time of DNA synthesis (24 h). This biphasic pattern in reductase activity was also found when the cells were cultured in the presence of high levels of LDL, suggesting that the increase in reductase activity may reflect both a requirement for cholesterol and also for some other mevalonate product(s). It is possible that the early (4–6 h) increase in HMG-CoA reductase activity may help to provide the mevalonate, which we previously[20] had shown to be required between 10–18 h for DNA synthesis to occur.

In studies reported here, we utilized ^{3}H-mevalonic acid made available to cells either at a noncritical time period (0–8 h) or at a critical time period (10–18 h) to address the question of the metabolism of mevalonic acid in mitogenically stimulated cells during a critical time, as compared to a nonessential time with regard to cell growth. As described, we found no significant difference in the amount of ^{3}H-mevalonate-derived label incorporated into the cellular lipids, proteins, nucleic acids, or other water soluble compounds of the cells during the two time periods. In addition, we also found no difference in the incorporation of ^{3}H-mevalonate-derived products into the nuclear pellet or the postnuclear supernatants of cells during these two time periods. The finding of a marked incorporation of mevalonate-derived label into proteins during both time periods is an intriguing one. During further fractionation of the apparent protein-bound products of mevalonic acid by SDS-polyacrylamide gel electrophoresis, a major band of apparent molecular weight of 28–29K and a minor band at <14K were evident. The identity of these proteins and of the mevalonate product(s) bound to them, the type of bond involved, and the role of these proteins are questions which remain to be answered. In a similar manner, the rather large percentage of mevalonate-derived counts found in the nuclear pellet is also of interest. Whether these products could be playing a direct role in DNA synthesis in the nucleus remains to be determined. Further studies are clearly needed in order to explore the role that mevalonic acid and its products play in the regulation of cell proliferation.

ACKNOWLEDGMENT

The authors wish to thank Ms. Deardra Shuler for her help in preparing the manuscript.

REFERENCES

1. Ross, G. 1981. Arteriosclerosis: A problem of the biology of arterial wall cells and their interaction with blood components. Arteriosclerosis **1:** 293–311.
2. Rozengurt, E. & M. Collins. 1983. Molecular aspects of growth factor action: Receptors and intracellular signals. J. Pathol. **141:** 309–331.
3. Westermark, B., C-H. Heldin, B. Ek, A. Johnson, K. Mellstrom, M. Nister & A. Wasteson. 1983. Biochemistry and biology of platelet-derived growth factor. *In* Growth and Maturation Factors, vol. 1. G. Guroff, Ed.: 73–115. John Wiley and Sons. New York.
4. Stiles, C. D. 1983. The molecular biology of platelet-derived growth factor. Cell **33:** 653–655.
5. Carpenter, G. & S. Cohen. 1979. Epidermal growth factor. Ann. Rev. Biochem. **48:** 193–216.
6. Zapf, J., E. R. Froesch & R. E. Humbel. 1981. The insulin-like growth factors (IEF) of human serum: Chemical and biological characterization and aspects of their possible physiological role. Curr. Top. Cell. Regul. **19:** 257–309.
7. Mroczkowski, B., G. Mosig & S. Cohen. 1984. ATP-stimulated interaction between epidermal growth factor receptor and supercoiled DNA. Nature **309:** 270–273.
8. Berridge, M. 1983. Rapid accumulation of inositol triphosphate reveals that agonists hydrolyse polyphosphoinositidases instead of phosphatidylinositol. Biochem. J. **212:** 849–858.
9. Habenicht, A. J. R., J. A. Glomset, W. C. King, C. Nist, C. D. Mitchell & R. Ross. 1981. Early changes in phosphatidylinositol and arachidonic acid metabolism in quiescent Swiss 3T3 cells stimulated to divide by platelet-derived growth factor. J. Biol. Chem. **256:** 12329–12335.
10. Majerus, P. W., E. J. Neufeld & D. B. Wilson. 1984. Production of phosphoinositide-derived messengers. Cell **37:** 701–703.
11. Witte, L. D., J. A. Cornicelli, R. W. Miller & D. S. Goodman. 1982. Effects of platelet-derived and endothelial cell-derived growth factors on the low-density lipoprotein receptor pathway in cultured human fibroblasts. J. Biol. Chem. **257:** 5392–5401.
12. Chen, H. W. 1981. The activity of 3-hydroxy-3-methylglutaryl coenzyme A reductase and the rate of sterol synthesis diminished in cultures with high cell density. J. Cell. Physiol. **108:** 91–97.
13. Rodwell, V. W., J. L. Nordstrom & J. J. Mitschelen. 1976. Regulations of HMG-CoA reductase. Adv. Lipid Res. **14:** 1–74.
14. Brown, M. S. & J. L. Goldstein. 1974. Suppression of 3-hydroxy-3-methylglutaryl coenzyme A reductase activity and inhibition of growth of human fibroblasts by 7-ketocholesterol. J. Biol. Chem. **249:** 7306–7314.
15. Cornell, R. B. & A. F. Horwitz. 1980. Apparent coordination of the biosynthesis of lipids in cultured cells: Its relationship to the regulation of the membrane sterol: phospholipid ratio and cell cycling. J. Cell Biol. **86:** 810–819.
16. Kandutsch, A. A. & H. W. Chen. 1977. Consequences of blocked sterol synthesis in cultured cells: DNA synthesis and membrane composition. J. Biol. Chem. **252:** 409–415.
17. Brown, M. S. & J. L. Goldstein. 1980. Multivalent feedback regulation of HMG-CoA reductase, a control mechanism coordinating isoprenoid synthesis and cell growth. J. Lipid Res. **21:** 505–517.
18. Quesney-Huneeus, V., H. A. Galick, M. D. Siperstein, S. K. Erickson, T. A. Spencer & J. A. Nelson. 1983. The dual role of mevalonate in the cell cycle. J. Biol. Chem. **258:** 378–385.
19. Yachnin, S. 1982. Mevalonic acid as an initiator of cell growth: Studies using human lymphocytes and inhibitors of endogenous mevalonate biosynthesis. Oncodevel. Biol. Med. **3:** 111–123.
20. Fairbanks, K. P., L. D. Witte & D. S. Goodman. 1984. Relationship between mevalonate and mitogenesis in human fibroblasts stimulated with platelet-derived growth factor. J. Biol. Chem. **259:** 1547–1551.
21. Cornicelli, J. A., L. D. Witte & D. S. Goodman. 1983. Inhibition of LDL degradation in

cultured human fibroblasts induced by endothelial cell-conditioned medium. Arteriosclerosis **3:** 560–567.
22. LIBERTI, J. P. & M. S. MILLER. 1978. Stimulation of human fibroblasts protein, ribonucleic acid, and deoxyribonucleic acid synthesis by bovine growth hormone fragments. Endocrinology **102:** 1756–1760.
23. ALBERTS, A. W., J. CHEN, G. KURON, V. HUNT, J. HUFF, C. HOFFMAN, J. ROTHROCK, M. LOPEZ, H. JOSHUA, E. HARRIS, A. PATCHETT, R. MONAGHAN, S. CURRIE, E. STAPLEY, G. ALBERS-SCHONBERG, O. HENSENS, J. HIRSHFIELD, K. HOOGSTEEN, J. LIESCH & J. SPRINGER. 1980. Mevinolin: A highly potent competitive inhibitor of hydroxymethylglutaryl-coenzyme A reductase and a cholesterol-lowering agent. Proc. Natl. Acad. Sci. USA **77:** 3957–3961.
24. YANG, W-K. & G. D. NOVELLI. 1971. Analysis of isoaccepting tRNA's in mammalian tissues and cells. Methods Enzymol. **20:** 44–55.
25. SHEELER, P. 1981. *In* Centrifugation in Biology and Medical Sciences, p. 31–46. John Wiley and Sons. New York.
26. LAEMMLI, U. K. 1970. Cleavage of structural proteins during the assembly of the head of bacteriophage T_4. Nature **277:** 680–685.
27. LOWRY, O. H., N. J. ROSEBROUGH, A. L. FARR & R. J. RANDALL. 1951. Protein measurement with the folin phenol reagent. J. Biol. Chem. **193:** 265–275.

Atherogenic Regulation by Heparin-like Molecules[a]

ROBERT D. ROSENBERG, CHRISTOPHER REILLY, AND LINDA FRITZE

Department of Biology
Whitaker College
Massachusetts Institute of Technology
Cambridge, Massachusetts 02045
and
Department of Medicine
Harvard Medical School;
Beth Israel Hospital;
and
Dana Farber Cancer Center;
Boston, Massachusetts

The arterial wall consists of the intimal endothelial cells, which line the lumen, and the underlying medial smooth muscle cells, which usually remain in a quiescent growth state. Several investigators have observed that within minutes of experimental desquamation of the endothelium, platelets adhere to the denuded surface and release their alpha-granule content. Platelet proteins, such as platelet-derived growth factor (PDGF), appear on the surface of the exposed smooth muscle cells within the denuded area and are internalized within the first hour.[1–4] Smooth muscle cells also appear to be exposed to mitogenic factors released from endothelial cells and macrophages present at the site of injury. Vascular smooth muscle cells respond to these various mitogens by migrating from the media into the intima. Thereafter, the smooth muscle cells in the denuded area replicate their DNA within 24 to 48 hours and proliferate to eventually form a myointimal plaque.[5–8] Of course, at the periphery of the damaged site, uninjured endothelial cells multiply and migrate until the damaged area is re-endothelialized. Provided that the site of injury is sufficiently small, endothelial cells will completely cover this area and the proliferation of smooth muscle cells will cease. It is currently believed that repeated endothelial injury might lead to cycles of smooth muscle cell hyperplasia with subsequent lipid deposition and the eventual development of the atherosclerotic lesion.

The administration of commercial heparin to animals following denudation of intimal endothelial cells markedly reduced smooth muscle cell proliferation.[9] Cell types other than vascular smooth muscle cells appear to be much less sensitive to the action of heparin and heparin-like components.[10] We have studied the effect of heparin on the proliferation of cultured smooth muscle cells isolated from bovine and rat aortae.[11,12] The cells were plated at a density of 6000 cells/ml, growth-arrested in a medium supplemented with low concentrations of serum (0.4%) or platelet-poor plasma (2.0%), and released from the growth-arrested state by feeding them with medium supplemented with 5% to 20% serum in the absence or presence of heparin at

[a]This work was supported by grants from the National Institutes of Health HL-28625 and HL-17747, and the National Foundation for Cancer Research.

the desired concentrations. Growth was monitored by quantitating changes in cell number over a period of seven days (FIGURE 1). Commercial heparin was separated into anticoagulantly active and non-anticoagulantly active species by employing affinity fractionation with antithrombin, as we have previously reported.[13] Our results demonstrate that both anticoagulantly active and anticoagulantly inactive heparin significantly inhibit the growth of smooth muscle cells within the cell culture system. A 60%–90% inhibition of cell proliferation was observed with heparin doses that ranged between 1 and 10 micrograms.[11] As expected, removal of antithrombin from the serum did not significantly alter these results. It should be noted, though, that the antiproliferative effect of heparin does not appear to be the result of a direct interaction of the mucopolysaccharide with PDGF[11] since this complex carbohydrate is an effective inhibitor of cell proliferation when added twelve hours after the admixture of PDGF, which is known to be internalized and "trigger" the cells within one to three hours.[14]

We have also shown that the highly specific growth inhibitory effect does not occur

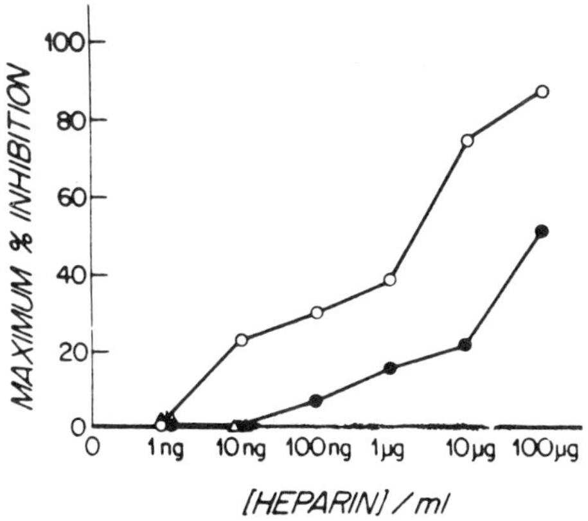

FIGURE 1. Effect of heparin on rat smooth muscle cells (SMC) growth. Exponential and growth-arrested cultures of rat SMC were obtained and exposed to heparin as described in the text: (O—O), growth-arrested rat SMC; (●—●), exponential rat SMC. Data are the average of five or more experiments.

in the presence of glycosaminoglycans other than heparin or heparin-like molecules such as heparan sulfate.[12] For example, chondroitin sulfate, dermatan sulfate, and hyaluronic acid exhibited no antiproliferative potency. However, dextran sulfate, which was similar to the heparin molecule in molecular weight and pattern of sulfation, appeared to possess some growth inhibitory activity (FIGURE 2). Thus, the secondary structure and/or charge distribution of the mucopolysaccharide play an important role in endowing heparin with antiproliferative potency. Indeed, the critical substituents present on the heparin molecule that are necessary for antiproliferative activity appear to be a cluster of O-sulfate groups and may involve negative charges about these positions.[15]

Given the fact that endothelial cells are in close contact with smooth muscle cells within the vascular tree, we have suggested that endothelial cells secrete a heparin-like substance which may regulate the growth of underlying smooth muscle cells.[12] To test this hypothesis, we examined bovine aortic endothelial cells in culture. Our data showed that conditioned medium from confluent endothelial cells inhibited the

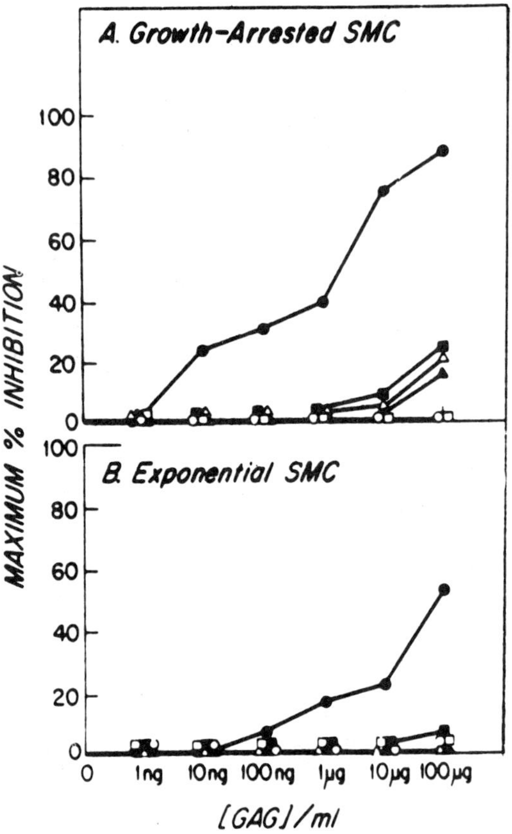

FIGURE 2. Effect of glycosaminoglycans (GAGs) on rat smooth muscle cells (SMC) growth. (A) Rat SMC were plated and growth-arrested as described in the text. The cells were then exposed to RPMI plus 20% containing the indicated concentrations of GAGs. Cell number was measured at daily intervals. Data are expressed as maximum percent inhibition. (B) Rat SMC were plated at $6 \times 10^3/16$ mm well. After 24 hours, the medium was aspirated and replaced with fresh RPMI plus 20% fetal calf serum (FCS) with or without the indicated concentrations of GAGs. Data are expressed as maximum percent inhibition. (○—○), heparin; (□—□), beef lung heparan sulfate; (△—△), dermatan sulfate; (▲—▲), chondroitin ABC sulfate; (●—●), hyaluronic acid. Data for the heparan sulfates are the average of three experiments; data for other GAGs are the average of five or more experiments.

proliferation of growth-arrested smooth muscle cells by approximately 70%, whereas conditioned medium from exponentially growing endothelial cells could not perform this function.

The inhibitory activity observed when utilizing conditioned medium from confluent bovine aortic endothelial cells appeared to be due to a heparin-like substance. This conclusion was supported by the fact that a crude isolate of glycosaminoglycans (TCA-soluble, ethanol-precipitable material) from endothelial cell-conditioned medium reconstituted in 20% serum inhibited smooth muscle cell growth, whereas glycosaminoglycans isolated from unconditioned medium had no effect on smooth muscle proliferation. In addition, neither exposure of the glycosaminoglycan preparation to 100° C for prolonged periods of time, nor treatment with proteases such as trypsin, chymotrypsin, hyaluronidase, or chondroitin sulfate ABC lyase, destroyed the growth inhibitory activity. However, the antiproliferative potency of these products was abolished by exposure to highly purified *Flavobacterium* heparinase. This highly specific enzyme cleaves heparin and heparan sulfate into tetrasaccharide and disaccharide units, which we have shown do not possess growth inhibitory activity.

We have, subsequently, demonstrated that bovine aortic endothelial cells release a heparin-like substance in the presence of 0.4% fetal calf serum. This substance inhibited the growth of smooth muscle cells *in vitro* by about 70%. Substitution of platelet-poor plasma for serum resulted in minimal liberation of inhibitory activity from the cells unless at least tenfold higher concentrations of platelet-poor plasma were utilized[12] (FIGURE 3). This indicated that a platelet product was involved in the release process.

This observation prompted us to develop the first procedure for isolating a potent platelet-derived endoglycosidase which is able to specifically cleave heparin and heparan sulfate into fragments of approximately ten monosaccharide units. It also helped to demonstrate that heparin-like mucopolysaccharides that possess antiproliferative activity are released from endothelial cells. To this end, an endoglycosidase was isolated from outdated human platelets by freeze-thaw solubilization, heparin-Sepharose chromatography, DEAE-cellulose chromatography, hydroxylapatite chromatography, octyl-agarose chromatography, Concanavalin A-Sepharose chromatography, and Sephacryl S-200 gel filtration.[16] The overall extent of purification of this

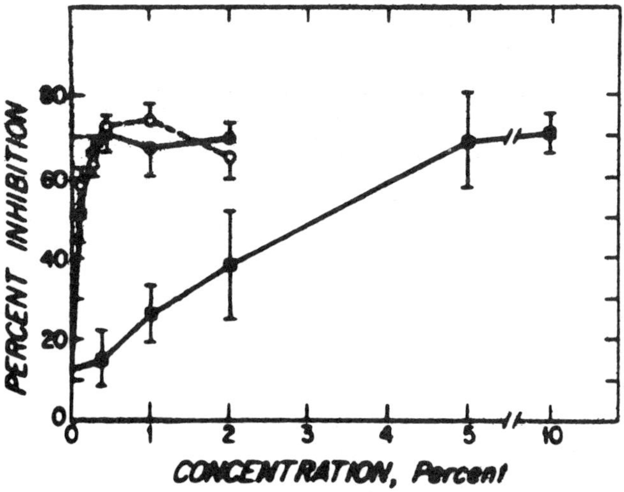

FIGURE 3. Ability of fetal calf serum, human serum, and platelet-poor plasma to release inhibitory activity from bovine aortic endothelial cells. The endothelial cells from three bovine aortas were pooled and plated into 60 mm dishes. Confluent primary cultures were washed and incubated in RPMI 1640 containing the indicated concentrations of fetal calf serum (O- - -O), human serum (●——●), or platelet-poor plasma (■——■) for 48 hours. The resulting medium was mixed with RPMI 1640 and fetal calf serum (final serum concentration, 20%) and tested for its ability to inhibit smooth muscle cell growth. Error bars indicate standard deviations.

platelet heparitinase is about 240,000-fold and the overall yield of the enzyme is about 5.6%, as compared to the initial freeze-thaw solubilization preparation. The final product is physically homogeneous as judged by disc gel electrophoresis at acidic pH, as well as by gel filtration chromatography, and exhibits an apparent molecular weight of approximately 134,000.[16] Furthermore, our results indicate that the above enzyme is present within platelet lysosomes.

The biologic potency of the endoglycosidase was examined as a function of pH. The data show that the platelet heparitinase is maximally active from pH 5.5 to pH 7.5. However, the enzyme possesses minimal ability to cleave heparin at pH less than 4.0 or greater than 9.0. The substrate specificity of the platelet endoglycosidase was determined by identifying susceptible linkages within the heparin molecule that can be

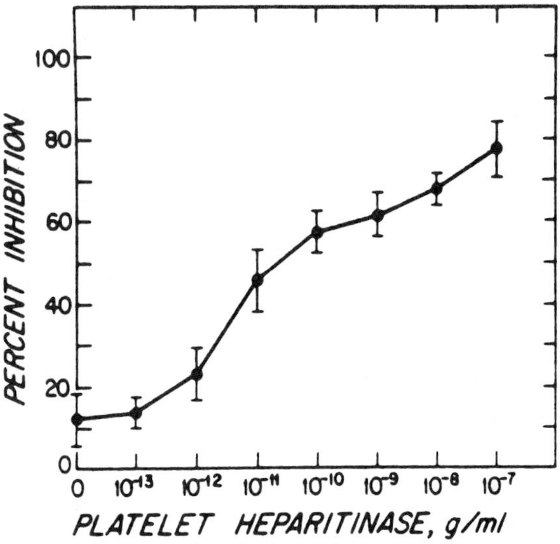

FIGURE 4. Ability of platelet heparitinase to release inhibitory activity from bovine aortic endothelial cells. Confluent primary cultures of endothelial cells were incubated in serum-free RPMI 1640 containing the indicated concentrations of platelet heparitinase for 4 hours at 37°C. The resulting medium was mixed with RPMI 1640 and fetal calf serum (final serum concentration, 20%) and tested for its ability to inhibit smooth muscle cell growth. Error bars indicate standard deviations.

cleaved by the above component. Our studies indicate that this enzyme is only able to hydrolyze glucuronsyl-glycosamine linkages. Furthermore, investigation of the structure of the disaccharide which lies on the nonreducing end of the cleaved glucuronic acid residue suggests that N-sulfation of the glucosamine moiety or ester sulfation of the adjacent iduronic acid groups are not essential for bond scission.[16]

We then examined the ability of the platelet heparitinase, described above, to release heparin-like species from cultured endothelial cells.[17] Our results show that when endothelial cells were exposed to serum-free medium containing 1 ng/ml of the purified platelet endoglycosidase, at least as much inhibitory activity was released as was obtained with 0.4% serum (FIGURE 4). Dose response experiments indicated that only 10 pg/ml of the enzyme were necessary to liberate 50% of the inhibitory activity from endothelial cells.[17] The heparin-like nature of the inhibitory substance was demonstrated by its sensitivity to *Flavobacterium* heparinase. Utilizing appropriate controls, the release of heparin-like material by the endoglycosidase was shown to be enzyme-specific and was not due to artifacts of experimental manipulation. In addition, this enzyme did not convert prereleased material to an active component, but directly liberated the active heparin-like species from endothelial cells.

Furthermore, we have recently shown that smooth muscle cells possess large quantities of antiproliferative heparin-like species which can also be liberated by the action of an endogenous endoglycosidase.[18] We have isolated a heparan sulfate from the medial region of the bovine aortic wall, and have shown that this mucopolysaccharide is able to inhibit the growth of SMCs.[23] Since SMCs are the predominant cell type within this segment of the vascular tissue, we thought it likely that these cells might also synthesize heparin-like molecules which could regulate their own growth potential. We investigated this possibility by isolating heparan sulfate from the cell surface, cell pellet, and culture medium of exponentially growing and post-confluent SMCs, and by determining their antiproliferative potencies. To accomplish this purpose, primary cultures of exponentially growing, as well as post-confluent SMCs were incubated with $Na_2S^{35}O_4$, and the radiolabeled glycosaminoglycans were obtained from the cell surface and cell pellet, as well as from the culture medium. These molecular species were freed of protein by extensive proteolytic digestion, and the resultant mucopolysaccharide chains were isolated by DEAE Sephadex and Sepharose 4B chromatography. The latter chromatographic techniques suggest that the average size and average charge density of either heparan sulfate or chondroitin sulfate are virtually identical and independent of cellular origin and growth stage. The bioassay of these components demonstrated that heparan sulfate from the cell surface, cell pellet, and culture medium of exponentially growing SMCs, as well as post-confluent SMCs, exhibits antiproliferative activity, whereas the similarly designated fractions of chondroitin sulfate possess no such biologic potency. Therefore, the anionic charge of the heparan sulfate cannot be the sole reason for the growth inhibitory potency of this component since the DEAE Sephadex chromatographic analyses clearly show that chondroitin sulfate has a higher average charge density than heparan sulfate. Indeed, the above findings indicate that certain specific structural elements of heparan sulfate, such as glycosidic bond configuration, sulfate position, or iduronic acid residues, are required for the observed antiproliferative effect.[11] The data indicate that heparan sulfate isolated from the surface of post-confluent SMCs exhibits about eight times the antiproliferative potency of the corresponding material obtained from the surface of exponentially growing SMCs. Heparan sulfate isolated from the cell pellet or culture medium of SMCs (in either growth state) possesses only minimal amounts of the growth inhibitory activity.

In order to prove that heparan sulfate, itself, was responsible for the antiproliferative phenomenon observed above, we exposed the post-confluent SMC mucopolysaccharide to either purified *Flavobacterium* heparinase or platelet endoglycosidase, separated the resultant species by HPLC/G 2000 SW, and assayed these components for growth inhibitory activity. On the one hand, our results indicated that degradation of the heparan sulfate to tetrasaccharides and disaccharides completely abolished antiproliferative potency. On the other hand, our data showed that cleavage of the heparan sulfate into larger fragments with molecular weights that ranged from 20,000 to 1300 had little effect on the growth inhibitory activity per 10^5 ^{35}S counts until a molecular weight of about 4000 (dodecasaccharide) was attained. Our demonstration that the antiproliferative potency of the heparan sulfate comigrates with the ^{35}S counts of large fragments of the mucopolysaccharide and that the growth inhibitory activity of the heparan sulfate can be eliminated by degradation of the mucopolysaccharide to tetrasaccharides and disaccharides strongly supports our contention that this glycosaminoglycan is responsible for the suppression of SMC proliferation.

The chemical masses of the various fractions of heparan sulfate were also determined by hexosamine analyses, and the specific antiproliferative activities of these glycosaminoglycans were calculated. The data showed that exponentially growing SMCs synthesize about 1.5 to 3.0 times the amount of heparan sulfate found in the corresponding fractions of post-confluent SMCs. Thus, the large amounts of antiproliferative activity present on the surface of post-confluent SMCs are not simply due to the augmented production of this glycosaminoglycan. Indeed, the heparan sulfate isolated from the surface of post-confluent SMCs had a specific inhibitory activity that is thirteen times that of the similarly designated mucopolysaccharide obtained from exponentially growing SMCs. This highly active heparan sulfate is able to dramatically inhibit SMC proliferation when added at a level as low as 20 ng/ml, and hence its potency is more than forty times greater than that of commercial heparin in suppressing the growth of these cells.[19]

We thought it possible that the reduced specific antiproliferative activity of heparan sulfate obtained from the surface of exponentially growing SMCs might be due to the degradation of the biologically active component by these cellular elements. To examine this hypothesis, we incubated radiolabeled heparan sulfate from the surface of post-confluent SMCs with exponentially growing SMCs for 24 hours, and showed by HPLC/G 2000 SW chromatography that minimal cleavage or desulfation had taken place. Thus, our data indicate that post-confluent SMCs are uniquely able to synthesize a heparan sulfate with remarkably potent antiproliferative activity and to place these components on their cell surface. This highly active heparan sulfate is likely to differ structurally to only a very minor extent when compared to mucopolysaccharides isolated from exponentially growing cells since both types of glycosaminoglycans appear to have similar average molecular sizes and average charge densities.[19]

Given that the surface of exponentially growing SMCs possess heparan sulfate with minimal growth inhibitory activity, we wondered whether the levels of this biologically potent mucopolysaccharide could represent residual highly active glycosaminoglycan generated by the primary post-confluent SMCs utilized to seed our cultures. To test this hypothesis, we harvested the surface glycosaminoglycans present on SMCs from the time of seeding to the period of post-confluence, isolated heparan sulfate by column chromatography, and ascertained the antiproliferative activity of the mucopolysaccharide per 10^6 cells. Our results indicate that exponentially growing SMCs retain small amounts of residual highly active heparan sulfate from the surface of primary post-confluent SMCs, but can produce little of the biologically active component. Indeed, we would suggest that the post-confluent SMCs and the SMCs at other stages of growth probably differ by as much as several hundredfold in regard to their ability to synthesize heparan sulfate with growth inhibitory potency and place these components on their surface. It is also of interest to note that the production of the biologically potent glycosaminoglycan appears to be abruptly induced at about four days after confluence is attained. The molecular signals needed to accomplish this end are unknown, but they could be similar to those required to express specific receptors on cell surfaces immediately after the cessation of growth.[19]

At the present time, it is difficult to completely explain the relative absence of the heparan sulfate with growth inhibitory activity from the culture medium and cell pellet of the post-confluent SMCs. These findings may be due to the differential placement of this component on the surface of the cells with an associated reduction in the sensitivity of this glycosaminoglycan to platelet endoglycosidase in the serum. With respect to the intracellular levels of heparan sulfate with antiproliferative activity, our observations are consistent with the presence of a large pool of minimally active heparan sulfate within the post-confluent SMCs and/or with an accelerated destruction of mucopolysaccharide with growth inhibitory potency within the SMCs. In this regard, it is of interest to note that other investigators have observed that secreted and cell surface heparan sulfate are handled as separate metabolic pools in other cell types.[20]

Based upon the above observations, we would propose a simple model for the possible role of heparin-like components and endoglycosidase in the regulation of SMC growth within the vessel wall. In the normal artery, endothelial cells, macrophages, and/or platelets serve as sources for mitogenic factors necessary for the growth of medial SMCs. However, SMCs also generate a specific type of heparan sulfate with antiproliferative activity that is positioned at the surface of the cell. The endoglycosidase, which can liberate the growth inhibitory mucopolysaccharide, is also available within the vessel wall. Under normal circumstances, the net effect of the mitogenic factors and the synthesis/release of the above heparan sulfate is to permit a small amount of SMC growth to compensate for the death of these cellular elements ($<0.1\%$ per day).

During damage to the endothelium, platelets and macrophages would appear at the site of injury and release high concentrations of growth factors. The SMCs might be able to respond to these pathologic alterations by augmenting the synthesis/release of the heparan sulfate with antiproliferative activity in a fashion identical to that noted when these cellular elements reach a post-confluent stage of cell growth. In this situation, the net balance between the elevated concentrations of mitogenic factors and the increased levels of free heparan sulfate with growth inhibitory activity would ultimately determine whether SMCs migrate to the luminal surface of the blood vessel wall and mount a proliferative response. Thus, this specific form of heparan sulfate would be positioned to act as a negative control element during the regulation of cell proliferation, which acts in a similar manner to that postulated for certain proteins isolated from the surface of 3T3 cells and endothelial cells.[21,22] It should be possible to test the above model once the structure of this unique heparan sulfate has been elucidated and the biosynthetic steps required to generate the mucopolysaccharide have been defined.

REFERENCES

1. Ross, R., B. Glomset, B. Kariya & L. Harker. 1974. Platelet and smooth muscle cell proliferation. Proc. Natl. Acad. Sci. USA **71:** 1207–1210.
2. Harker, L. A., R. Ross, S. J. Slichter & C. R. Scott. 1976. The role of endothelial cell injury and platelet response in its genesis. J. Clin. Invest. **58:** 731–741.
3. Heldin, C. H., A. Wasteson & B. Westermarke. 1977. Partial purification and characterization of platelet factors stimulating the multiplication of normal human glial cells. Exp. Cell. Res. **109:** 429–437.
4. Scher, C. D., W. J. Pledger, P. Martin, H. N. Antoniades & C. D. Stiles. 1978. Transforming viruses directly reduce the cellular growth requirement for a platelet-derived growth factor. J. Cell. Physiol. **97:** 371–380.
5. Gajdusek, C., P. DiCorleto, R. Ross & S. M. Schwartz. 1980. An endothelial cell-derived growth factor. J. Cell Biol. **85:** 467–472.
6. Friedman, R. J., M. B. Stemerman, B. Wenz, S. Moore, J. Galudie, M. Gent, M. L. Tiell & T. H. Spaet. 1977. The effect of thrombocytopenia on experimental arteriosclerotic lesion formation in rabbits: Smooth muscle cell proliferation and re-endothelialization. J. Clin. Invest. **60:** 1191–1201.
7. Groves, H. M., R. L. Kinlough-Rathbone, M. Richardson, S. Moore & J. F. Mustard. 1979. Platelet interaction with damaged rabbit aorta. Lab. Invest. **40:** 194–200.
8. Moore, S., R. J. Friedman, D. J. Singal, J. Galudie, M. A. Blajchman & R. S.

ROBERTS. 1976. Inhibition of injury induced thromboatherosclerotic lesions by antiplatelet serum in rabbits. Thromb. Haemostas. **35:** 70–81.

9. CLOWES, A. W. & M. J. KARNOVSKY. 1977. Suppression of heparin of smooth muscle cell proliferation in injured arteries. Nature **265:** 625–626.
10. CASTELLOT, J. J., JR., M. J. KARNOVSKY & R. D. ROSENBERG. The biology of endothelial cells. E. Jaffe, Ed. In press.
11. HOOVER, R. L., R. D. ROSENBERG, W. HAERING & M. J. KARNOVSKY. 1980. Inhibition of rat arterial smooth muscle cell proliferation by heparin. Part II. *In vitro* studies. Cir. Res. **47:** 578–583.
12. CASTELLOT, J. J., JR., M. L. ADDONIZIO, R. D. ROSENBERG & M. J. KARNOVSKY. 1981. Cultured endothelial cells produce a heparin-like inhibitor of smooth muscle cell growth. J. Cell Biol. **90:** 372–379.
13. LAM, L. H., J. E. SILBERT & R. D. ROSENBERG. 1976. The separation of active and inactive forms of heparin. Biochem. Biophys. Res. Commun. **69:** 570–577.
14. PLEDGER, W. J., C. D. STILES, H. N. ANTONIADES & C. D. SCHER. 1977. Induction of DNA synthesis in BALB/c 3T3 cells by serum components: Reevaluation of the commitment process. Proc. Natl. Acad. Sci. USA **74:** 4481–4485.
15. CASTELLOT, J. J., JR., M. J. KARNOVSKY, R. D. ROSENBERG & D. L. BEELER. 1984. Structural determinants of the capacity of heparin to inhibit the proliferation of vascular smooth muscle cells. J. Cell. Physiol. In press.
16. OOSTA, G. M., L. V. FAVREAU, D. L. BEELER & R. D. ROSENBERG. 1982. Purification and properties of human platelet heparitinase. J. Biol. Chem. **257:** 11249–11255.
17. CASTELLOT, J. J., JR., L. V. FAVREAU, R. D. ROSENBERG & M. J. KARNOVSKY. 1982. Inhibition of vascular smooth muscle cell growth by endothelial cell-derived heparin: Possible role of a platelet endoglycosidase. J. Biol. Chem. **257:** 11256–11260.
18. KARNOVSKY, M. J., J. J. CASTELLOT, JR., R. D. ROSENBERG & G. M. OOSTA. 1984. Effects of heparin on vascular smooth muscle cell proliferation. Clin. Physiol. Series. American Physiol. Society. Washington, D.C. In press.
19. FRITZE, L. M. S., C. F. REILLY & R. D. ROSENBERG. 1985. An antiproliferative heparan sulfate species produced by post-confluent smooth muscle cells. J. Cell Biol. **100:** 1041–1049.
20. VOGEL, K. G., V. F. KENDALL & R. E. SAPIEN. 1981. Glycosaminoglycan synthesis and composition in human fibroblasts during *in vitro* cellular aging (IMR–90). J. Cell Physiol. **107:** 271–281.
21. WHITTENBERGER, B., D. RABEN, M. A. LIEBERMAN & L. GLASER. 1978. Inhibition of growth of 3T3 cells by extract of surface membranes. Proc. Natl. Acad. Sci. USA **75:** 5457–5461.
22. HEIMARK, R. L. & S. M. SCHWARTZ. 1983. Inhibition of endothelial cell growth by a membrane preparation from confluent endothelial cells. J. Cell Biol. **97:** 90a, abs. 344.
23. REILLY, C. & R. D. ROSENBERG. Manuscript in preparation.

Physiologic Functions of Normal Endothelial Cells

ERIC A. JAFFE

Division of Hematology-Oncology
Department of Medicine
Cornell University Medical College
New York, New York 10021

Endothelial cells (EC) line the insides of all blood vessels and occupy a surface area of more than 1000 m^2. Assuming individual endothelial cells are approximately 20 × 50 $microns^2$, the body contains about 1000 m^2/1000 $microns^2$ or 10^{12} endothelial cells which weigh in excess of 100 grams. Because of their location and contact with the flowing bloodstream, endothelial cells are perfectly positioned to modulate the various biologic systems in blood, particularly the coagulation system. The development in the early 1970's of methods for culturing EC[1] made possible the study of EC cell biology. In this article, I will review briefly the normal physiologic functions of EC.

SYNTHESIS OF CONNECTIVE TISSUE COMPONENTS

EC *in vivo* rest on a basement membrane which anchors the EC to the blood vessel wall and which forms a secondary barrier to the passage of fluid and formed elements into the extravascular compartment. Basement membranes contain one or more types of collagen, elastin, microfibrils, laminin, and mucopolysaccharides, along with some fibronectin and thrombospondin. *In vitro,* EC synthesize and secrete several types of collagen. Cultured human umbilical vein and vena cava EC secrete type IV collagen into their culture medium, while they secrete both types IV and V into their underlying extracellular matrix.[2] In contrast, bovine aortic, pulmonary artery, and mesenteric vein EC secrete types III and "EC" (a newly described collagen type) into their post-culture medium, while they secrete types III, IV, and V collagen into their underlying extracellular matrix.[3–6] Bovine adrenal capillary EC secrete types I and III collagen into both their post-culture medium and into their extracellular matrix, but also, they secrete type V collagen into their extracellular matrix.[6] It is not clear if these differences are due to the fact that the EC were cultured from different species or that the cells tested originated from different sites within one specie. This subject has recently been reviewed in detail.[7]

Elastin which exists *in vivo* as a highly cross-linked protein is initially synthesized *in vitro* by EC as a single chain molecule, tropoelastin, which has a molecular weight 75 kD.[8,9] Soon after tropoelastin is secreted, it starts to become cross-linked as shown by the appearance of the elastin cross-link specific amino acids, desmosine and isodesmosine.[10]

Fibronectin and thrombospondin, while present in only small amounts *in vivo* in the basement membrane when compared to other basement membrane proteins, are two of the major proteins secreted by cultured EC. In human EC, fibronectin makes up about 17% and thrombospondin about 14% of the protein secreted into the post-culture medium.[2,11,12] Both proteins are incorporated into the EC extracellular matrix and form fibrillar meshworks. These proteins are also synthesized by bovine aortic endothelial cells.[13–15]

Mucopolysaccharides are present on both EC membranes and in extracellular matrix. The cell surface pool is predominantly heparan sulfate and the extracellular pool contains heparan sulfate, dermatan sulfate, and chondroitin sulfate.[16–22] These mucopolysaccharides may play a role in the activation of antithrombin III (see below).

Laminin, another component of basement membrane, is also secreted by EC, but its production rate varies markedly over a 20-fold range with the level of cell confluency. It is secreted in greatest quantities when the EC are subconfluent. In confluent cultures, laminin is associated primarily with the extracellular matrix and codistributes with type IV collagen.[23]

EC can also remodel basement membranes since, when stimulated, they release and/or contain collagenases that can digest types I, II, III, IV, and V collagen.[24–26]

PROPERTIES OF ENDOTHELIAL CELLS

Procoagulant Properties of EC

The subendothelium synthesized by EC is ordinarily covered by EC, and unstimulated platelets do not adhere to intact EC. However, removal or contraction of EC exposes the subendothelium, which rapidly becomes covered with a layer of platelets that soon degranulates.[27,28] Subendothelial collagen types IV and V and microfibrils cause platelet aggregation and thromboxane A_2 release,[29–33] whereas laminin, elastin, and heparan sulfate proteoglycan do not.[28,31]

Adhesion of platelets to the subendothelium is dependent on factor VIII-von Willebrand factor (VIII–vWF).[34–39] EC synthesize VIII–vWF (MW 220–225K) in a "pro" form, which has a MW 240–260 kD.[40,41] This "pro" form is cleaved and aggregates into the large MW multimers that are active in supporting platelet adhesion.[42] VIII–vWF binds *in vitro* to types I, III, IV, and V collagen,[39] and is found *in vivo* in the subendothelium.[43,44] Since platelets contain a surface receptor for VIII–vWF,[45–48] it is likely that platelets adhere to the subendothelium via VIII–vWF. This concept is consistent with findings that platelet adhesion to the subendothelium is decreased in von Willebrand's disease[34,36] and is corrected by exogenous VIII–vWF.[36]

Factor V functions to accelerate the activation of prothrombin by factor X_a. Recently, EC have been shown to synthesize factor V,[49] though other studies have also demonstrated synthesis of factor V by hepatocytes.[50] In addition, EC also bind exogenous factor V with a $K_d = 2$ n*M*. Each cell binds about 20–25,000 factor V molecules, and this factor V is active in coagulation assays.[51]

Tissue factor reacts with factor VII and calcium, and markedly accelerates the ability of factor VII to activte factor X. Intact EC possess little or no tissue factor activity.[52–54] However, when EC are exposed to thrombin or endotoxin, their tissue factor activity increases ten- to fortyfold. The additional presence of washed platelets enhanced tissue factor activity by up to 170-fold.[55,56] The presence of either lymphocytes, granulocytes, or macrophages also stimulated tissue factor activity two- to sevenfold.[57]

Recently, two groups have demonstrated that factors IX_a and X_a bind to EC. Factor IX_a binds to EC with a K_d of 2.3 n*M* and a B_{max} of 20,000 molecules/cell.[58,59] Binding is calcium-dependent and is blocked by unlabeled factors IX or IX_a, but not by factor X, prothrombin, or thrombin. Cell-bound factor IX_a is at least threefold more active than factor IX_a in solution,[58] and EC-bound factor IX can be activated.[60] Similar studies have shown that factors X and X_a also bind to EC and that binding is up to sixfold greater in sparse EC.[59,61] Binding of these two coagulation proteins probably serves to localize the coagulation process.

The mechanism of the initial activation of Hageman factor (factor XII) *in vivo* is still not clear, but rabbit EC have been shown to activate factor XII by proteolytic cleavage.[62] The enzyme responsible for the activation is apparently membrane-bound and does not directly cleave either factor XI nor prekallikrein, though the factor XII_a produced will cleave both factor XI and prekallikrein.[62]

Antiplatelet Properties of EC

EC *in vivo* are intrinsically non-thrombogenic since unstimulated platelets do not adhere to the surface of intact confluent monolayers of endothelial cells *in vivo*,[28,63] and they adhere only minimally to intact monolayers *in vitro*.[64–67] *In vitro*, platelets that appear to adhere to EC actually adhere to exposed subendothelium and not to the cells themselves.[64] This non-thrombogenic property seems to be intrinsic to the EC plasma membrane and is unrelated to prostacyclin production since inhibition of prostacyclin production does not increase the adhesion of unstimulated platelets.[63,65–67] In contrast, the inhibition of adhesion of stimulated platelets to EC is highly prostacyclin-dependent.[65,67,68]

Prostacyclin (PGI_2) is a potent vasodilator and inhibitor of platelet function.[69–73] EC synthesize PGI_2 from arachidonic acid, an essential fatty acid, and secrete it into the adjacent fluid.[68,74,75] PGI_2 has a short half-life (6 min in whole blood), and is synthesized and secreted when the cells are stimulated. PGI_2 synthesis is markedly stimulated by thrombin and trypsin,[76] histamine,[77,78] bradykinin,[79] lipoproteins (especially HDL),[80,81] serum factors produced during coagulation,[82] selenium,[83] and immunologic injury.[84] Other stimulators of EC PGI_2 synthesis include adenine nucleotides (particularly ATP),[85] enkephalins,[86] leukotriene C,[87] $MgSO_4$,[88] and platelet-derived growth factor.[81] Synthesis of PGI_2 is inhibited by aspirin[89] and several nonsteroidal anti-inflammatory agents such as indomethacin;[74] both types of agents inhibit the enzyme cyclooxygenase. Nicotine also inhibits the release of PGI_2,[90] as does feeding the cells linoleic acid, the predominant fatty acid in diets high in polyunsaturated fats.[91] EC can also convert prostaglandin endoperoxides secreted by platelets into PGI_2;[92] this mechanism is probably most important in the microvasculature where the EC/platelet ratio is $> = 1{:}1$. Treatment of EC with human platelet calcium-activated protease inhibits thrombin-induced PGI_2 synthesis,[93] suggesting that activated platelets have a mechanism for modulating EC PGI_2 synthesis. Both 6-keto-PGF_{1a}, the stable, but inactive end product of PGI_2, and PGI_2, itself, can be converted to 6-keto-PGE_1, a stable and active vasodilator and inhibitor of platelet function.[94] While measurable levels of 6-keto-PGE_1 are found in normal plasma, it is unclear what role, if any, 6-keto-PGE_1 plays *in vivo*. Interestingly, not all EC synthesize PGI_2 as their major arachidonic acid metabolite since recent studies have demonstrated that human foreskin capillary EC synthesize mainly PGE_2 and PGF_{2a}.[95]

Aggregating platelets release ADP, which recruits nearby platelets into the developing platelet plug, and ATP, a vasodilator. EC can modulate the effects of the released ADP and ATP because they possess ectoenzymes, which rapidly metabolize ADP and ATP to AMP, and adenosine, a strong inhibitor of platelet function. EC can take up exogenous adenosine and convert it to ATP, and can also release ATP.[96–101] Adenosine is a vasodilator, and is considered to be a local hormone which can regulate blood flow.

Anticoagulant Properties of EC

In vivo, plasma antithrombin III rapidly inactivates thrombin by forming a covalent thrombin-antithrombin complex, which circulates in plasma until cleared by the liver.[102] *In vitro,* the process proceeds slowly, but the inactivation of thrombin by antithrombin III is dramatically accelerated by heparin, heparan sulfate, or EC.[103] The acceleratory effect of EC is probably due to heparan sulfate on the cell membrane.[16,17,102,103] EC may also support the ability of antithrombin III to inactivate factors IX_a, X_a, and XII_a. During aggregation, platelets release both an endoglycosidase that degrades EC surface heparan sulfate[19] and platelet factor 4, which blocks the ability of EC to accelerate the inactivation of thrombin by antithrombin III.[103] Exogenous heparin also binds to EC[104,105] and appears to promote the inactivation of thrombin by antithrombin III.[106]

Protein C is a vitamin K dependent protein synthesized by the liver that inactivates factors V and VIII by proteolysis.[107–112] Protein C is activated only by thrombin, and this activation proceeds very slowly unless it takes place in the presence of EC. EC contain on their surface a protein called thrombomodulin, which binds thrombin and markedly enhances the ability of thrombin to activate protein C.[110,111,113] Interestingly, thrombin bound to thrombomodulin cannot activate platelets or cleave fibrinogen.[114,115] Unlike the antithrombin III-EC interaction, the acceleration of protein C activation by EC is not blocked by platelet factor 4.[111] Protein C, therefore, must play an important role *in vivo* because congenital deficiency of protein C is associated with thrombotic disease.[116–119]

EC secrete protease nexin, a protein of M_r 40,000 daltons, which inactivates thrombin by forming a covalent complex at its active site, and which is unrelated to antithrombin III.[120,121] The thrombin-protease nexin complex then binds to the EC, is internalized, and is degraded by lysosomal enzymes.[121] Protease nexin also binds and inactivates trypsin, urokinase, and plasmin.[121] Since almost all of the thrombin injected into animals rapidly complexes with antithrombin III,[102] the role of protease nexin in inhibiting thrombin *in vivo* is unclear.

Fibrinolytic Properties of EC

Plasminogen activator exists in two forms; the urokinase type activates plasminogen in the fluid phase, whereas the tissue type is active only when bound to fibrin. *In vivo,* EC apparently only synthesize tissue plasminogen activator, while in tissue culture, both types are made.[122–124] EC also secrete an M_r 55,000 inhibitor of plasminogen activator.[122,125] In tissue cultures with low-cell densities, EC secrete small amounts of plasminogen activator and high amounts of plasminogen activator inhibitor, whereas at confluency, the secretion of plasminogen activator by the cells rises while the inhibitor activity falls.[126] In addition, thrombin causes a rapid and profound decrease in the secretion of plasminogen activator by the cells.[127]

EC-Derived Growth Regulators

EC play an important role in regulating the growth of underlying smooth muscle cells. EC secrete a platelet-derived growth factor-like protein that binds to PDGF receptors on both 3T3 cells and smooth muscle cells.[128] The binding of the EC-derived growth factor (ECDGF) to the cells is blocked by treating the ECDGF with antiserum to human PDGF.[128] EC also secrete a heparin-like inhibitor of smooth muscle cell growth that is active at concentrations as low as 10 ng/ml.[129] Interestingly, secreting platelets release a endoglycosidase that can cleave EC surface heparin-like species from cultured EC.[130] Lastly, EC secrete an activity which can support the growth of other EC, and which is different from the PDGF-like material described above.[131]

Metabolic Properties of EC

Lipoprotein lipase hydrolyzes the di- and triacylglycerol constituents of very low-density lipoproteins (VLDL) and chylomicrons. Several groups have demonstrated that while EC do not synthesize lipoprotein lipase, they do bind the enzyme avidly to heparan sulfate or heparan sulfate-like molecules on their surfaces.[132,133] Lipoprotein lipase, itself, is synthesized by macrophages and smooth muscle cells, and presumably is transferred from these cell types to EC.[134]

EC possess receptors for beta-LDL, HDL, acetyl-LDL (the scavenger receptor), and chylomicrons.[135–137] While rapidly growing EC bind and internalize LDL, confluent EC bind, but do not internalize LDL.[138] EC also can modify LDL molecules and generate a form that is more rapidly degraded by macrophages and that is recognized by the macrophage receptor for acetylated LDL.[139]

Like many other cells, EC also bind insulin.[140] Arterial EC bind 2.5 times more insulin/cell than venous EC.[141] In addition, there is a difference in the insulin effect among EC from different anatomical locations. Insulin increases glucose incorporation into glycogen and thymidine incorporation into DNA in retinal EC, but not in aortic EC.[142] These data suggest that a differential response to insulin may exist between the endothelium of large and small vessels.

EC contain on their surface angiotensin converting enzyme (ACE), which converts vasoinactive angiotensin I to the vasoconstrictor angiotensin II and inactivates the vasodilator bradykinin.[143,144] EC also contain angiotensinases A and C, which inactivate angiotensin II.[144,145]

Interactions of EC with White Cells

Polymorphonuclear leukocytes (PMN) adhere to the surfaces of EC *in vivo* (50% of PMN are in the marginal pool), and they must traverse across the EC barrier before reaching the extravascular space. Chemotactic factors stimulate PMN adherence to EC,[146,147] and there are high-affinity binding sites for formyl-methionyl-leucyl-phenylalanine (FMLP) on the surface of EC.[148] However, it is not clear if FMLP exerts its effect by interacting with EC rather than with PMN.[149] Platelet-release products enhance PMN-EC interaction, and this effect appears to be due to serotonin.[150] Monocytes also selectively interact with EC, though the biochemical mechanism involved is unknown.[151] Lastly, lymphocytes adhere to cultured EC, and this adherence seems to be greater for stimulated lymphocytes than for naive cells.[152,153]

EC synthesize and release colony stimulating activity (CSA) that is active on granulocyte-macrophage colonies.[154] Synthesis of this material is enhanced by treating the EC with endotoxin.[154] Recent work shows that this material has a molecular weight of 15–30,000.[155] In addition, EC released material that stimulated the growth of BFU-E.[155] Synthesis of CSA by EC is, in turn, stimulated by a monokine whose own release is suppressed by lactoferrin.[156] Thus, there seems to be a circular control mechanism for regulating the production of PMN and CSA.

Immunologic Properties of EC

Human EC contain ABO blood group and HLA-A,B antigens.[1,157] In contrast, only a small percentage of unstimulated EC contain Ia antigens.[158] However, when human EC are stimulated with gamma-interferon or by activated T cells, Ia antigens are induced on the surface of all EC exposed to the stimulus after an exposure of 72 hours.[159] This observation is compatible with and supports the observation that EC can act as antigen-presenting cells.[160,161]

REFERENCES

1. JAFFE, E. A., R. L. NACHMAN, C. G. BECKER & C. R. MINICK. 1973. Culture of human endothelial cells derived from umbilical cord veins. Identification by morphologic and immunologic criteria. J. Clin. Invest. **52:** 2745–2756.
2. SAGE, H. & P. BORNSTEIN. 1982. Endothelial cells from umbilical vein and a hemangioendothelioma secrete basement membrane largely to the exclusion of interstitial collagens. Arteriosclerosis **2:** 27–36.
3. SAGE, H., E. C. CROUCH & P. BORNSTEIN. 1979. Collagen synthesis by bovine aortic endothelial cells in culture. Biochemistry **18:** 5433–5442.
4. SAGE, H., P. PRITZL & P. BORNSTEIN. 1980. A unique, pepsin-sensitive collagen synthesized by aortic endothelial cells in culture. Biochemistry **19:** 5747–5755.
5. SAGE, H., P. PRITZL & P. BORNSTEIN. 1981. Characterization of cell matrix-associated collagens synthesized by aortic endothelial cells in culture. Biochemistry **20:** 436–442.
6. SAGE, H., P. PRIZTL & P. BORNSTEIN. 1981. Secretory phenotypes of endothelial cells in culture: Comparison of aortic, venous, capillary, and corneal endothelium. Arteriosclerosis **1:** 427–442.
7. SAGE, H. 1984. Collagen synthesis by endothelial cells in culture. *In* Biology of Endothelial Cells. E. A. Jaffe, Ed.: 161–177. Martinus-Nijhoff. Boston.
8. MECHAM, R. P., J. MADARAS, J. A. MCDONALD & U. RYAN. 1983. Elastin production by cultured calf pulmonary artery endothelial cells. J. Cell. Physiol. **116:** 282–288.
9. CARNES, W. H., P. A. ABRAHAM & V. BUONASSISI. 1979. Biosynthesis of elastin by an endothelial cell culture. Biochem. Biophys. Res. Commun. **90:** 1393–1399.
10. CANTOR, J. O., S. KELLER, M. S. PARSHLEY, T. V. DARNULE, A. T. DARNULE, J. M. CERRETA, G. M. TURINO & I. MANDL. 1980. Synthesis of cross-linked elastin by an endothelial cell culture. Biochem. Biophys. Res. Commun. **95:** 1381–1386.
11. MOSHER, D. F., M. J. DOYLE & E. A. JAFFE. 1982. Synthesis and secretion of thrombospondin by cultured endothelial cells. J. Cell Biol. **93:** 343–348.
12. JAFFE, E. A. & D. F. MOSHER. 1978. Synthesis of fibronectin by cultured human endothelial cells. J. Exp. Med. **147:** 1779–1791.
13. MCPHERSON, J., H. SAGE & P. BORNSTEIN. 1981. Isolation and characterization of a glycoprotein secreted by aortic endothelial cells in culture. Apparent identity with platelet thrombospondin. J. Biol. Chem. **256:** 11330–11336.
14. BIRDWELL, C. R., D. GOSPODAROWICZ & G. L. NICOLSON. 1978. Identification, localization, and role of fibronectin in cultured bovine endothelial cells. Proc. Natl. Acad. Sci. USA **75:** 3273–3277.
15. MACARAK, E. J., E. KIRBY, T. KIRK & N. A. KEFALIDES. 1978. Synthesis of cold-insoluble globulin by cultured calf endothelial cells. Proc. Natl. Acad. Sci. USA **75:** 2621–2625.
16. BUONASSISI, V. 1973. Sulfated mucopolysaccharide synthesis and secretion in endothelial cell cultures. Exp. Cell Res. **76:** 363–368.
17. BOUNASSISI, V. & M. ROOT. 1975. Enzymatic degradation of heparin-related mucopolysaccharides from the surface of endothelial cell cultures. Biochim. Biophys. Acta **385:** 1–10.
18. SAMPSON, P., M. S. PARSHLEY, I. MANDL & G. M. TURINO. 1975. Glycosaminoglycans produced in tissue culture by rat lung cells. Isolation from a mixed cell line and a derived endothelial clone. Connect. Tissue Res. **4:** 41–49.

19. WASTESON, A., B. GLIMELIUS, C. BUSCH, B. WESTERMARK, C-H. HELDIN & B. NORLING. 1977. Effect of platelet endoglycosidase on cell surface associated heparan sulfate of human cultured endothelial and glial cells. Thrombos. Res. **11:** 309–321.

20. BIHARI-VARGA, M., E. CSONKA & H. JELLINEK. 1980. Endothelial glycosaminglycans—*in vitro* studies. Artery **8:** 355–361.

21. OOHIRA, A., T. N. WIGHT & P. BORNSTEIN. 1983. Sulfated proteoglycans synthesized by vascular endothelial cells in culture. J. Biol. Chem. **258:** 2014–2021.

22. GAMSE, G., H. G. FROMME & H. KRESSE. 1978. Metabolism of sulfated glycosaminoglycans in cultured endothelial cells from bovine aorta. Biochim. Biophys. Acta **544:** 514–528.

23. GOSPODAROWICZ, D., G. GREENBURG, J. M. FOIDART & N. SAVION. 1981. The production and localization of laminin in cultured vascular and corneal endothelial cells. J. Cell. Physiol. **107:** 171–183.

24. MOSCATELLI, D., E. A. JAFFE & D. B. RIFKIN. 1980. Tetradecanoyl phorbol acetate stimulates latent collagenase production by cultured human endothelial cells. Cell **20:** 343–351.

25. GROSS, J. L., D. MOSCATELLI, E. A. JAFFE & D. B. RIFKIN. 1982. Plasminogen activator and collagenase production by cultured capillary endothelial cells. J. Cell. Biol. **95:** 974–981.

26. KALEBIC, T., S. GARBISA, B. GLASER & L. A. LIOTTA. 1983. Basement membrane collagen: Degradation by migrating endothelial cells. Science **221:** 281–283.

27. WARREN, B. A. & O. VALES. 1972. The release of vesicles from platelets following adhesion to vessel walls *in vitro*. Br. J. Exp. Pathol. **53:** 206–215.

28. STEMERMAN, M. B. 1974. Vascular intimal components: Precursors of thrombosis. *In* Progress in Hemostasis and Thrombosis, vol. 2. T. H. Spaet, Ed.: 1–47. Grune & Stratton. New York.

29. CHIANG, T. M., C. L. MAINARDI, J. M. SEYER & A. H. KANG. 1980. Collagen platelet interaction. Type V (A–B) collagen induces platelet aggregation. J. Lab. Clin. Med. **95:** 99–107.

30. BARNES, M. J., A. J. BAILEY, J. L. GORDON & D. E. MACINTYRE. 1980. Platelet aggregation by basement membrane-associated collagens. Thrombos. Res. **18:** 375–388.

31. TRYGGVASON, K., J. OIKARINEN, L. VIINIKKA & O. YLIKORKALA. 1981. Effects of laminin, proteoglycan, type IV collagen, and components of basement membranes on platelet aggregation. Biochem. Biophys. Res. Commun. **100:** 233–239.

32. LEGRAND, Y., F. FAUVEL, N. GUTMAN, J. P. MUH, G. TOBELEM, H. SOUCHON, A. KARNIGUIAN & J. P. CAEN. 1980. Microfibrils (MF) platelet interaction: Requirement of von Willebrand factor. Thrombos. Res. **19:** 737–739.

33. FAUVEL, F., M. E. GRANT, Y. J. LEGRAND, H. SOUCHON, G. TOBELEM, D. S. JACKSON & J. P. CAEN. 1983. Interaction of blood platelets with a microfibrillar extract from adult bovine aorta: Requirement for von Willebrand factor. Proc. Natl. Acad. Sci. USA **80:** 551–554.

34. TSCHOPP, T. B., H. J. WEISS & H. R. BAUMGARTNER. 1974. Decreased adhesion of platelets to subendothelium in von Willebrand's disease. J. Lab. Clin. Med. **83:** 296–300.

35. BAUMGARTNER, H. R., T. B. TSCHOPP & D. MEYER. 1980. Shear rate dependent inhibition of platelet adhesion/aggregation on collagenous surfaces by antibodies to human factor VIII/von Willebrand factor. Br. J. Haematol. **44:** 127–139.

36. WEISS, H. J., H. R. BAUMGARTNER, T. B. TSCHOPP, V. T. TURITTO & D. COHEN. 1978. Correction by factor VIII of the impaired platelet adhesion to subendothelium in von Willebrand's disease. Blood **51:** 267–279.

37. SAKARIASSEN, K. S., P. A. BOLHUIS & J. J. SIXMA. 1979. Human blood platelet adhesion to artery subendothelium is mediated by factor VIII-von Willebrand factor bound to the subendothelium. Nature **279:** 636–638.

38. BOLHUIS, P. A., K. S. SAKARIASSEN, H. J. SANDER, B. N. BOUMA & J. J. SIXMA. 1981. Binding of factor VIII-von Willebrand factor to human arterial subendothelium

precedes increased platelet adhesion and enhances platelet spreading. J. Lab. Clin. Med. **97:** 568–576.
39. MEYER, D. & H. R. BAUMGARTNER. 1983. Role of von Willebrand factor in platelet adhesion to the subendothelium. Br. J. Haematol. **54:** 1–9.
40. WAGNER, D. D. & V. J. MARDER. 1983. Biosynthesis of von Willebrand protein by human endothelial cells. Identification of a large precursor polypeptide chain. J. Biol. Chem. **258:** 2065–2067.
41. LYNCH, D. C., R. WILLIAMS, T. S. ZIMMERMAN, E. P. KIRBY & D. M. LIVINGSTON. 1983. Biosynthesis of the subunits of factor VIIIR by bovine aortic endothelial cells. Proc. Natl. Acad. Sci. USA **80:** 2738–2742.
42. LYNCH, D. C., T. S. ZIMMERMAN, E. P. KIRBY & D. M. LIVINGSTON. 1983. Subunit composition of oligomeric human von Willebrand factor. J. Biol. Chem. **258:** 12757–12760.
43. BLOOM, A. L., J. C. GIDDINGS & C. J. WILKS. 1973. Factor VIII on the vascular intima: Possible importance in haemostasis and thrombosis. Nature (New Biol.) **24:** 217–219.
44. RAND, J. H., R. E. GORDON, I. I. SUSSMAN, S. V. CHU & V. SOLOMON. 1982. Electron microscopic localization of factor-VIII-related antigen in adult human blood vessels. Blood **60:** 627–634.
45. FUJIMOTO, T., S. OHARA & J. HAWIGER. 1982. Thrombin-induced exposure and prostacyclin inhibition of the receptor for factor VIII-von Willebrand factor on human platelets. J. Clin. Invest. **69:** 1212–1222.
46. KAO, K. J., S. V. PIZZO & P. A. MCKEE. 1979. Demonstration and characterization of specific binding sites of factor VIII-von Willebrand factor on human platelets. J. Clin. Invest. **63:** 656–664.
47. KAO, K. J., S. V. PIZZO & P. A. MCKEE. 1979. Platelet receptor for human factor VIII-von Willebrand protein: Functional correlation of receptor occupancy and ristocetin-induced platelet aggregation. Proc. Natl. Acad. Sci. USA **76:** 5317–5320.
48. MORISATO, D. K. & H. R. GRALNICK. 1980. Selective binding of the factor VIII-von Willebrand factor protein to human platelets. Blood **55:** 9–15.
49. CERVENY, T. J., D. N. FASS & K. G. MANN. 1984. Synthesis of coagulation factor V by cultured aortic endothelium. Blood **63:** 1467–1474.
50. WILSON, D. B., H. H. SALEM, J. S. MRUK, I. MARUYAMA & P. W. MAJERUS. 1984. Biosynthesis of coagulation factor V by a human hepatocellular carcinoma cell line. J. Clin. Invest. **73:** 654–658.
51. MARUYAMA, I., H. H. SALEM & P. W. MAJERUS. 1984. Coagulation factor V_a binds to human umbilical vein endothelial cells and accelerates protein C activation. J. Clin. Invest. **74:** 224–230.
52. MAYNARD, J. R., B. E. DREYER, M. B. STEMERMAN & F. A. PITLICK. 1977. Tissue-factor coagulant activity of cultured human endothelial and smooth muscle cells and fibroblasts. Blood **50:** 387–396.
53. COLUCCI, M., G. BALCONI, R. LORENZET, A. PIETRA, D. LOCATI, M. B. DONATI & N. SEMARARO. 1983. Cultured human endothelial cells generate tissue factor in response to endotoxin. J. Clin. Invest. **71:** 1893–1896.
54. RODGERS, G. M., C. S. GREENBERG & M. A. SHUMAN. 1983. Characterization of the effects of cultured vascular cells on the activation of blood coagulation. Blood **61:** 1155–1162.
55. JOHNSEN, U. L. H., T. LYBERG, K. S. GALDAL & H. PRYDZ. 1983. Platelets stimulate thromboplastin synthesis in human endothelial cells. Thromb. Haemostas. **49:** 69–72.
56. BROX, J. H., B. OSTERUD, E. BJORKLID & J. W. FENTON II. 1984. Production and availability of thromboplastin in endothelial cells: The effects of thrombin, endotoxin, and platelets. Br. J. Haematol. **57:** 239–246.
57. LYBERG, T., K. S. GALDAL, S. A. EVENSEN & H. PRYDZ. 1983. Cellular cooperation in endothelial cell thromboplastin synthesis. Br. J. Haematol. **53:** 85–95.
58. STERN, D. M., M. DRILLINGS, H. L. NOSSEL, A. HURLET-JENSEN, K. LAGAMMA & J. OWEN. 1983. Binding of factors IX and IX_a to cultured vascular endothelial cells. Proc. Natl. Acad. Sci. USA **80:** 4119–4123.
59. HEIMARK, R. L. & S. M. SCHWARTZ. 1983. Binding of coagulation factors IX and X to the endothelial surface. Biochem. Biophys. Res. Commun. **111:** 723–731.

60. STERN, D. M., M. DRILLINGS, W. KISIEL, P. NAWROTH, H. L. NOSSEL & K. S. LAGAMMA. 1984. Activation of factor IX bound to cultured bovine aortic endothelial cells. Proc. Natl. Acad. Sci. USA **81:** 913–917.
61. RODGERS, G. M. & M. A. SHUMAN. 1983. Prothrombin is activated on vascular endothelial cells by factor X_a and calcium. Proc. Natl. Acad. Sci. USA **80:** 7001–7005.
62. WIGGINS, R. C., D. J. LOSKUTOFF, C. G. COCHRANE, J. H. GRIFFIN & T. S. EDGINGTON. 1980. Activation of rabbit Hageman factor by homogenates of cultured rabbit endothelial cells. J. Clin. Invest. **65:** 197–206.
63. DEJANA, E., J-P. CAZENAVE, H. M. GROVES, R. L. KINLOUGH-RATHBONE, M. A. PACKHAM & J. F. MUSTARD. 1980. The effect of aspirin inhibition of PGI_2 production on platelet adherence to normal and damaged rabbit aortae. Thrombos. Res. **17:** 453–464.
64. BOOYSE, F. M., S. BELL, B. SEDLAK & M. E. RAFELSON. 1975. Development of an *in vitro* vessel wall model for studying certain aspects of platelet-vessel (endothelial) interactions. Artery **1:** 518–539.
65. CZERVIONKE, R. L., J. C. HOAK & G. L. FRY. 1978. Effect of aspirin on thrombin-induced adherence of platelets to cultured cells from the blood vessel wall. J. Clin. Invest. **62:** 847–856.
66. CURWEN, K. D., M. A. GIMBRONE, JR. & R. I. HANDIN. 1980. *In vitro* studies of thromboresistance. The role of prostacyclin (PGI_2) in platelet adhesion to cultured normal and virally transformed human vascular endothelial cells. Lab. Invest. **42:** 366–374.
67. FRY, G. L., R. L. CZERVIONKE, J. C. HOAK, J. B. SMITH & D. L. HAYCRAFT. 1980. Platelet adherence to cultured vascular cells: Influence of prostacyclin (PGI_2). Blood **55:** 271–275.
68. CZERVIONKE, R. L., J. B. SMITH, G. L. FRY, J. C. HOAK & D. L. HAYCRAFT. 1979. Inhibition of prostacyclin by treatment with aspirin. Correlation with platelet adherence. J. Clin. Invest. **63:** 1089–1092.
69. MONCADA, S., R. GRYGLEWSKI, S. BUNTING & J. R. VANE. 1976. An enzyme isolated from arteries transforms prostaglandin endoperoxides to an unstable substance that inhibits platelet aggregation. Nature **263:** 663–665.
70. GRYGLEWSKI, R., S. BUNTING, S. MONCADA & J. R. VANE. 1976. Arterial walls are protected against deposition of platelet thrombi by a substance (prostaglandin X) which they make from prostaglandin endoperoxides. Prostaglandins **12:** 685–714.
71. BUNTING, S., R. J. GRYGLEWSKI, S. MONCADA & J. R. VANE. 1976. Arterial walls generate from prostaglandin endoperoxides a substance which relaxes strips of mesenteric and coeliac arteries, and inhibits platelet aggregation. Prostaglandins **12:** 897–913.
72. KULKARNI, P. S., R. ROBERTS & P. NEEDLEMAN. 1976. Paradoxical endogenous synthesis of a coronary dilating substance from arachidonate. Prostaglandins **12:** 337–353.
73. RAZ, A., P. C. ISAKSON, M. S. MINKES & P. NEEDLEMAN. 1977. Characterization of a novel metabolic pathway of arachidonate in coronary arteries which generates a potent coronary vasodilator. J. Biol. Chem. **252:** 1123–1126.
74. WEKSLER, B. B., A. J. MARCUS & E. A. JAFFE. 1977. Synthesis of prostaglandin I_2 (prostacyclin) by cultured human and bovine endothelial cells. Proc. Natl. Acad. Sci. USA **74:** 3922–3926.
75. MARCUS, A. J., B. B. WEKSLER & E. A. JAFFE. 1978. Enzymatic conversion of prostaglandin endoperoxide H_2 and arachiodonic acid to prostacyclin by cultured human endothelial cells. J. Biol. Chem. **253:** 7138–7141.
76. WEKSLER, B. B., C. W. LEY & E. A. JAFFE. 1978. Stimulation of endothelial prostacyclin production by thrombin, trypsin, and the ionophore A23187. J. Clin. Invest. **62:** 923–930.
77. BAENZIGER, N. L., L. E. FORCE & P. R. BECHERER. 1980. Histamine stimulates prostacyclin synthesis in cultured human endothelial cells. Biochem. Biophys. Res. Commun. **92:** 1435–1440.
78. BAENZIGER, N. L., F. J. FOGERTY, L. F. MERTZ & L. F. CHERNUTA. 1981. Regulation of histamine-mediated prostacyclin synthesis in cultured human vascular endothelial cells. Cell **24:** 915–923.

79. Hong, S. L. 1980. Effect of bradykinin and thrombin on prostacyclin synthesis in endothelial cells from calf and pig aorta and human umbilical vein. Thrombos. Res. **18:** 787–795.
80. Fleisher, L. N., A. R. Tall, L. D. Witte, R. W. Miller & P. J. Cannon. 1982. Stimulation of arterial endothelial cells prostacyclin synthesis by high-density lipoproteins. J. Biol. Chem. **257:** 6653–6655.
81. Coughlin, S. R., M. A. Moskowitz, B. R. Zetter, H. N. Antoniades & L. Levine. 1980. Platelet-dependent stimulation of prostacyclin synthesis by platelet-derived growth factor. Nature **288:** 600–602.
82. Ritter, J. M., M-A. Ongari, M. A. Orchard & P. J. Lewis. 1983. Prostacyclin synthesis is stimulated by a serum factor formed during coagulation. Thromb. Haemostas. **49:** 58–60.
83. Schiavon, R., G. E. Freeman, G. C. Guidi, G. Perona, M. Zatti & V. V. Kakkar. 1984. Selenium enhances prostacyclin production by cultured endothelial cells: Possible explanation for increased bleeding times in volunteers taking selenium as a dietary supplement. Thrombos. Res. **34:** 389–396.
84. Goldsmith, J. C. & J. J. McCormick. 1984. Immunologic injury to vascular endothelial cells: Effects on release of prostacyclin. Blood **63:** 984–989.
85. Pearson, J. D., L. L. Slakey & J. L. Gordon. 1983. Stimulation of prostaglandin production through purinergic receptors on endothelial cells and macrophages. Biochem. J. **214:** 273–276.
86. Boogaerts, M. A., J. Vermylen, H. Deckmyn, C. Roelant, R. L. Verwilgen, H. S. Jacob & C. F. Moldow. 1983. Enkephalins modify granulocyte-endothelial interactions by stimulating prostacyclin production. Thrombos. Haemostas. **50:** 572–575.
87. Cramer, E. B., L. Pologe, N. A. Pawlowski, Z. A. Cohn & W. A. Scott. 1983. Leukotriene C promotes prostacyclin synthesis by human endothelial cells. Proc. Natl. Acad. Sci. USA **80:** 4109–4113.
88. Watson, K. V., C. F. Moldow, P. Ogburn & H. S. Jacob. 1984. Mg_2SO_4 promotes the release of prostacyclin (PGI_2) by endothelial cells: A rationale for its use in preeclampsia. Clin. Res. **32:** 341A.
89. Jaffe, E. A. & B. B. Weksler. 1979. Recovery of endothelial cell prostacyclin production after inhibition by low doses of aspirin. J. Clin. Invest. **63:** 532–535.
90. Busacca, M., E. Dejana, G. Balconi, S. Olivieri, A. Pietra, M. Vergara-Dauden & G. de Gaetano. 1982. Reduced prostacyclin production by cultured endothelial cells from umbilical arteries of babies born to women who smoke. Lancet **2:** 609–610.
91. Spector, A. A., J. C. Hoak, G. L. Fry, G. M. Denning. L. L. Stoll & J. B. Smith. 1980. Effect of fatty acid modification on prostacyclin production by cultured human endothelial cells. J. Clin. Invest. **65:** 1003–1012.
92. Marcus, A. J., B. B. Weksler, E. A. Jaffe & M. J. Broekman. 1980. Synthesis of prostacyclin from platelet-derived endoperoxides by cultured human endothelial cells. J. Clin. Invest. **66:** 979–986.
93. Yoshida, N., B. Weksler & R. Nachman. 1983. Purification of human platelet calcium-activated protease. Effect on platelet and endothelial function. J. Biol. Chem. **258:** 7168–7174.
94. Wong, P. Y-K., W. H. Lee, P. H-W. Chao, R. F. Reiss & J. C. McGiff. 1980. Metabolism of prostacyclin by 9-hydroxyprostaglandin dehydrogenase in human platelets. J. Biol. Chem. **255:** 9021–9024.
95. Charo, I. F., S. Shak, M. A. Karasek, P. M. Davison & I. M. Goldstein. 1984. Prostaglandin I_2 is not a major metabolite of arachidonic acid in cultured endothelial cells from human foreskin microvessels. J. Clin. Invest. **74:** 914–919.
96. Dieterle, Y., C. Ody, A. Ehrensburger, H. Stalder & A. F. Junod. 1978. Metabolism and uptake of adenosine triphosphate and adenosine by porcine aortic and pulmonary endothelial cells and fibroblasts in culture. Circ. Res. **42:** 869–876.
97. Dosne, A. M., C. Legrand, B. Bauvois, E. Bodevin & J. P. Caen. 1978. Comparative degradation of adenyl-nucleotides by cultured endothelial cells and fibroblasts. Biochem. Biophys. Res. Commun. **85:** 183–189.

98. Dosne, A. M., B. Escoubet, E. Bodevin & J. P. Caen. 1979. Adenosine diphosphate metabolism by cultured human endothelial cells. FEBS Lett. **105:** 286–290.
99. Pearson, J. D., J. S. Carleton & J. L. Gordon. 1980. Metabolism of adenosine nucleotides by ectoenzymes of vascular endothelial and smooth muscle cells in culture. Biochem. J. **190:** 421–429.
100. Crutchley, D. J., U. S. Ryan & J. W. Ryan. 1980. Effects of aspirin and dipyridamole on the degradation of adenosine diphosphate by cultured cells derived from bovine pulmonary artery. J. Clin. Invest. **66:** 29–35.
101. Pearson, J. D. & J. L. Gordon. 1979. Vascular endothelial and smooth muscle cells in culture selectively release adenine nucleotides. Nature **281:** 384–386.
102. Lollar, P. & W. G. Owen. 1980. Clearance of thrombin from circulation in rabbits by high-affinity binding sites on endothelium. Possible role in the inactivation of thrombin by antithrombin III. J. Clin. Invest. **66:** 1222–1230.
103. Busch, C. & W. G. Owen. 1982. Identification *in vitro* of an endothelial cell surface cofactor for antithrombin III. Parallel studies with isolated perfused rat hearts and microcarrier cultures of bovine endothelium. J. Clin. Invest. **69:** 726–729.
104. Hiebert, L. M. & L. B. Jacques. 1976. The observation of heparin on endothelium after injection. Thrombos. Res. **8:** 195–204.
105. Glimelius, B., C. Busch & M. Hook. 1978. Binding of heparin on the surface of cultured endothelial cells. Thrombos. Res. **12:** 773–782.
106. Bjorck, C., R. Larsson, P. Olsson & U. Rothman. 1981. Uptake and inactivation of thrombin by the fresh, glutardialdehyde or heparin treated human umbilical cord. Thrombos. Res. **21:** 603.
107. Kisiel, W., W. M. Canfield, L. H. Ericsson & E. W. Davie. 1977. Anticoagulant properties of bovine plasma protein C following activation by thrombin. Biochemistry **16:** 5824–5831.
108. Walker, F. J., P. W. Sexton & C. T. Esmon. 1979. The inhibition of blood coagulation by activated protein C through the selective inactivation of activated factor V. Biochim. Biophys. Acta **571:** 333–342.
109. Vehar, G. A. & E. W. Davie. 1980. Preparation and properties of bovine factor VIII (antihemophilic factor). Biochemistry **19:** 401–410.
110. Esmon, C. T. & W. G. Owen. 1981. Identification of an endothelial cell cofactor for thrombin-catalyzed activation of protein C. Proc. Natl. Acad. Sci. USA **78:** 2249–2252.
111. Owen, W. G. & C. T. Esmon. 1981. Functional properties of an endothelial cell cofactor for thrombin-catalyzed activation of protein C. J. Biol. Chem. **256:** 5532–5535.
112. Marlar, R. A., A. J. Kleiss & J. H. Griffin. 1982. Mechanism of action of human activated protein C, a thrombin-dependent anticoagulant enzyme. Blood **59:** 1067–1072.
113. Esmon, N. L., W. G. Owen & C. T. Esmon. 1982. Isolation of a membrane-bound cofactor for thrombin-catalyzed activation of protein C. J. Biol. Chem. **257:** 859–864.
114. Esmon, C. T., N. L. Esmon & K. W. Harris. 1982. Complex formation between thrombin and thrombomodulin inhibits both thrombin-catalyzed fibrin formation and factor V activation. J. Biol. Chem. **257:** 7944–7947.
115. Esmon, N. L., R. C. Carroll & C. T. Esmon. 1983. Thrombomodulin blocks the ability of thrombin to activate platelets. J. Biol. Chem. **258:** 12238–12242.
116. Griffin, J. H., B. Evatt, T. S. Zimmerman, A. J. Kleiss & C. Wideman. 1981. Deficiency of protein C in congenital thrombotic disease. J. Clin. Invest. **68:** 1370–1373.
117. Broekmans, A. W., J. J. Veltkamp & R. M. Bertina. 1983. Congenital protein C deficiency and venous thromboembolism. N. Engl. J. Med. **309:** 340–344.
118. Branson, H. E., J. Katz, R. Marble & J. H. Griffin. 1983. Inherited protein C deficiency and coumarin-responsive chronic relapsing purpura fulminans in a newborn infant. Lancet **2:** 1165–1168.
119. Seligsohn, U., A. Berger, M. Abend, L. Rubin, D. Attias, A. Zivelin & S. I. Rapaport. 1984. Homozygous protein C deficiency manifested by massive venous thrombosis in the newborn. N. Engl. J. Med. **310:** 559–562.

120. ISAACS, J., N. SAVION, D. GOSPODAROWICZ & M. A. SHUMAN. 1981. Effect of cell density on thrombin binding to a specific site on bovine vascular endothelial cells. J. Cell Biol. **90:** 670–674.
121. KNAUER, D. J. & D. D. CUNNINGHAM. 1984. Protease nexins: Cell-secreted proteins which regulate extracellular serine proteases. Trends Biochem. Sci. **9:** 231–233.
122. LOSKUTOFF, D. J. & T. S. EDGINGTON. 1977. Synthesis of a fibrinolytic activator and inhibitor by endothelial cells. Proc. Natl. Acad. Sci. USA **74:** 3903–3907.
123. LEVIN, E. G. & D. J. LOSKUTOFF. 1982. Cultured bovine endothelial cells produce both urokinase and tissue-type plasminogen activators. J. Cell Biol. **94:** 631–636.
124. BOOYSE, F. M., G. OSIKOWICZ, S. FEDER & J. SCHEINBUKS. 1984. Isolation and characterization of a urokinase-type plasminogen activator (M_r = 54,000) from cultured human endothelial cells indistinguishable from urinary urokinase. J. Biol. Chem. **259:** 7198–7205.
125. LOSKUTOFF, D. J., J. A. VAN MOURIK, L. A. ERICKSON & D. LAWRENCE. 1983. Detection of an unusually stable fibrinolytic inhibitor produced by bovine endothelial cells. Proc. Natl. Acad. Sci. USA **80:** 2956–2960.
126. LEVIN, E. G. & D. J. LOSKUTOFF. 1979. Comparative studies of the fibrinolytic activity of cultured vascular cells. Thrombos. Res. **15:** 869–878.
127. LOSKUTOFF, D. J. 1979. Effect of thrombin on the fibrinolytic activity of cultured bovine endothelial cells. J. Clin. Invest. **64:** 329–332.
128. DICORLETO, P. E. & D. F. BOWEN-POPE. 1983. Cultured endothelial cells produce a platelet-derived growth factor-like protein. Proc. Natl. Acad. Sci. USA **80:** 1919–1923.
129. CASTELLOT, J. J., JR., M. L. ADDONIZO, R. ROSENBERG & M. J. KARNOVSKY. 1981. Cultured endothelial cells produce a heparin-like inhibitor of smooth muscle cell growth. J. Cell Biol. **90:** 372–379.
130. CASTELLOT, J. J., JR., L. V. FAVREAU, M. J. KARNOVSKY & R. D. ROSENBERG. 1982. Inhibition of vascular smooth muscle cell growth by endothelial cell-derived heparin. Possible role of a platelet endoglycosidase. J. Biol. Chem. **257:** 11256–11260.
131. GAJDUSEK, C. M. & S. M. SCHWARTZ. 1982. Ability of endothelial cells to condition culture medium. J. Cell. Physiol. **110:** 35–42.
132. CHENG, C-F., G. M. OOSTA, A. BENSADOUN & R. D. ROSENBERG. 1981. Binding of lipoprotein lipase to endothelial cells in culture. J. Biol. Chem. **256:** 12893–12898.
133. SHIMADA, K., P. J. GILL, J. E. SILBERT, W. H. DOUGLAS & B. L. FANBURG. 1981. Involvement of cell surface heparin sulfate in the binding of lipoprotein lipase to cultured bovine endothelial cells. J. Clin. Invest. **68:** 995–1002.
134. KHOO, J. C., E. M. MAHONEY & J. L. WITZTUM. 1981. Secretion of lipoprotein lipase by macrophages in culture. J. Biol. Chem. **256:** 7105–7108.
135. BAKER, D. P., B. J. VAN LENTEN, A. M. FOGELMAN, P. A. EDWARDS, C. KEAN & J. A. BERLINER. 1984. LDL, scavenger, and β-VLDL receptors on aortic endothelial cells. Arteriosclerosis **4:** 248–255.
136. FIELDING, C. J., I. VLODAVSKY, P. E. FIELDING & D. GOSPODAROWICZ. 1979. Characteristics of chylomicron binding and lipid uptake by endothelial cells in culture. J. Biol. Chem. **254:** 8861–8868.
137. BRINTON, E. A., R. D. KENAGY, J. F. ORAM & E. L. BIERMAN. 1983. Up-regulation of high-density lipoprotein receptor activity of bovine endothelial cells by acetylated low-density lipoproteins. Clin. Res. **31:** 170A.
138. FIELDING, P. E., I. VLODAVSKY, D. GOSPODAROWICZ & C. J. FIELDING. 1979. Effect of contact inhibition on the regulation of cholesterol metabolism in cultured vascular endothelial cells. J. Biol. Chem. **254:** 749–755.
139. HENRIKSEN, T., E. M. MAHONEY & D. STEINBERG. 1981. Enhanced macrophage degradation of low-density lipoprotein previously incubated with cultured endothelial cells: Recognition by receptors for acetylated low-density lipoproteins. Proc. Natl. Acad. Sci. USA **78:** 6499–6503.
140. BAR, R. S., J. C. HOAK & M. L. PEACOCK. 1978. Insulin receptors in human endothelial cells: Identification and characterization. J. Clin. Endocrinol. Metab. **47:** 699–702.
141. BAR, R. S., M. L. PEACOCK, R. G. SPANHEIMER, R. VEENSTRA & J. C. HOAK. 1980.

Differential binding of insulin to human arterial and venous endothelial cells in primary culture. Diabetes **29:** 991–995.

142. King, G. L., S. M. Buzney, C. R. Kahn, N. Hetu, S. Buchwald, S. G. Macdonald & L. I. Rand. 1983. Differential responsiveness to insulin of endothelial and support cells from micro- and macrovessels. J. Clin. Invest. **71:** 974–979.

143. Ody, C. & A. F. Junod. 1977. Converting enzyme activity in endothelial cells isolated from pig pulmonary artery and aorta. Am. J. Physiol. **232:** C95–C98.

144. Johnson, A. R. & E. G. Erdos. 1977. Metabolism of vasoactive peptides by human endothelial cells in culture. Angiotensin I converting enzyme (kininase II) and angiotensinase. J. Clin. Invest. **59:** 684–695.

145. Kumamoto, K., T. A. Stewart, A. R. Johnson & E. G. Erdos. 1981. Prolylcarboxypeptidase (angiotensinase C) in human lung and cultured cells. J. Clin. Invest. **67:** 210–215.

146. Beesley, J. E., J. D. Pearson, J. S. Carleton, A. Hutchings & J. L. Gordon. 1978. Interactions of leukocytes with vascular cells in culture. J. Cell Sci. **33:** 85–101.

147. Pearson, J. D., J. S. Carleton, J. E. Beesley, A. Hutchings & J. L. Gordon. 1979. Granulocyte adhesion to endothelium in culture. J. Cell Sci. **38:** 225–235.

148. Hoover, R. L., R. Folger, W. A. Haering, B. R. Ware & M. J. Karnovsky. 1980. Adhesion of leukocytes to endothelium: Roles of divalent cations, surface charge, chemotactic agents, and substrate. J. Cell Sci. **45:** 73–86.

149. Tonneson, M. G., L. Smedley & P. M. Henson. 1984. Neutrophil-endothelial cell interactions. Modulation of neutrophil adhesiveness induced by complement fragments C5a and C5a des arg and formyl-methionyl-leucyl-phenylalanine *in vitro.* J. Clin. Invest. **74:** 1581–1592.

150. Boogaerts, M. A., O. Yamada, H. S. Jacob & C. F. Moldow. 1982. Enhancement of granulocyte-endothelial cell adherence and granulocyte-induced cytotoxicity by platelet release products. Proc. Natl. Acad. Sci. USA **79:** 7019–7023.

151. Pawlowski, N. A., W. A. Scott, E. L. Araham & Z. A. Cohn. 1984. The selective interaction of human monocytes with vascular endothelium. Clin. Res. **32:** 507A.

152. de Bono, D. 1976. Endothelial-lymphocyte interactions *in vitro.* I. Adherence of nonallergised lymphocytes. Cell. Immunol. **26:** 78–88.

153. de Bono, D. 1979. Endothelium-lymphocyte interactions *in vitro.* II. Adherence of allergised lymphocytes. Cell. Immunol. **44:** 64–70.

154. Quesenberry, P. J. & M. A. Gimbrone, Jr. 1980. Vascular endothelium as a regulator of granulopoiesis: Production of colony-stimulating activity by cultured human endothelial cells. Blood **56:** 1060–1067.

155. Ascensao, J. L., G. M. Vercellotti, H. S. Jacob & E. D. Zanjani. 1984. Role of endothelial cells in human hematopoiesis: Modulation of mixed colony growth *in vitro.* Blood **63:** 553–558.

156. Bagby, G. C., Jr., E. McCall, K. A. Bergstrom & D. Burger. 1983. A monokine regulates colony-stimulating activity production by vascular endothelial cells. Blood **62:** 663–668.

157. Gibofsky, A., E. A. Jaffe, M. Fotino & C. G. Becker. 1975. The identification of HL–A antigens on fresh and cultured human endothelial cells. J. Immunol. **115:** 730–733.

158. Pober, J. S. & M. A. Gimbrone, Jr. 1982. Expression of Ia-like antigens by human vascular endothelial cells is inducible *in vitro:* Demonstration by monoclonal antibody binding and immunoprecipitation. Proc. Natl. Acad. Sci. USA **79:** 6641–6645.

159. Pober, J. S., M. A. Gimbrone, Jr., R. S. Cotran, C. S. Reiss, S. J. Burakoff, W. Fiers & K. A. Ault. 1983. Ia expression by vascular endothelium is inducible by activated T cells and by human gamma-interferon. J. Exp. Med. **157:** 1339–1353.

160. Hirschberg, H., O. J. Bergh & E. Thorsby. 1980. Antigen-presenting properties of human vascular endothelial cells. J. Exp. Med. **152:** 249s–255s.

161. Hirschberg, H., T. Hirschberg, E. Jaffe & E. Thorsby. 1981. Antigen-presenting properties of human vascular endothelial cells: Inhibition by anti-HLA–DR antisera. Scand. J. Immunol. **14:** 545–553.

Kinetics of Atherosclerosis: A Stem Cell Model

STEPHEN M. SCHWARTZ,[a] MICHAEL R. REIDY,[a]
AND ALEXANDER CLOWES[b]

[a]*Department of Pathology SJ–60*
[b]*Department of Surgery RF–25*
University of Washington
Seattle, Washington 98195

There is a famous story of a committee of three blind men examining an elephant. The first man, holding the ear, described a large leaf; the second committee member, holding a leg, described a tree trunk; the chairman, holding the tail, recognized a vine. A banana tree was decided on by committee consensus.

Like the elephant, atherosclerosis has been viewed variously as a clinical problem in lipid metabolism, an epidemiologic issue of clinical risk factors for myocardial infarction, a cell biologist's fascination with cellular proliferation seen in models of atherosclerotic injury, or as thrombosis, probably the major final event in the disease. The composite of these and other points of view has produced many definitions of this disease. The consensus usually appears as a complex, difficult to describe, "multifactorial" elephant (FIGURE 1).

The only real solution to analysis of this sort of problem may be by attempting to understand one of the processes at a time. Several components of the atherosclerotic process are already well-established and beginning to be understood. The best example is lipid metabolism. Brown and Goldstein's review, elsewhere in this volume, greatly enhances our extensive knowledge about mechanisms of lipid accumulation. It seems likely that we will soon know why and how lipid accumulates in the vessel wall. The relationship of that process to lesions becoming clinically significant, however, remains totally unclear.

Platelet interaction, reviewed by Baumgartner in this volume, is obviously important for final occlusion of the vessel, and great progress is being made in understanding the physiology of platelet adhesion and thrombosis at this critical stage of the disease. In addition, as will be discussed later, platelets may be important in the initiation of the disease because of their role in stimulation of smooth muscle proliferation. Monocytes may also be important at this stage. Monocytosis is a prominent feature of the initial stages of atherosclerosis in fat-fed animals.[1–8] Fat-fed monocytes comprise a major portion of the foam cells in the lesion, and monocytes can contribute growth factors able to stimulate smooth muscle growth.[6] Here again, important questions arise concerning the accumulation of monocytes, their kinetics in the vessel wall, and their involvement in the evolution of the lesion. The possible role of other components of the immune system has only now begun to be explored.

Finally, a great deal of attention has been given to the interconnections between endothelial denudation, thrombosis, and smooth muscle proliferation, which is the "response to injury" hypothesis reviewed by Russell Ross in this volume. In many ways, the "response to injury" model has formed a unifying hypothesis. Its central feature is the relationship of endothelial injury to smooth muscle proliferation. In this article, we will concentrate on the narrow problem of smooth muscle proliferation as seen in one model involving the response of animal vessel walls to trauma, particularly the removal of the endothelium by the balloon catheter technique. We will attempt to review this model and address two issues:

1. Response of the vessel wall to endothelial cell loss;
2. The temporal sequence of response that might occur in the evolution of the human lesion.

NONDENUDING DESQUAMATION

The ability of denudation, via the balloon catheter, to stimulate smooth muscle proliferation has led to considerable interest in the possibility that focal areas of

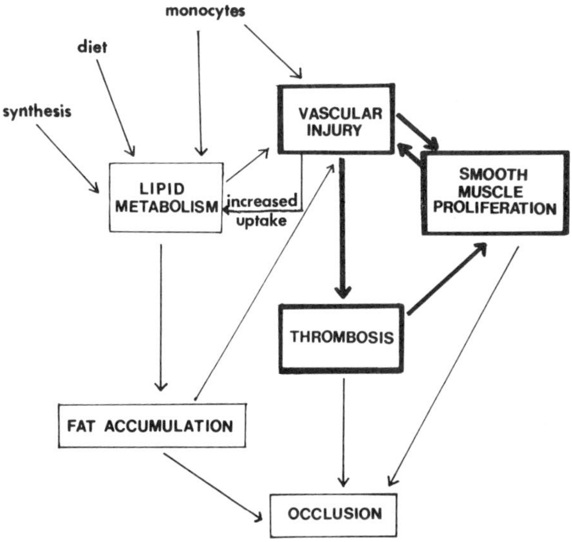

FIGURE 1. Schematic diagram of complex hypotheses for atherosclerosis. The various concepts of atherosclerosis are usually summarized in multifactorial diagrams such as this one. While apparently confusing, each of the individual boxes may, in and of themselves, be relatively well understood. The focus of this review is in the box labeled smooth muscle proliferation, and in the relation of that box to vascular injury and thrombosis.

spontaneous denuding injury might have a similar effect. There are, in fact, focal areas where endothelial cell turnover is quite high.[9] These areas, however, do not become denuded. Apparently, both in focal areas of high turnover in normal animals and in increased turnover in response to hypertension or endotoxemia, the rate of regeneration is sufficient to replace cells as they desquamate.[10]

This does not obviate the possibility that denudation plays an important role in the pathogenesis of lesions.[5,6] In animals fed high fat diets, endothelial denudation does occur over as lesions advance.[8] This event may be critical to rapid progression. If this is true, it is reasonable to believe that the well-studied and simple model of proliferation following balloon denudation will provide clues to understanding common mechanisms involved in proliferative responses of the vessel wall.

BALLOON DENUDATION

FIGURE 2 summarizes the present state of our knowledge of the smooth muscle proliferative response to denudation. Total denudation, via the balloon, is followed immediately by platelet adherence. This is followed by medial smooth muscle DNA synthesis, beginning about two to three days after manipulation.[11–14] While the stimulated smooth muscle cells continue to replicate for a number of weeks, recruitment of cells into the growth fraction is largely completed by three days.[15] Heparin infusion inhibits the proliferative response, but only if heparin is given within the first two days.[16] This suggests that heparin acts by preventing some as yet undefined early event that is critical to this response.

One of the most important aspects of this injury model is the selective accumulation of cells in the intima. This is also true of atherosclerotic lesions. One possible

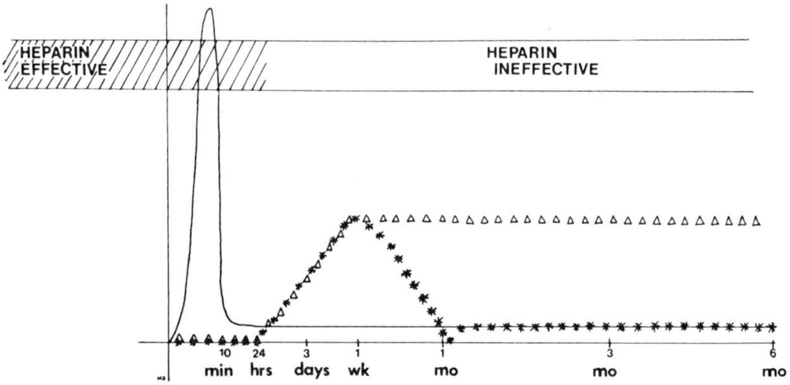

FIGURE 2. Kinetics in response of vessel wall to injury. This figure is a diagrammatic summary of data gathered from a number of different sources. The data suggest that some relatively acute event, occurring shortly after balloon catheter denudation, is a necessary event for the commitment of the lesion to proliferate. Perhaps more impressive is the observation that continuation of proliferation of the cells comprising the lesion after three to seven days depends upon a fixed population of cells which enters the growth fraction within the first three days. (— = Platelet adhesion; * = Replication rate (smooth muscle); ΔΔΔ = Cumulative growth fraction for smooth muscle).

explanation is that lesions arise from preexisting intimal smooth muscle cells. There is evidence for this from autopsy studies comparing the histology of arteries in children with the pathology of arteries in adults.[17] Benditt has also presented evidence that human lesions arise by multiple replications of single cells. This monoclonal mechanism would also seem to imply origin of human lesions from affected cells in the intima since lesions are not seen in the media.[18] There is some evidence to support this sequence in fat-fed swine, as well as in ballooned swine.[19–21] Cell kinetic studies of these models imply that lesions arise from multiplication of multiple cells already present in the normal intima. In the rat, however, the intima has few smooth muscle cells prior to balloon denudation, and none are evident immediately after the balloon.[22] Thus, migration must play a major role in formation of lesions in this animal. More direct evidence using 3-thymidine autoradiography and cell kinetic analysis support this argument.[11,15] Morphologic studies of fat-fed animals also support the idea that at least some migration occurs in other models.[8,23]

SMOOTH MUSCLE KINETICS IN RESPONSE TO BALLOON DENUDATION

An understanding of the relationship of endothelial denudation to smooth muscle proliferation requires that we expand on the discussion of the temporal sequence of events following balloon denudation. The most immediate adherence of platelets to the surface with release of platelet granule products into the vessel wall occurs within ten minutes.[24,25] After this, the surface rapidly becomes nonthrombogenic, with few new platelets adhering after these first ten minutes and with a return to low levels of thrombogenicity by 24 hours. If platelet release is important, this period may be critical to the later sequence of events. Other blood cells are also found adherent to the surface of ballooned vessels, including neutrophils and mononuclear cells. While these cells may play a role in some species, they are not found in the rat, and therefore, are not, at least in this species, required for stimulation of smooth muscle proliferation.[22]

The data on smooth muscle cell replication in FIGURE 2 represent a composite of data gained by two methods. Animals receiving a single pulse of 3-thymidine will only label those cells in the S (DNA synthesis) phase of the cell cycle within 30 minutes of the time of injection. This is because of the rapid rate of catabolism of thymidine *in vivo*. Since S is about eight hours long, three doses at eight-hour intervals will, approximately, label all cells entering S over one day.[26] This daily labeling rate is a direct measure of the number of cells passing through the cell cycle over one day. The daily labeling rate does not provide a direct measure of the rate of entry into the cell cycle, the proportion of cells capable of synthesizing DNA, or the total increase in cell number. To gather these values, a different type of labeling is required. Continuous labeling, using an osmotic minipump, allows us to label all cells entering the cell cycle over a period of as much as one month.[15] By combining this measure with measurement of total DNA content, one can obtain values for cell number, change in cell number, and fraction of cells growing over the labeling interval.

FIGURE 2 shows some interesting facts about this process. Smooth muscle cells begin to enter the cell cycle between one and three days after the injury. The daily labeling rate data show a continuation of cell replication over a period of one month.[12] Similarly, DNA content of the intima continues to increase over this interval. In contrast, the cumulative growth fraction, that is, the proportion of the original population that goes from a nonreplicating state into the cell cycle, rises rapidly over the interval between one and three days, as expected, but then remains essentially constant after day 7. In other words, those cells that are going to contribute to lesion growth become committed to replicate very early after injury. This committed population, about 30% of the cells in a carotid artery, is then responsible for the bulk of the growth of the ballooned vessel. Interestingly, not all of the cells that enter the intima replicate. About one out of nine intimal smooth muscle cells are not labeled, even with continuous labeling. Based on an estimate of the number of divisions in each cell, we estimate that 50% of the cells that cross the internal elastic lamina never divide.[15]

It is reasonable to speculate that the commitment of cells to enter the growth fraction may correlate with migration of smooth muscle cells from the media into the wounded intima. As shown by morphologic and by cytokinetic studies,[6,11,15,19,27] smooth muscle cells migrate across the vessel wall. The first arrival of cells in the intima does not occur until after cell replication, as measured by 3-thymidine autoradiography, has begun.[12] This is important because it rules out the possibility that the initial entry of cells into the cell cycle, as described above, requires relocation of smooth muscle cells into the intima. However, the possibility remains that continuation of replication, i.e., division of committed cells, may depend on this translocation. If this is true, then one might speculate on the possibility that migration is critical to the maintenance of a proliferative state in the ballooned wall.

PERSISTENT DENUDATION

While studies in other species have claimed that endothelial regeneration goes to completion, most of these studies have lacked careful scanning electron microscopic surveys of the extent of recovery or have failed to demonstrate that the initial denudation was complete. In our own studies with aortic balloon injury, we found some rabbits that completely regenerated their endothelium. We then looked at animals two weeks after denudation. Despite the absence of evident endothelial cells in freshly denuded vessels, the presence of patches of regenerated cells at many places on the vessel surface suggested incomplete denudation. The available literature[28] supports the idea that endothelial regeneration occurs only from the edge of preexisting sheets of endothelium. Since circulating cells do not appear to give rise to endothelium,[29] we concluded that denudation had not been complete. When we increased the number of passages of the balloon up and down the aorta, the patches disappeared and regeneration was seen to be limited (Reidy and Schwartz, unpublished results).

Regeneration in the rat aorta appears to follow a slightly different pattern since the ballooned aorta does form lesions despite complete regeneration of the endothelium.[30] We have shown, however, that regeneration in this species is limited when a large surface without branches, the carotid artery,[31] is denuded. Probably, the completion of regeneration in the aorta reflects the relatively small distance between branches. This is important because of the apparent distribution of the lesion in the ballooned rat aorta.[30] Virtually all the lesion is found at the ventral margin of the vessel, that is, the region of the vessel at the greatest possible distance from the endothelium regenerating from the intercostal arteries.

These results suggest that persistent, if not permanent, denudation is required for localization of the lesion in the rat. However, it is also possible that the inverse correlation of endothelial regeneration with absence of smooth muscle replication in the rat could be circumstantial. The ventral aorta could well respond to injury differently than the dorsal aorta. This could be due to differences in mechanical stretch of the two portions of the aorta since the dorsal aorta is closely applied to the vertebral bodies and is supported by retroperitoneal connective tissue. Other more subtle differences in response of ventral and dorsal aorta could reflect the distribution of cells in the intima described by Thomas and his colleagues.[21]

In 1979, Minick and his colleagues reported an apparently different result. They looked at the distribution of intimal thickening as a function of the extent of regeneration of endothelium in the ballooned rabbit aorta and found *maximal* thickening of the intima at the edge of the regenerated sheet of endothelium.[32] These observations might be explained in a number of ways. One might imagine that the regenerating endothelial cells in the rabbit have some special "atherogenic" properties, such as production of endothelial cell-derived growth factor,[33] altered metabolism of lipids by regenerating cells,[34-36] or production of an altered extracellular matrix.[37]

Attempts to relate this finding to endothelial replication turned out, however, to be misleading. When we looked at cell replication in this model, endothelial regeneration was complete by one month. This left the surface with large areas of persistent denudation. Therefore, the data represent an accentuation of lesion formation at a static interface defined by the edge of the regenerated sheet and a denuded surface which is now covered by altered smooth muscle cells.[22,31,38] Before interpreting these results in terms of smooth muscle growth, it is important to realize that Minick and his collaborators measured only thickening of the intima. This does not necessarily correlate with cellular proliferation. Later studies by Wight *et al.*[37] have shown that the increased intimal thickening under regenerating endothelium is due to deposition of connective tissue without an increase of cell number above that seen in the denuded surface. In summary, the available data on the rabbit response to denuding injury does not contradict the rat model.

Finally, it is important to point out that cells can also be lost from a developing lesion. This issue was raised by the results of a series of experiments employing the ballooned rat carotid.[12,31,39] A long extent of this vessel never becomes recovered by the endothelium. Hence, smooth muscle cells in the intima are exposed to blood for periods up to one year. We found that smooth muscle cells at the intimal surface continued to replicate even at very late times; however, this continued replication does not produce an increase in the size of the intimal lesion or the number of smooth muscle cells. This finding suggests that the replicating cells die or are lost.[12,39]

In summary, localization of smooth muscle proliferation after denuding injury is consistent with the hypothesis that denudation is necessary to elicit smooth muscle replication.

SELECTIVE DENUDATION

While denudation may be necessary, there is also experimental evidence opposing the idea that persistence of a denuded surface is sufficient to produce intimal cell proliferation. Some years ago, we showed that the normal endothelium contained focal areas with quite high levels of cell turnover. This and similar studies from other laboratories were correlated with the denudation hypothesis to support the idea that spontaneous endothelial injury could function as the initiating event in atherogenesis via denudation and release of PDGF.[26,27,40–42] For spontaneous turnover to participate in this process, however, one would have to equate turnover and denudation. This equation now appears to be false. Scanning electron microscopy of these normal surfaces, as well as surfaces of cholesterol-fed animals in the early stages of fat-fed atherosclerosis, shows no evident denudation.[5,6,27,43–47] Similarly, if one increases turnover by hypertension or by endotoxemia, cell loss increases. This is evidenced by changes in turnover without any loss in continuity of the cell layer. Thus, it seems unlikely that endothelial turnover, even focal turnover, can account for release of platelet-derived mitogens into the vessel wall (FIGURE 3).

A better analogy to the balloon may be selective denudation. In a series of experiments in our group and by others,[48–50] narrow regions of endothelium have been removed. In the initial study, regions as narrow as a cell or as wide as five cells were removed. The five-cell lesion required two days to heal and no smooth muscle cell replication was seen. Given the kinetics of smooth muscle replication described above, this time course could be consistent with the idea that endothelial regeneration inhibits smooth muscle proliferation. To test this hypothesis, we selectively denuded regions of the aorta large enough to require one week or more for regeneration. As with the earlier selective lesions, these wider lesions failed to produce smooth muscle proliferation. Since the surface was exposed during the critical interval for commitment of smooth muscle cells to replication, it appears that denudation, by itself, is not sufficient to initiate replication. These observations do not rule out the possibility that endothelial regeneration can inhibit proliferation in the balloon model. Factors other than denudation, however, must be required to stimulate growth.

ROLE OF THROMBOSIS

As we have already discussed, the thrombotic response to denudation is extremely transitory. By 48 hours, the number of platelets adhering to the denuded vessel is less than half the number observed acutely after injury.[51] This low level of ^{111}In uptake persists for several months, perhaps related to the persistence, as mentioned above, of denudation. If this initial platelet response is critical to proliferation, then we would

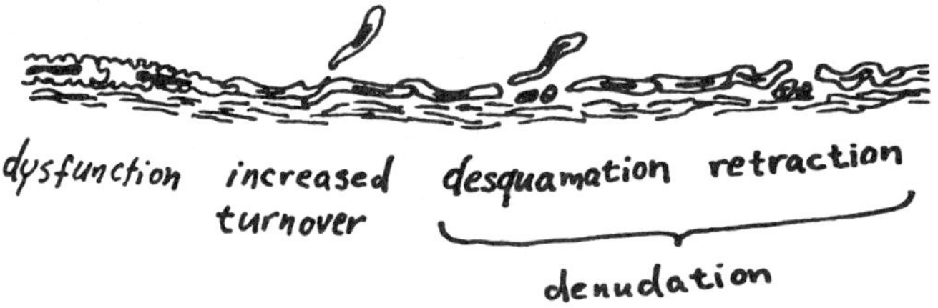

FIGURE 3. Classification of endothelial injury. Advances in our understanding of the biology of the endothelial cell have led us to posit a wide variety of forms of injury. It is important to note that endothelial cells can undergo complete cell death without exposure of the subendothelium to blood. Thus, even endothelial death need not be a stimulus for thrombosis. On the other hand, exposure to the subendothelium could, at least in theory, occur even without cell death.

expect smooth muscle proliferation even with a narrow endothelial wound. A critical role of platelets in the response to the balloon is supported by the observation that antiplatelet serum inhibits proliferation in the injury model.[52–55] Since proliferation does not occur with selective injury, the acute thrombotic response is not a sufficient stimulus. The possibility remains that persistence of low levels of platelet interaction is sufficient. As noted above, however, even substantial denudation fails to stimulate smooth muscle proliferation, unless other as yet undefined effects of the balloon are present.

The argument for a critical role for denudation and thrombosis in the later stages of the disease is more compelling. Ballooning a vessel a second time produces a more persistent thrombotic response with formation of a clot, as well as platelet aggregation.[56] The reason for this difference in behavior is not known, but it is not unreasonable to consider the possibility that platelet interaction at sites over a plaque where denudation results from breakdown of the underlying vessel wall may be much higher and more persistent than the changes observed following a single use of the balloon catheter to denude a healthy wall.

POSSIBLE COMMITMENT EVENTS FOLLOWING BALLOON INJURY

If we return to the balloon model, the studies of kinetics of smooth muscle proliferation leave one question open. Some event occurring in the first three days appears to commit the smooth muscle cell to replication. The simplest possibility is that PDGF could remain in the vessel wall long after the initial release, or that the persistent, though low, levels of release of its denuded surface could provide a critical continued stimulus.

Alternatively, the acute events induced by injury of platelet release or other factors could induce a persistent change in the proliferative potential of the smooth muscle cells themselves. For example, we know that migration is an early event. Migration of dividing cells into the intima could be required for subsequent proliferation if cells in the intima are released from density-dependent controls present in the densely populated tunica media. In turn, this hypothesis would require either some sustained change in the smooth muscle cells in the intima or in their environment that would permit these cells to continue growing long after the initial thrombotic response has been ended.

Other hypotheses need to be considered. We have recently shown that dead smooth muscle cells release a cytoplasmic factor that is mitogenic for other smooth muscle cells.[57] In our hands, the balloon is considerably more traumatic than the narrow scratch catheter. Indeed, trauma sufficient to cause total endothelial denudation always appears to be associated with smooth muscle cell death.[39] It is also interesting to note that Imai and his collaborators showed that oxidized dietary cholesterol was a more effective atherogen than unoxidized cholesterol, and that this difference could be correlated with occurrence of smooth muscle cell death in animals receiving the oxidized material. Putting these observations together, one might posit that mitogens released from dying cells are required for stimulation of smooth muscle replication *in vivo*.

Platelet factors released as part of the injury response might have several effects related to the important question of localization of cells to the intima. PDGF is not only mitogenic, it is chemotactic for smooth muscle cells.[58] Platelets also contain beta-TGF, a polypeptide that is not mitogenic, but when presented with a mitogen, promotes growth of normal cells in soft agar.[59] Beta-TGF could be required for growth of smooth muscle cells outside the media. Smooth muscle cell movement into the intima and growth in that location could require both a chemotactic stimulus, e.g., PDGF, a stimulus to growth without anchorage and breakdown of the extracellular matrix that perhaps results from a combination of release of proteases from necrotic cells, and a mechanical disruption by distension.

Finally, an alternative possibility for the maintenance of growth is offered by recent studies in our laboratories. We attempted to determine the cell cycle status of quiescent cultures of smooth muscle cells of the newborn rat by placing these cells in plasma-deficient serum. To our surprise, growth of these cells could not be arrested under these conditions (FIGURE 4). When the conditioned medium was examined for mitogenicity, the culture medium was able to stimulate 3T3 cell and smooth muscle cell replication. The mitogen responsible for this activity is inactivated by anti-PDGF antibody and the conditioned medium competes for the PDGF receptor. Thus, it appears likely that fetal smooth muscle cells, at least in one species, can make this important mitogen.[60] Furthermore, there is also evidence that adult smooth muscle cells can be induced to produce similar material. Cultured rat arterial smooth muscle cells from adult animals produce low or absent levels of PDGF-like material. However, when cells were derived from a ballooned vessel two weeks after injury, these cells also produced PDGF-like material.[61] It is important to point out that these observations were only made on cells placed in culture; we have no direct evidence for comparable levels of production *in vivo*. Nonetheless, the appearance of activity in cells derived from the balloon-injured vessel implies that some dramatic change has occurred in the capabilities of the smooth muscle cells making up the injured vessel wall. It is intriguing to consider the possibility that this change could be responsible for both the commitment to replication and the maintenance of replication during the days and weeks after injury.

At this point, we would like to offer a speculation. Commitment of smooth muscle cells in the ballooned vessel to continued replication and the behavior of cultured cells derived from these ballooned intima could be accounted for in one of two ways. First,

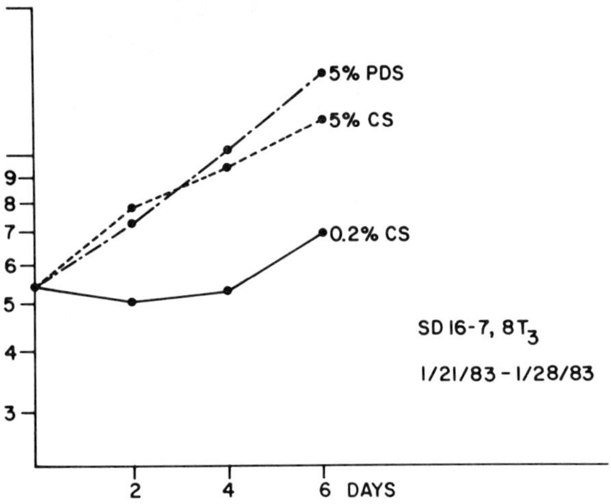

FIGURE 4. Growth of fetal smooth muscle cells and serum in medium. These data represent typical growth data obtained from smooth muscle cells placed in culture after isolation from the aortas of newborn rats. These cells, unlike cells obtained from adult rats, are able to grow even in the absence of platelet-derived growth factor. The figure shows equally good growth in the presence of fetal calf serum (CS), containing platelet-derived growth factor, or plasma-derived serum (PDS), prepared in the absence of platelet release.

the balloon might activate some property of all vessel wall smooth muscle cells, so that these cells maintain or develop the ability to produce PDGF. Alternatively, the balloon could selectively activate a subpopulation of cells that retain the properties of the immature smooth muscle cells found in the pup aorta. This latter idea is attactive for several reasons. A small population of residual immature "blast" cells is known to exist in skeletal muscle and to play a role in regeneration of this muscle.[62,63] If, as a response to the balloon, a few widely scattered immature smooth muscle "blast" cells were stimulated to migrate into the intima, the cells could be released from controls of proliferation imposed by neighboring more mature cells. In the intima, these cells might not only proliferate, but also, they might produce mitogens for other cells. This form of selective proliferation of a subset of cells is consistent with our kinetic evidence that only 50% of cells crossing the intima in response to the balloon go on to proliferate.

More importantly, selection amongst a smooth muscle population to a subpopulation already having a proliferative advantage could account for both the monoclonal phenotype of chronic human atherosclerotic lesions[18] and the suggestions from others that monoclonality arises gradually as the human lesion evolves.[21,64] Obviously, the idea that stem cells exist at all is highly speculative. The idea that such a phenomenon might be important in atherosclerosis depends on knowing whether the proposed blast cells exist in man and, if they do, what proportion of cells forming this lesion has these properties.

IMPLICATIONS OF THIS HYPOTHESIS

It may be worth returning to the elephant. A "residual stem cell" hypothesis provides no insight into the mechanism of accumulation of lipid or the reasons that a relatively innocuous proliferative response eventuates in vascular occlusion. On the other hand, the proliferative response of the vessel wall has been viewed as a simple question of stimulus and response. If more than one population of smooth muscle cell is present, then we may need to consider other issues, particularly the mechanisms involved in embryogenesis of blood vessels. In this regard, it is disturbing to realize that very little is known about the developmental biology of arteries. The stem cell hypothesis raises the possibility that intrinsic properties of the vessel wall may predispose to development of atherosclerotic lesions. The possible contribution of such phenomena to the focal development of lesions and to the variations in propensity of different individuals to develop disease is intriguing.

REFERENCES

1. Shio, H., N. J. Haley & S. Fowler. 1979. Characterization of lipid-laden aortic cells from cholesterol-fed rabbits. II. Morphometric analysis of lipid-filled lysosomes and lipid droplets in aortic cell populations. Lab. Invest. **39:** 390–397.
2. Schaffner, T., K. Taylor, E. J. Bartucci, K. Fisher-Dzoga, J. H. Beeson, S. Glagov & R. W. Wissler. 1980. Arterial foam cells with distinctive immunomorphologic and histochemical features of macrophages. Am. J. Pathol. **100:** 57–74.
3. Schwartz, C. J. & J. R. A. Mitchell. 1962. Cellular infiltration of the human arterial adventitia associated with atheromatous plaques. Circulation **26:** 73–78.
4. Still, W. J. S. & P. R. Marriott. 1964. Comparative morphology of the early atherosclerotic lesion in man and cholesterol-atherosclerosis in the rabbit. An electron microscopic study. J. Atheroscler. Res. **4:** 373–386.
5. Faggiotto, A., R. Ross & L. Harker. 1984. Studies of hypercholesterolemia in the nonhuman primate. I. Changes that lead to fatty streak formation. Arteriosclerosis **4:** 323–340.
6. Faggiotto, A. & R. Ross. 1984. Studies of hypercholesterolemia in the nonhuman primate. II. Fatty streak conversion to fibrous plaques. Arteriosclerosis **4:** 341–356.
7. Gerrity, R. G., H. K. Naito, M. Richardson & C. J. Schwartz. 1979. Dietary induced atherogenesis in swine. Morphology of the intima in prelesion stage. Am. J. Pathol. **95:** 775–792.
8. Massman, J. & H. Jellinek. 1980. Hematogenic infiltration of the aortic intima in normal and hypercholesterolemic swine. Studies on *en face* endothelium-intima preparations. Exp. Pathol. **18:** 11–24.
9. Schwartz, S. M., C. M. Gajdusek, M. A. Reidy, S. C. Selden III & C. C. Haudenschild. 1980. Maintenance of integrity in aortic endothelium. Fed. Proc. **39:** 2618–2625.

10. REIDY, M. A. & S. M. SCHWARTZ. 1983. Endothelial injury and regeneration. IV. Endotoxin: A nondenuding injury to aortic endothelium. Lab. Invest. **48:** 25–34.
11. HASSLER, O. 1970. The origin of the cells constituting arterial intimal thickening. An experimental autoradiographic study. Lab. Invest. **22:** 286–295.
12. CLOWES, A. W., M. A. REIDY & M. M. CLOWES. 1983. Kinetics of cellular proliferation after arterial injury. I. Smooth muscle growth in the absence of endothelium. Lab. Invest. **49:** 327–332.
13. BURNS, E. R., T. H. SPAET & M. B. STEMERMAN. 1978. Response of the arterial wall to endothelial removal: An autoradiographic study. Proc. Soc. Exp. Biol. Med. **159:** 473–377.
14. WEBSTER, W. A., S. P. BISHOP & J. C. GEER. 1974. Experimental aortic intimal thickening. I. Morphology and source of intimal cells. Am. J. Pathol. **76:** 245–264.
15. CLOWES, A. W. & S. M. SCHWARTZ. 1985. Significance of quiescent smooth muscle migration in the injured rat carotid artery. Circ. Res. **56:** 139–145.
16. CLOWES, A. W. & M. M. CLOWES. 1984. Heparin inhibits injury induced arterial smooth muscle migration and proliferation. Fed. Proc. **43:** 1022.
17. VELICAN, C. & D. VELICAN. 1980. The precursors of coronary atherosclerotic plaques in subjects up to 40 years old. Atherosclerosis **37:** 33–46.
18. BENDITT, E. P. & A. M. GOWN. 1980. Atheroma: The artery wall and the environment. Int. Rev. Exp. Pathol. **21:** 55–118.
19. THOMAS, W. A., R. A. FLORENTIN, J. M. REINER, W. M. LEE & K. T. LEE. 1976. Alterations in population dynamics of arterial smooth muscle cells during atherogenesis. IV. Evidence for polyclonal origin of hypercholesterolemic diet-induced atherosclerotic lesions in young swine. Exp. Mol. Pathol. **24:** 244–260.
20. THOMAS, W. A., J. M. REINER, K. JANAKIDEVI, R. A. FLORENTIN & K. Y. LEE. 1979. Population dynamics of arterial cells during atherogenesis. X. Study of monotypism in atherosclerotic lesions of black women heterozygous for glucose-6-phosphate dehydrogenase (G-6-PD). Exp. Mol. Pathol. **31:** 367–386.
21. THOMAS, W. A. & D. N. KIM. 1983. Atherosclerosis as a hyperplastic and/or neoplastic process. Lab. Invest. **48:** 245–255.
22. SCHWARTZ, S. M., M. B. STEMERMAN & E. P. BENDITT. 1975. The aortic intima. II. Repair of the aortic lining after mechanical denudation. Am. J. Pathol. **81:** 15–42.
23. FAGGIOTTO, A., R. ROSS & L. A. HARKER. 1982. Early arterial changes in the hypercholesterolemic nonhuman primate. Circulation **66:** II–225.
24. MUSTARD, J. F. & M. A. PACKHAM. 1975. The role of blood and platelets in atherosclerosis and the complications of atherosclerosis. Thromb. Diath. Haemorrh. **33:** 444–456.
25. GOLDBERG, I. D., M. B. STEMERMAN & R. I. HANDIN. 1980. Vascular permeation of platelet factor IV after endothelial injury. Science **209:** 610–612.
26. SCHWARTZ, S. M. & E. P. BENDITT. 1976. Clustering of replicating cells in aortic endothelium. Proc. Natl. Acad. Sci. USA **73:** 651–653.
27. GERRITY, R. G. 1981. The role of the monocyte in atherogenesis. I. Transition of blood-borne monocytes into foam cells in fatty lesions. Am. J. Pathol. **103:** 181–190.
28. FRENCH, J. E. 1965. Atherosclerosis in relation to the structure and function of the arterial intima with special reference to the endothelium. Int. Rev. Exp. Pathol. **5:** 253–353.
29. HALPERT, B., R. M. O'NEAL, G. L. JORDAN & M. E. DE BAKEY. 1966. "Vasa vasorum" of dacron prosthesis in canine aorta. Arch. Pathol. **81:** 412–417.
30. HAUDENSCHILD, C. C. & S. M. SCHWARTZ. 1979. Endothelial regeneration. II. Restitution of endothelial continuity. Lab. Invest. **41:** 407–418.
31. REIDY, M. A., A. W. CLOWES & S. M. SCHWARTZ. 1983. Endothelial regeneration. V. Inhibition of endothelial regrowth in arteries of rat and rabbit. Lab. Invest. **49:** 569–575.
32. MINICK, C. R., M. B. STEMERMAN & W. INSULL, JR. 1979. Role of endothelium and hypercholesterolemia in intimal thickening and lipid accumulation. Am. J. Pathol. **95:** 131–151.
33. GAJDUSEK, C., P. DICORLETO, R. ROSS & S. SCHWARTZ. 1980. An endothelial cell-derived growth factor. J. Cell Biol. **85:** 467–472.
34. VLODAVSKY, I., P. E. FIELDING, C. J. FIELDING & D. GOSPODAROWICZ. 1978. Role of contact inhibition in the regulation of receptor-mediated uptake of low-density lipoprotein in cultured vascular endothelial cells. Proc. Natl. Acad. Sci. USA **75:** 356–360.

35. KENAGY, R., E. L. BIERMAN & S. SCHWARTZ. 1983. Regulation of low-density lipoprotein metabolism by cell density and proliferative state. J. Cell. Physiol. **116:** 404–408.
36. ALBERS, J. J. & E. L. BIERMAN. 1976. The influence of lipoprotein composition on binding, uptake, and degradation of different lipoprotein. Artery **2:** 337–348.
37. WIGHT, T. N., K. D. CURWEN & C. R. MINICK. 1983. The effect of endothelium on glycosaminoglycan accumulation in the rabbit aorta. Am. J. Pathol. **113:** 156–164.
38. CLOWES, A. W. & M. J. KARNOVSKY. 1977. Failure of certain antiplatelet drugs to affect myointimal thickening following arterial endothelial injury in the rat. Lab. Invest. **36:** 452–464.
39. CLOWES, A. W., M. A. REIDY & M. M. CLOWES. 1983. Mechanisms of stenosis after arterial injury. Lab. Invest. **49:** 208–215.
40. SCHWARTZ, S. M. & E. P. BENDITT. 1977. Aortic endothelial cell replication. I. Effects of age and hypertension in the rat. Circ. Res. **41:** 248–255.
41. WRIGHT, H. P. 1972. Mitosis patterns in aortic endothelium. Atherosclerosis **15:** 93–100.
42. ROSS, R. & L. HARKER. 1976. Hyperlipidemia and atherosclerosis. Science **193:** 1044–1099.
43. DAVIES, P., M. REIDY, T. GOODE & D. BOWYER. 1976. Scanning electron microscopy in the evaluation of endothelial integrity of the fatty lesion in atherosclerosis. Atherosclerosis **25:** 125–130.
44. TAYLOR, K., S. GLAGOV, J. LAMBERTI, D. VESSELINOVITCH & T. SCHNAFFNER. 1978. Surface configuration of early atheromatous lesions in controlled pressure perfusion-fixed monkey aortas. Scanning Electron Microsc. **11:** 449–457.
45. REIDY, M. A. & D. E. BOWYER. 1978. Scanning electron microscopy studies of rabbit aortic endothelium in areas of haemodynamic stress during induction of fatty streaks. Virchow Arch. A. Pathol. **377:** 237–248.
46. JORIS, I., T. ZAND, J. J. NUNNARI, F. J. KROLIKOWSKI & G. MAJNO. 1983. Studies on the pathogenesis of atherosclerosis. I. Adhesion and emigration of mononuclear cells in the aorta of hypercholesterolemic rats. Am. J. Pathol. **113:** 341–358.
47. SCOTT, R. F. 1979. Distribution of intimal smooth muscle cell masses and their relationship to early atherosclerosis in the abdominal aortas of young swine. Atherosclerosis **34:** 291–301.
48. HIRSCH, E. Z. & A. L. ROBERTSON. 1977. Selective acute arterial endothelial injury and repair. I. Methodology and surface characteristics. Atherosclerosis **28:** 271–287.
49. REIDY, M. A. & S. M. SCHWARTZ. 1981. Endothelial regeneration. III. Intimal changes after small defined injury to rat aorta. Lab. Invest. **44:** 301–308.
50. RAMSAY, M. M., L. N. WALKER & D. E. BOWYER. 1982. Narrow superficial injury to rabbit aortic endothelium. The healing process as observed by scanning electron microscopy. Atherosclerosis **43:** 233–243.
51. GROVES, H. M., R. L. KINLOUGH-RATHBONE, M. RICHARDSON, S. MOORE & J. F. MUSTARD. 1979. Platelet interaction with damaged rabbit aorta. Lab. Invest. **40:** 194–206.
52. MOORE, S. 1979. Endothelial injury and atherosclerosis. Exp. Mol. Pathol. **31:** 182–190.
53. TIELL, M. L., I. I. SUSSMAN, R. MOSS, L. C. DROUET & T. H. SPAET. 1982. Production of experimental arteriosclerosis in fawn-hooded rats with platelet storage pool deficiency. Artery **10:** 329–340.
54. MOORE, S., R. J. FRIEDMAN, D. P. SINGAL, J. GAULDIE, M. A. BLAJCHMAN & R. S. ROBERTS. 1976. Inhibition of injury induced thromboatherosclerotic lesions by antiplatelet serum in rabbits. Thromb. Haemost. **35:** 70–81.
55. FRIEDMAN, R. J., M. B. STEMERMAN, B. WENZ, S. MOORE, J. GAULDIE, M. GENT, M. L. TIELL & T. H. SPAET. 1977. The effect of thrombocytopenia on experimental arteriosclerotic lesion formation in rabbits. Smooth muscle cell proliferation and re-endothelialization. J. Clin. Invest. **60:** 1191–1201.
56. GROVES, H. M., R. L. KINLOUGH-RATHBONE, M. RICHARDSON, L. JØRGENSEN, S. MOORE & J. F. MUSTARD. 1982. Thrombin generation and fibrin formation following injury to rabbit neointima. Studies of vessel wall reactivity and platelet survival. Lab. Invest. **46:** 605–612.
57. GAJDUSEK, C. M. & S. M. SCHWARTZ. 1984. Comparison of intracellular and extracellular mitogen activity. J. Cell. Physiol. In press.

58. GROTENDORST, G. R., H. E. J. SEPPA, H. K. KLEINMAN & G. R. MARTIN. 1981. Attachment of smooth muscle cells to collagen and their migration toward platelet-derived growth factor. Proc. Natl. Acad. Sci. USA **78:** 3669–3672.
59. ASSOIAN, R. K., C. A. FROLIK, A. B. ROBERTS, D. M. MILLER & M. B. SPORN. 1984. Transforming growth factor-beta controls receptor levels for epidermal growth factor in NRK fibroblasts. Cell **36:** 35–41.
60. SEIFERT, R. A., S. M. SCHWARTZ & D. F. BOWEN-POPE. 1984. Developmentally regulated production of platelet-derived growth factor-like molecules. Nature **311:** 669–671.
61. WALKER, L. N., D. BOWEN-POPE & M. A. REIDY. 1984. Secretion of platelet-derived growth factor (PDGF)-like activity in arterial smooth muscle cells is induced as a response to injury. J. Cell Biol. **99**(abstract): 416a.
62. DIENTSMAN, S. R. & H. HOLTZER. 1975. Myogenesis: A cell lineage interpretation. *In* Cell Cycle and Cell Differentiation. J. Reinert & H. Holtzer, Eds.: 1–25. Springer-Verlag. New York.
63. KONIGSBERG, U. R., B. H. LIPTON & I. R. KONIGSBERG. 1975. The regenerative response of single mature muscle fibers isolated *in vitro.* Dev. Biol. **45:** 260–275.
64. PEARSON, T. A., J. M. DILLMAN & R. H. HEPTINSTALL. 1983. The clonal characteristics of human aortic intima. Comparison with fatty streaks and normal media. Am. J. Pathol. **113:** 33–40.

Cell Population Kinetics in Atherogenesis

Cell Births and Losses in Intimal Cell Mass-Derived Lesions in the Abdominal Aorta of Swine[a]

W. A. THOMAS, K. T. LEE, AND D. N. KIM

Department of Pathology
Albany Medical College
Albany, New York 12208

Studies in experimental animals have shown that atherosclerotic lesions can originate in a number of different ways (TABLE 1). Gerrity[1,2] has demonstrated lesions in the thoracic aortas of hyperlipidemic (HL) swine that appear to arise from penetration of the endothelium by monocytes from the blood to form collections in the intima. Lewis *et al.*[3] have studied lesions in the aortas of pigeons that appear to arise from monocytes in a similar fashion. Others have produced intimal lesions in several species of experimental animals by removing the endothelium, which appear to arise by migration of smooth muscle cells (SMC) from the media. We have demonstrated lesions in the abdominal aortas of HL swine that appear to originate by hyperplasia of normally occurring intimal cell masses (ICM).[4,5] Cell population kinetics in atherosclerotic lesions arising in these different ways are likely to be different also.

This presentation is limited to the origin and development of ICM-derived atherosclerotic lesions in the abdominal aortas of HL swine. We suspect that information obtained from this swine model has much wider application and, in particular, that most human atherosclerotic lesions are derived from ICM in a similar fashion. However, this remains to be proved and will not be dealt with here.

We shall begin with a discussion of ICM as a normal structure in control swine, followed by descriptions of the origin and early development of atherosclerotic lesions in the ICM. We shall end with a brief description of the progression of the early ICM-derived lesions to the advanced stage characterized by large atheromatous lesions with extensive foci of lipid-rich calcific necrotic debris.

ICM AS NORMAL STRUCTURES IN CONTROL SWINE FED LOW FAT, LOW CHOLESTEROL MASH DIETS

Terms

Many other terms have been used for the structures we are calling ICM. When they are around branch orifices, they are usually called branch cushions or pads. When they are away from orifices and involve extensive portions of intima, they are frequently referred to as diffuse intimal thickening. The term ICM encompasses both of these forms. Stary[6] has suggested that since they are a normal part of the intima, they do not need a special name; that is, it is enough to say that the intima is thicker in some places than in others. We have no serious objection to this point of view, but it

[a]This work was supported by USPHS grant no. HL–20993.

does seem more convenient to have a name for them. The term ICM emphasizes the cellular aspect, but these structures also contain collagen, elastic tissue, glycosoaminoglycans, and other extracellular components.

Location and Extent

The ICM are found in fairly specific locations, probably related to hemodynamic forces. In the proximal portion of the swine abdominal aorta, they are predominantly on the dorsal surface, while in the distal portion, they predominate on the ventral aspect.[4]

Size and Cell Numbers in Relation to the Media at Various Ages

At two months of age, ICM constitute about 2% of the arterial wall (intima plus media) and about the same proportion of total cells.[5] At one year of age, the proportions are about the same, but ICM do grow larger as the swine gets older. We have studied ICM in swine up to twelve years of age, and by that age, ICM may constitute as much as 15% of the aortic wall.[7]

TABLE 1. Atherosclerotic Lesions May Originate by:

1.	Monocyte infiltration of intima from blood.
2.	SMC migration to intima from media.
3.	Excessive growth of normal intimal cell masses (ICM) to form ICM-lesions.
4.	Other means.

Cell Types

Differential cell counts by transmission electron microscopy (TEM) of cells in the ICM at ages from newborns to twenty weeks of age have been done.[8] About 90–95% of the cells at these ages have basement membranes and other features characterizing them as SMC. In the newborn, many of the SMC are the synthetic type described by Campbell *et al.*[9] However, within a few weeks, most SMC are the contractile type with abundant myofilaments. Some 3–5% of the cells in the ICM at all ages studied are monocytes or at least moncyte-like cells. Approximately 3–4% do not show specialized features that permit easy classification. We have tended to lump these unidentified cells with the monocytes although we cannot eliminate the possibility that they are modified SMC.

INITIATION AND EARLY DEVELOPMENT OF ICM-DERIVED ATHEROSCLEROTIC LESIONS IN HL SWINE

For this part of the presentation, we are, in large part, summarizing some of the data from a specific experiment[10] although we have supporting data from many other experiments. Eight-week-old male Yorkshire swine were placed on an HL diet for up to 90 days. Sacrifices of these and control mash-fed swine were made on diet days 0, 14, 49, and 90. Comparisons between HL and mash swine of ICM in the abdominal aorta

TABLE 2. ICM and ICM-Lesion Areas per Cross Section (mm^2)[a]

	0-day	14	49	90
Mash	0.05(10)	0.06(5)	0.09(6)	0.10(13) *
HL	—	0.04(6)	0.11(6)	0.89(9)

[a]Numbers in parentheses are the number of swine. Asterisks in this and subsequent tables indicate statistically significant differences between Mash and HL.

were made at the sequential time points in regard to size, cell numbers, cell types, intracellular lipid, tritiated thymidine labeling indices, cell losses, and endothelial integrity. When the ICM begin to show characteristics of atherosclerotic lesions, we are referring to them, herein, as ICM-lesions.

ICM and ICM-Lesion Sizes

ICM area was measured with an eyepiece micrometer on H & E stained slides from multiple cross sections of the abdominal aorta as an index of size. Data are shown in TABLE 2. It is apparent that through the 49th day, ICM and ICM-lesion sizes are not significantly different between the HL and mash groups. However, by day-90, the ICM-lesions in the HL swine have become 8–9 times larger than the mash ICM.

ICM and ICM-Lesion Cell Numbers

Data presented in TABLE 3 are expressed as average numbers of nuclear profiles in cross sections, which is used here as an index of cell numbers. This does not take into account growth in aortic length, which will be included in another type of index presented later on. Results in this table parallel those regarding size in TABLE 2. The big increase in cell numbers in the ICM-lesions of the HL group is between days 49 and 90.

Necrosis with Accumulation of Lipid-rich Calcific Debris

There were virtually no necrotic foci at this stage in atherogenesis.

Cell Types in ICM and ICM-Lesions

The predominant cell type (90–95% of total) in mash swine was the SMC as already described above. In the ICM-lesions of the HL swine at 49 and 90 days, many

TABLE 3. ICM and ICM-Lesion Nuclear Profiles per Cross Section

	0-day	14	49	90
Mash	137	185	202	287 *
HL	—	124	275	2383

TABLE 4. Changes in Lipid Quantity in ICM-Lesions of HL Swine (%)

Cells	HL–14	HL–49	HL–90
Non-vacuolated	96	57	48
Vacuolated			
Rounded	1	27	33
Elongated	3	16	19

of the cells were rounded and packed with lipid droplets. By light microscopy, these were thought to be monocyte-macrophages. However, by electron microscopy, most of these cells had basement membranes, which eliminate them from the monocyte-macrophage category. They appear to be SMC of the synthetic type described by Campbell *et al.* in cell cultures.[9] In changing from the contractile to the synthetic type, these SMC have been shown in cell cultures to lose much of their cholesteryl esterase activity and to accumulate far more lipid than contractile type SMC. Differential counts on ICM-lesions by TEM at 49 and 90 days on HL diet showed 95% or more of the cells to be SMC, with monocytes being no more numerous than in the ICM of mash-fed controls.

Numbers of Lipid Containing Cells

Data are presented in TABLE 4 as percentages of vacuolated cells. Oil-red-0 stains on appropriate material showed that the vacuoles corresponded to lipid droplets. Data on the mash swine are not shown since only a small percentage contained lipid droplets. At 14 days, the values for the HL swine are not significantly different from controls. However, by 49 days, nearly 50% of the cells were vacuolated, with a somewhat greater number by 90 days. Of interest is the big increase in percentage of ICM-lesion cells containing lipid, which precedes the big increase in cell numbers.

Tritiated Thymidine Labeling Indices (LI)

The tritiated thymidine LI were used as an index of cell division. We have shown in previous studies that practically all labeled cells in the aorta go on to divide. LI in the ICM-lesions of the HL swine were four times greater than those in the mash swine by 49 days, and this difference was maintained at 90 days (TABLE 5). Note that the large increase in the LI of the HL swine precedes the large increase in cell numbers.

n-Fold Increase in Cells in ICM and ICM-Lesions from 0 to 90 Days Observed and That Expected on the Basis of the Average LI

Data are given in TABLE 6. The observed n-fold increase is obtained by dividing a value reflecting the number of cells present in ICM or ICM-lesions at 90 days, by a

TABLE 5. Tritiated Thymidine Labeling Indices in ICM and ICM-Lesions (%)

	0-day	14	49	90
Mash	0.91	0.62	0.69	0.49
			*	*
HL	—	1.00	2.84	1.86

TABLE 6. n-Fold Increases 0–90 Days in Cells in ICM and ICM-Lesions Observed versus That Expected with LI Observed Assuming No Cell Loss

	Observed	Expected
Mash	2.8-fold	3.2-fold
	*	*
HL	24.4-fold	44.4-fold

corresponding value reflecting the number present on 0-day. The expected n-fold increase from divisions among resident cells present at 0-day (assuming no cell loss) is obtained by calculations based on the average LI for the 90-day period and the average length of the DNA synthesis (S) period (about twelve hours in these cells). Details are given in the original paper. It is apparent from TABLE 6 that divisions among resident cells can more than account for the observed increase in numbers and that input from other sources (such as the underlying media) is not required. We are showing here the expected input from divisions of resident cells only. If there is additional input by migration of SMC from the media, it would have to be offset by greater losses.

Estimation of Cell Losses per S Period

Data are given in TABLE 7. The LI observed is the weighted average of the values at 0, 14, 49, and 90 days. The LI required to provide the observed fold increase in cells is calculated to be quite small between observed and required values (equivalent to about 10% of the observed LI for mash, and 15% for HL), and they actually do not reach statistically significant differences from zero. These results suggest that lesion cell deaths are not an important factor in the initiation and early development of ICM-derived lesions in this model. The additional observation that we found almost no accumulation of necrotic debris by light microscopy tends to support this conclusion.

Endothelium

Studies of the endothelium by scanning electron microscopy (SEM) revealed no evidence for loss of integrity even in the HL swine at 90 days. Studies of endothelial cell losses in the HL swine, based on tritiated thymidine labeling indices (and using the same mathematical methods as for lesion cells mentioned above), suggested a significant loss equivalent to 50% of their LI per S period over the 90-day HL diet period. However, a similar loss was calculated for the endothelial cells in the control mash-fed swine. However, other types of comparisons involving tritiated thymidine LI of EC did bring out differences between mash and HL swine. Thus, a role of EC in the initiation and early development of the ICM-derived lesions cannot be eliminated.

TABLE 7. Estimation of Cell Losses per S Period Using Average LI Observed and LI Required for Observed n-Fold Increases (%)

	LI observed	LI required	Difference
Mash	0.64	0.58	0.06
	*	*	
HL	2.13	1.79	0.34

Conclusions Regarding Initiation and Early Development of ICM-Derived Atherosclerotic Lesions in the Abdominal Aortas of HL Swine

(a) The ICM-lesions appear to arise from resident SMC stimulated to excessive multiplication, as indicated by the calculations based on the tritiated thymidine LI.

(b) Monocytes are few in number in the ICM-lesions in the early stage of development where there is little or no necrosis, and, at least on the basis of numbers, they do not appear to be an important factor. However, we cannot entirely eliminate the possibility that they are making some contribution such as supplying monocyte-derived growth factor (MDGF).

(c) Endothelial cell integrity is, at least, not grossly impaired at this early stage in lesion development as seen by SEM. Thus, no simple basis for increased platelet interactions has been demonstrated. However, some differences between HL and control swine have been demonstrated by tritiated thymidine autoradiography studies of EC, and we cannot eliminate the possibility that platelets and platelet-derived growth factor (PDGF) are involved in some more subtle fashion.

(d) The calculations regarding lesion cell losses based on the tritiated thymidine LI data suggest that cell deaths are relatively small in number in early lesion development. Thus, they are probably not playing a major role in pathogenesis at this stage. However, the caveat that they cannot be completely dismissed must once more be invoked.

(e) After all of these relatively negative conclusions, we arrive at the observations that strike us as the most significant. The large increase in the number of resident ICM cells containing lipid and the accompanying large increase in tritiated thymidine labeling indices both immediately precede the large increase in ICM-lesion cell numbers. We are inclined to link the lipid increase and the division activity increase, and to suggest that the lipid is the most likely source of the putative SMC growth stimulatory factor. Some support for this suggestion is provided by SMC culture studies[11] in which HL serum is shown to stimulate more rapid cell multiplication than normolipidemic serum. The stimulation could be by the lipid *per se,* or by substances which may be associated with the lipid, e.g., MDGF or PDGF. If it is the lipid *per se,* it will be of interest to know the relative stimulatory effects of various lipid subclasses. In this regard, Fless *et al.*[12] have shown in SMC culture studies that an abnormally large species of LDL is especially stimulatory to *in vitro* SMC multiplication.

TRANSFORMATION OF THE EARLY PROLIFERATIVE ICM-LESION TO THE ADVANCED ATHEROMATOUS PHASE CHARACTERIZED BY EXTENSIVE FOCI OF LIPID-RICH CALCIFIC NECROTIC DEBRIS OVER THE PERIOD 90–300 DAYS ON HL DIET

For this part of the presentation, we are summarizing some observations on the abdominal aorta of a group of swine fed an HL diet for approximately 300 days,[13] and then, comparing these with the observations at 90 days on HL diet given above.

ICM-Lesion Sizes

By 300 HL diet days, the aggregate lesion volume has increased about tenfold over that of 90 days. In many places, the lesions are far thicker than the underlying media.

It should be noted that this tremendous growth of the ICM-derived lesions in the abdominal aortas is in striking contrast to that of the monocyte-derived lesions in the thoracic aortas, which are still quite thin in the same swine.

ICM-Lesion Cell Numbers

The increase in cells from 90 to 300 days was only about threefold.

Necrosis with Accumulation of Lipid-rich Calcific Debris

The most striking difference between the lesions at 90 and 300 days was that in the latter, there were extensive regions of accumulation of lipid-rich calcific necrotic debris. These regions occupied about 65% of the aggregate lesion volume, as compared to their virtual absence at 90 days. This accounts for the discrepancy between increases in lesion volumes and increases in lesion cell numbers.

Cell Types in ICM-Lesions

We have not carried out extensive cell differential counts by TEM as we have at 90 days (where 95% or more of the cells were SMC). However, we have done some preliminary counts. SMC are still abundant, but there are many foci in which there are numerous monocyte-macrophages which are generally associated with sites of necrosis.

Number of Lipid Containing Cells

We have not carried out counts on the relative numbers of vacuolated cells as we did at 90 days. However, they are numerous in many areas and appear to be in greater numbers than at 90 days.

Tritiated Thymidine LI

The LI appeared to be somewhat lower than those at 90 days. However, they are still significantly high compared to the normal media.

n-Fold Increases in ICM and ICM-Lesions from 90 to 300 Days Observed and That Expected on the Basis of Average LI

The observed n-fold increase in ICM-lesion cells in these particular experiments between 90 and 300 diet days was only about threefold. The increase expected on the basis of the LI with no cell deaths would be greatly more than that (50-fold or more), indicating extensive cell losses.

Estimation of Cell Losses per S Period

We have an adequate data base for this type of calculation only for the period 270–345 days on HL diet. The difference between observed and required LI's reflecting cell losses was quite large, being equivalent to about 65% of the observed LI (compared to about 15% of the observed LI for 0–90 days on HL diet).

Endothelium

We have not carried out SEM studies on endothelium at 300 days on HL diet. However, we do have some limited data on tritiated thymidine LI at this stage. These data suggest endothelial cell loss rates about fourfold greater over ICM-lesions in HL swine compared with cells over ICM in mash swine. Recall that at 90 days, losses appeared to be similar over HL ICM-lesions and mash ICM. These data are, thus, consistent with endothelial cell damage associated with the HL diet at this stage. This putative endothelial cell damage could well be associated with increased platelet-arterial wall interactions although we have no specific data on this point.

Conclusions Regarding Progressive Development of ICM-Derived Atherosclerotic Lesions between HL Diet Days 90 and 300 in the Abdominal Aortas of HL Swine

(a) The lesions increase greatly in size over the 90–300 day period, though only modestly in cell numbers.
(b) The major reason for the size increase is the accumulation of large amounts of lipid-rich calcific necrotic debris in the lesions; this material was virtually absent at 90 days.
(c) By 300 days, monocyte-macrophages, which were few in number at 90 days, are numerous in many areas, perhaps coming as a homeostatic response to the necrotic debris, extracellular lipid, and calcium deposits.
(d) Whatever the basis for the appearance of the monocyte-macrophages, they are not able to carry out successfully their physiological function of clearing away the pathological extracellular material. It is of interest to note that in regression studies in swine where the HL diet is replaced by a low fat, low cholesterol mash diet, much of the extracellular lipid and necrotic debris is cleared away, although the calcific deposits may remain.
(e) There is evidence for endothelial cell damage as the lesions progress to advanced stages, and this may enhance the pathologic process through platelet interactions or otherwise.
(f) Lesion cell deaths, which were small at 90 days, appear to have become a great deal larger by 300 days. This is consistent with and probably accounts for the extensive accumulation of necrotic debris.
(g) The above conclusions indicate that the progressive growth of ICM-derived atherosclerotic lesions from the early, largely proliferative phase to the late, necrotic phase is a much more complex process than initiation and early development.

SUMMARY

Atherosclerotic lesions may arise in a number of different ways. The two most notable, perhaps, are by monocyte infiltration of the intima and by hyperplasia of normally occurring intimal cell masses. This report is limited to the ICM-derived lesion type induced by a hyperlipidemic diet in the abdominal aorta of swine. The HL diet results, by 49 days, in accumulation of lipid in about 50% of the ICM cells and increases in cell division activity, as indicated by tritiated thymidine LI fourfold greater than in ICM of control swine. Cell numbers are not significantly increased over controls at 49 days, but by 90 HL diet days, they have increased to eightfold over control values. Throughout the 90 days, about 95% of the cells in the ICM or ICM-lesions are smooth muscle cells. Monocytes appear to constitute no more than 5% of the cells. Calculated lesion cell deaths are small during the 90 days, and foci of necrosis are rarely found. By scanning electron microscopy, the endothelial cell integrity appears to be maintained even over the ICM-lesions at 90 days. Calculations from tritiated thymidine LI indicate endothelial cell losses equivalent to 50% of the LI, but they are not significantly greater for the HL swine than for controls. We suggest, then, that the lipid in the ICM (or something associated with it) is the most likely candidate for the SMC growth stimulatory agent accounting for the increased tritiated thymidine LI and the great increase in ICM-lesion cell numbers between HL diet days 49 and 90. Platelet- and/or monocyte-derived growth factors may also be involved in some subtle fashion, but this study provides no positive evidence to support this hypothesis.

Progression of the ICM-derived lesions to the advanced atheromatous phase by 300 days on HL diet appears to be a much more complex process. By 300 days in the specific experiment cited, approximately 65% of the atherosclerotic lesion volume consisted of lipid-rich calcific necrotic debris; calculated death rates of lesion cells were very high compared to that at 90 days; calculated endothelial cell loss rates were considerably higher than in controls; and, large numbers of monocyte-macrophages were present in many areas generally associated with necrotic foci. These changes in the aggregate suggest a much more complex mode of pathogenesis for progression to advanced stages than for initiation and early development.

QUESTIONS THAT MIGHT BE ANSWERED IN FUTURE STUDIES WITH THIS MODEL

1. What are the characteristics of the agent(s) that stimulate excessive multiplication of SMC in the ICM? The major feature of the first 90 days on HL diet, in regard to atherogenesis, appears to be the proliferation of these cells. Other features prominent later on (such as endothelial cell damage, excessive deaths among lesion cells, extensive monocyte infiltration, and massive accumulations of lipid-rich calcific necrotic debris) appear to be minimal during this early 90-day period on HL diet, providing a relatively simple situation for study of the putative growth stimulatory agent. Specific questions could include:

(a) Is the stimulatory agent lipid *per se,* or some substance associated with the lipid, e.g., PDGF or MDGF?
(b) Are some lipid classes more stimulatory than others, e.g., LDL, VLDL, etc.?
(c) Are saturated fats more stimulatory than unsaturated fats?

2. What are the characteristics of the agent(s) that account for the necrosis and accumulation of lipid-rich calcific necrotic debris? This type of study would need to be done between 90 and 300 days on HL diet, and preliminary work is needed to identify the optimum times on HL diet. Candidates for necrotizing agents would include cholesterol oxidation products such as 25-hydroxycholesterol.

3. What is the role of the monocyte-macrophage in the progression of the lesions to advanced necrotic stages? This type of study would also need to be done after 90 days on diet. The monocyte-macrophage might be acting in a protective role and slowing the

progression of the lesion. It might, in addition, be contributing to the pathogenesis by incidentally releasing harmful substances into the tissues such as degradative enzymes.

4. As a corollary to #3, we can ask questions regarding the differences and similarities between the monocyte-derived lesions in the thoracic aorta and the ICM-derived lesions in the abdominal aorta.

5. Are there functional changes in the endothelium in the first 90 days on diet, even though we found no loss of integrity by SEM nor endothelial cell losses greater than in controls by tritiated thymidine autoradiography? For example, the endothelium might become more leaky to macromolecules such as lipoproteins.

6. What role does endothelial damage play in the progression of lesions in the 90–300 day HL diet period? We know from tritiated thymidine autoradiographic studies that, by 300 days, the endothelial cell loss rate is considerably greater than in controls.

7. What is the role of platelets in the progression of the ICM-derived atherosclerotic lesions? In the absence of gross evidence of loss of endothelial cell integrity in the first 90 days on diet, it seems unlikely that platelets are playing an important role in this early stage. Nonetheless, the possibility of some involvement cannot be eliminated. However, we do have evidence for endothelial cell damage by 300 days on HL diet, and it probably begins to occur long before the 300 days. During the period of endothelial cell damage, we might well have increased platelet-arterial wall interactions, and these might contribute to lesion progression.

REFERENCES

1. GERRITY, R. G. 1981. The role of the monocyte in atherogenesis. I. Transition of blood-borne monocytes into foam cells in fatty lesions. Am. J. Pathol. **103**: 181–190.
2. GERRITY, R. G. 1981. The role of the monocyte in atherogenesis. II. Migration of foam cells from atherosclerotic lesions. Am. J. Pathol. **103**: 191–200.
3. LEWIS, J. C., R. C. TAYLOR & M. S. WHITE. 1983. Monocyte (MC) migration and endothelial (EC) turnover: Simultaneous events at the edge of atherosclerotic lesions. Circulation **68** (supp. III): 300.
4. SCOTT, R. F., W. A. THOMAS, W. M. LEE, J. M. REINER & R. A. FLORENTIN. 1979. Distribution of intimal smooth muscle cell masses and their relationship to early atherosclerosis in the abdominal aortas of young swine. Atherosclerosis **34**: 291–301.
5. THOMAS, W. A., J. M. REINER, R. A. FLORENTIN & R. F. SCOTT. 1979. Population dynamics of arterial cells during atherogenesis. VIII. Separation of the roles of injury and growth stimulation in early aortic atherogenesis in swine originating in preexisting intimal smooth muscle cell masses. Exp. Mol. Pathol. **31**: 124–144.
6. STARY, H. C. 1983. Structure and ultrastructure of the coronary artery intima in children and young adults up to age 29. *In* Atherosclerosis VI: Proceedings of Sixth International Symposium. F. G. Schettler, A. M. Gotto, G. Middelhoff, A. J. R. Habenicht & K. R. Jurutka, Eds.: 82–86. Springer-Verlag. Berlin, Heidelberg, New York.
7. KIM, D. N., J. SCHMEE, K. T. LEE & W. A. THOMAS. 1985. Intimal cell masses in the abdominal aortas of swine fed a low-fat, low-cholesterol diet for up to twelve years of age. Atherosclerosis **55**: 151–159.
8. IMAI, H., C. E. CONNELL, K. T. LEE, D. N. KIM & W. A. THOMAS. 1985. Differential counts by electron microscopy of cell types in normal intimal cell masses in swine abdominal aorta. Exp. Mol. Pathol. **42**: 377–388.
9. CAMPBELL, J. H., L. POPADYNEC, P. J. NESTEL & G. R. CAMPBELL. 1983. Lipid accumulation in arterial smooth muscle cells. Influence of phenotype. Atherosclerosis **47**: 279–295.
10. KIM, D. N., H. IMAI, J. SCHMEE, K. T. LEE & W. A. THOMAS. 1984. Intimal cell mass-derived atherosclerotic lesions in the abdominal aorta of hyperlipidemic swine: Cell

of origin, cell divisions, and cell losses in first 90 days on diet. Atherosclerosis. Accepted for publication.
11. FLORENTIN, R. A., B. H. CHOI, K. T. LEE & W. A. THOMAS. 1969. Stimulation of DNA synthesis and cell division *in vitro* by serum from cholesterol-fed swine. J. Cell Biol. **41**: 641–645.
12. FLESS, G. M., T. KIRCHHAUSEN, K. FISCHER-DZOGA, R. W. WISSLER & A. M. SCANU. 1982. Serum low-density lipoprotein with mitogenic effect on cultured aortic smooth muscle cells. Atherosclerosis **41**: 171–183.
13. THOMAS, W. A., K. T. LEE, J. M. REINER, D. N. KIM, R. A. FLORENTIN, R. F. SCOTT & J. SCHMEE. 1983. Population dynamics of arterial cells during atherogenesis. XIII. Mitogenic and cytotoxic effects of a hyperlipidemic (HL) diet on cells in advanced lesions in the abdominal aorta of swine fed an HL diet for 270–345 days. Exp. Mol. Pathol. **39**: 257–270.

Summary and New Directions

ROBERT W. WISSLER

Specialized Center of Research on Atherosclerosis
and
Department of Pathology
University of Chicago
Chicago, Illinois 60637

This conference has been a rich and stimulating experience. As expected, the monograph which it is yielding is packed with information and new directions for research. All of us must be grateful for the remarkable initiative and work that the Albany group, led by K. T. Lee, has invested in this program.

In spite of very thoughtful and careful planning by all of us who were involved, there are a few areas related to pathogenesis which probably should have had more emphasis. I point them out now, only so that we won't forget them next time this subject is reviewed. I am referring to the role of hemodynamic factors, which may alter artery wall susceptibility, the involvement of the viral genome in some animal and human atheromatous plaques, and the mechanisms which may control and alter arterial endothelial permeability to macromolecules, especially the influence of the glycocalyx as well as the transport vesicles with their diaphragms.

In this summary and projection, I am going to review the highlights of some of the presentations on pathogenesis and try to give a prospectus of the research tasks for the immediate future.

The outline presented in TABLE 1 is designed to call attention to the multiple factors that may contribute to the progression of atherosclerotic plaques. These factors in no way detract from the dominant contribution, and perhaps even the primary one, of elevated blood cholesterol levels in plaque formation. What it does is to add a number of other factors that may contribute to pathogenesis in addition to the possible contribution of circulating immune complexes, which are reviewed in my presentation. Many of these factors require further development of clinical laboratory methods in order to evaluate their contribution. In my presentation, I tried to indicate the remarkable effects that immune complexes have on plaque morphology, which may, in turn, be reflected in resistance to lesion regression, greater artery dilatation, more tendency for thrombosis, and less tendency for artery spasm.

Identified in this table are several of the newer aspects of our knowledge of abnormal lipoprotein metabolism, not all of which are manifest by elevated cholesterol levels, and several of which may exert a strong influence on rate of plaque progression. It also reflects the subtle alterations in cholesterol metabolism and excretion, which may be expressed in many ways. It recognizes the important variations in atherogenesis which are produced by various food fats and their effects on gastrointestinal, hepatic, and arterial wall metabolism. These are likely to be reflected by influencing HDL and LDL levels as well as LCAT activity or by injuring the artery wall in such a way as to alter endothelial integrity or to change the lesion components.

Other factors which are listed can also alter endothelial integrity or platelet stickiness. Hypertension, a commonly recognized and powerful risk factor is included, but cigarette smoking is not, since we are not yet certain of the mechanism by which it augments atherogenesis.

This outline calls attention to the numerous "promoters" of the process of

TABLE 1. The Variety of Promoters of Atherogenesis which may Account for Some of the Evident Variations and Paradoxes which Are Observed when the Major Risk Factors Are Studied

1. Lipoprotein patterns in response to atherogenic rations:		
a. H–LDL and its fractions	d. Apo E levels	g. LPa
b. Apo B rich LDL	e. β–VLDL	h. HDL heterogeneity
c. HDL–C levels	f. Remnant disorders	i. Apoprotein genetic variants
2. Alterations in cholesterol metabolism and excretion:		
a. Apoprotein (including hepatic) receptors	c. RES storage	
b. LP lipases and LCAT activity	d. Macrophage involvement	
3. Effects of dietary lipids on:		
a. Gastrointestinal metabolism	c. HDL and LCAT levels	e. Lesion components
b. LDL levels	d. Endothelial integrity	
4. Factors with potential to alter endothelial-intimal integrity:		
a. Hypertension	c. Endotoxins	e. von Willebrand, etc.
b. Viremia	d. Homocystine	f. Ag–Ab complexes

atherogenesis, but in my opinion, based on the current evidence, hyperlipidemia is still the major factor.

It is clear that we have had many marvelous presentations on pathogenesis, and I will recount only a few highlights.

We are indebted to Gardner McMillan who again demonstrated his keen perception and his exceptional perspective regarding the pathogenesis of atherosclerosis. He recounted the recent contributions of cellular and molecular biology to our understanding of respective roles of cell proliferation, endothelial structure and function, and the molecular genetics of lipoprotein disorders. He emphasized the recent contributions of the study of primate models and the newer studies of the development of human lesions using modern methods, along with the current divergent views concerning the contribution of diffuse intimal thickening to the development of the plaque.

He called for new initiatives and new directions in the study of the differences in the pathogenesis of human atherosclerotic disease in order to expand our knowledge of male and female contrasts in coronary disease progression, the role of the macrophage, and the contribution of proteoglycans.

Speaking from his extensive experience with primate models, Tom Clarkson emphasized the broad range of arterial responses observed in monkeys when their levels of elevated serum cholesterol are similar. These studies illustrate that factors in the artery wall may be responsible for pathogenetic differences. The recent Bowman-Gray studies of the role of behavioral modification, based on a dominant or a submissive response to unstable social situations, demonstrate that the reaction to psychosocial stress may be of paramount importance in determining its effect on atherogenesis. Protection from the development of atherosclerosis in the female monkey, long associated with elevated HDL levels, appears to be most readily demonstrated in the dominant female.

William Wagner reviewed the newer knowledge of proteoglycans with an emphasis on the contribution of the pigeon model to our understanding of these complex and somewhat unstable macromolecules. His emphasis on the changes seen in chondroitin sulfate and the importance of proteoglycan aggregate size in atherogenesis add new dimensions to the ways in which these substances may influence and be influenced by the developing atherosclerotic plaque.

The importance of macrophages and their enzymes in atherogenesis as presented by Stanley Fowler and discussed by Jon Lewis and Colin Schwartz focused on their role in smooth muscle cell proliferation, which paved the way for a detailed consideration by Assaad Daoud of these cells in experimental swine lesions undergoing regression. Ultimately, these studies may provide new insights into the contribution of macrophages to both progression and regression of atherosclerosis.

The inclusion of prostaglandin metabolism in the program gave Salvador Moncada the opportunity to implicate the lipid peroxides as influential in inhibiting prostacyclin synthesis, as well as prostacyclin activity. He also emphasized the remarkable influence of platelet activity in prostacyclin synthesis and the important lessons learned from studies of the effects of colchicine on the prostacyclin metabolic process. These and other studies have led to the discovery of further functions of prostacyclin in atherogenesis, including its cytoprotective effects and its fibrinolytic effects. These recent studies suggest that prostacyclin may be a major regulator of platelet-artery wall interaction.

The presentation by Fujio Numano concentrated on some of the subtle effects of aspirin. He emphasized the salicylate effects on the response of the coronary vessels and the aorta to the prostaglandins and to serotonin. Aspirin also produces important changes in the cyclic nucleotides. He summarized recent studies of aspirin's promising effects on the progress of Takayasu's disease.

These two stimulating presentations of Salvador Moncada and Fujio Numano emphasize the probability that we are entering an era in which it will be important to be able to document chronic and sustained changes in artery wall metabolism in relation to the prostaglandin system and the cyclic nucleotide system. We need new ways to measure these effects if we are to understand the profound effects that relatively simple therapies, such as aspirin, exert on the atherosclerotic process.

The powerful presentation by Sean Moore signaled the shifting of the focus of the conference to the ancient question of the role of thrombosis in the pathogenesis of atherosclerosis. His presentation served to underscore the as yet unsolved problems about the role of small mural thrombi in the development of the atherosclerotic plaque in the human. Do they have an influence in the development of "gelatinous lesions" or "diffuse intimal thickening"? It is also clear from his very well-organized presentation that there needs to be more study of the long-standing and still unanswered question as to whether hypercholesterolemia *per se* injures endothelium and promotes thrombus formation.

The remarkable indwelling catheter lesions reported by his group in animals with normal cholesterol levels are fascinating. This simple traumatic maneuver produces highly developed plaques with many of the features of advanced human atherosclerosis. They represent the single best example of lipid- and cholesterol-containing advanced plaques, which develop in the absence of hypercholesterolemia and with only severe arterial injury as the major etiologic factor. This area of research certainly needs further detailed study with special emphasis on pathogenetic mechanisms.

In the final presentation of this series, H. R. Baumgartner described the beautiful *in vitro* system he is now using. This endothelial cell-coated coverslip technique makes it possible to study, under highly controlled conditions, the phenomena of platelet sticking, spreading, aggregation, and thrombosis.

With this system, which certainly seems promising enough to be exploited, it is possible to study human diseases that have abnormal platelets and to document the altered sticking and spreading in these disorders. In addition, it is possible to use modern cell biology approaches to observe, study, and illustrate what is happening at the ultrastructural level.

This part of the symposium on pathogenesis ended with a discussion by Daria Haust. She augmented the discussion by illustrating the human counterpart of many of these phenomena with ultrastructural evidence of lipid containing modified arterial smooth muscle cells in organizing mural thrombi. Further discussion by Peter Alaupovic supported the previous evidence that the indwelling catheter lesions develop with no substantial changes in the circulating lipoproteins. Furthermore, Colin Schwartz described the development of foam cells from monocytes that migrate into thrombi and use phagocytosed platelet membrane lipids to produce the visible lipid droplets.

Perhaps more than any other consideration of pathogenesis in recent times, this program made it possible to carefully assess the combined roles of many pathogenetic mechanisms. It should help to prepare us for the task of synthesis and the immense challenge of developing the necessary clinical laboratory tests that are needed if we are ever to be able to evaluate many of these promoters of atherogenesis in the patient or in the person at risk.

Cellular Mechanisms in Atherosclerosis

Theories and Therapies

STEPHEN M. SCHWARTZ

Department of Pathology SJ-60
University of Washington
Seattle, Washington 98195

I would like to suggest that our ability to understand atherosclerosis would be advanced greatly by concentrating on understanding simple parts of the processes rather than trying to tie everything together in one large "multifactorial" hypothesis. Current theories of atherosclerosis deal with quite different and independent processes in the vessel wall. For example, the "monoclonal" and "response to injury" hypotheses attempt to explain mechanisms of cellular proliferation, while the lipid hypothesis focuses on lipid accumulation. Since there is no obvious relationship between lipid accumulation and cell replication, attempts at unitary explanations of this complex disease are usually too complex. Three independent phenomena stand out as intrinsic to atherosclerosis:

(i) Lipid accumulation;
(ii) Smooth muscle cell proliferation;
(iii) Thrombosis.

All of these are essential to development of clinically significant lesions, and all are relatively well understood as single mechanisms. By itself, however, no mechanism provides a satisfactory model.

For example, the so-called fatty streaks seen in young adults are certainly not clinically significant. Pure fatty lesions, to the best of my knowledge, never encroach upon a vessel and never produce clinical symptoms. At the same time, the significance of lipid in the evolution of the later lesion is an area that is of considerable importance. For example, we simply do not know what effect the accumulation of lipid in the lesion has on clinical effects of the lesion. Does lipid contribute to thrombosis? Does lipid contribute to smooth muscle cell proliferation? Does lipid alter the propensity of lesions to produce spasm?

While we do not know why lipid in the lesion is harmful, we are learning how lipid accumulates. The most important hypothesis is based upon the work of Brown and Goldstein. Their work, in combination with work by Alan Fogelmann, Dan Steinberg, Guy Chisholm, and others, suggests that some kind of alteration of low-density lipoprotein (LDL) or of the ability of the cell to interact with LDL will ultimately explain the accumulation of lipid in foam cells in lesions. It is, however, quite important to note that at least a portion of that lipid appears to be in mononuclear cells rather than in smooth muscle cells. Thus, an understanding of lipid accumulation in the lesion may depend not only on the understanding of lipid metabolism by vessel wall cells, but on how monocytes accumulate in the lesion. Finally, there have been suggestions, so far not backed up by extensive evidence, that these monocytes are also able to remove lipid from the lesion. This could be a very important idea.

It seems likely that soon we will have enough understanding of the mechanisms of lipid metabolism by smooth muscle cells and monocytes to explain why lipid accumulates in lesions. The open question, then, will be what effect does that lipid have on the clinical effects of the lesion, particularly on thrombosis. Understanding of thrombosis is also progressing rapidly. Research undertaken in a large number of laboratories has begun to define the surface proteins of the platelet, the mechanism of interactions of those platelets with the connective tissue of the vessel wall, the series of events leading to activation of the platelet towards thrombosis, and the release of alpha-granule contents into the vessel wall. It seems likely, therefore, that the next five to ten years will see a sufficient understanding of the biology of the platelet so as to allow pharmacological intervention in the formation of the thrombus. This seems to me to be a very important prediction since the role of the thrombus in the evolution of vascular occlusion is quite clear. I am quite confident that this sort of therapy will become a routine adjunct to vascular surgery and angioplasty. It may also play a role in medical attempts to treat advanced vascular disease without surgery or angioplasty.

Even with this progress, a great deal remains unknown about the interactions of thrombosis and the other two major processes with each other. For example, we need to know why lipid stimulates proliferation, why lesions become thrombogenic, and why some lesions kill, while others remain silent toxins of disease. Perhaps most intriguing to the experimental pathologist, we do not yet know how lesions begin.

In my opinion, smooth muscle proliferation is probably the critical event in formation of the disease. As discussed by W. Thomas and by myself, there is evidence that focal, abnormal accumulations of smooth muscle cells can eventuate in lesions. This is consistent with a reasonable body of evidence from more than one laboratory suggesting that smooth muscle proliferation is the underlying ground upon which lesions develop. While the "fatty streak" made up of lipid-foam cells may be capable of producing a proliferative response, it is quite clear that lipid tends to preferentially accumulate in intimal cell masses. Thus, localization of intimal cells may be critical to localization of lesions, even for lipid accumulation. Finally, proliferation is always seen in advanced disease. I am unaware of any clinically significant occlusive disease that does not contain a rather large component of smooth muscle proliferation, and I have seen total lesions where proliferation is a predominant feature.

Currently, there are two major hypotheses of smooth muscle proliferation, namely, the response to injury hypothesis and the monoclonal hypothesis. The naming of these two hypotheses obscures their major differences and similarities. The monoclonal hypothesis, as originally offered by Benditt, suggests that lesions begin by a mutagenic event, which implies that the atherosclerotic lesion is a tumor. The atherosclerotic lesion fulfills the general textbook definition of a benign smooth muscle tumor, that is, a focal cellular overgrowth. If the atherosclerotic lesion is not a leiomyoma, i.e., not a benign smooth muscle tumor of the vessel wall, then we are left with the conclusion that there are no leiomyomas of the vessel wall. No other form of benign smooth muscle cell arterial tumor has been described.

This concept, however, begs the question of etiology. Defining the lesion as a tumor does not explain how it starts. Far more important in Benditt's hypothesis is the idea of a mutational or viral event. The possibility of exploring this hypothesis seemed relatively remote until the advent of recombinant DNA technology. It seems highly likely now that it will become possible to look within the atherosclerotic plaque for the steps required for commitment of a cell to a replicative state. Progress in this area is going to depend a great deal on progress in tumor research. If it becomes possible to define specific events involved in the transition from a normal to a benign transformed state, then the essential ingredient of a monoclonal hypothesis will become testable.

In the meantime, the possibility of specific therapeutic approaches to the problem of smooth muscle proliferation will depend on whether the processes uncovered in the vessel wall are tissue specific or more general. Certainly, one doesn't want to imagine a need for antiproliferative therapy of the magnitude required for the treatment of cancer. Russell Ross's suggestions about specific PDGF antagonists are of obvious importance, as is work by Robert Rosenberg on heparin as a growth inhibitor.

Some Future Directions for Research on Atherogenesis

DANIEL STEINBERG

Department of Medicine
University of California, San Diego
La Jolla, California 92093

For investigators interested in the basic mechanisms involved in atherogenesis, the past decade has been "the decade of cell biology." Largely through the application of cell culture techniques, we have learned an enormous amount about the behavior of the individual cell types involved, which are endothelial cells, smooth muscle cells, and monocyte/macrophages. We know that each of these cells, as well as the blood platelets, can produce growth factors and that these may contribute to the characteristic cellular proliferation of the developing atheroma. We understand a great deal about the manner in which these cells interact with lipoproteins, including the several specific membrane receptors involved (the LDL receptor, the beta-VLDL receptor, the acetyl LDL receptor), and how their metabolism of lipoproteins is regulated. While much has been learned, much remains unknown.

We still cannot write down the sequence of events intervening between the interaction of a growth factor with its receptor and the "turning on" of cell growth and multiplication. That remains a central problem for the cell biologist. It will probably be solved, in large part, by application of the powerful techniques of modern molecular biology over the next decade. Similarly, we still cannot spell out in detail how the several lipoprotein receptors are synthesized and inserted into the membrane, nor exactly how their numbers are regulated. The successful cloning of the LDL receptor by Goldstein, Brown, and their collaborators should soon make it possible to specify just how "down-regulation" is effected, and then to devise ways to control the number of LDL receptors. It may not be too extreme to predict that most of what we need to know about the behavior of individual cells as it relates to atherogenesis (but certainly, not everything there is to know about cells!) will be established over the next decade or two. However—and this is the major point I should like to make—even with all that information in hand, it seems most unlikely to me that we will be able to sketch out in detail and with certainty the train(s) of events involved in atherogenesis.

A complete picture of the atherogenic process can only come from an understanding of the interactions among cells. For example, substances produced by one cell type can importantly modify the metabolism of neighboring cells. Some of these factors may be labile and difficult to isolate for later study. A number of laboratories have recognized this and have begun the study of mixed cultures. Again, metabolites may be acted on and modified by one cell type to a form that can then influence the growth and metabolism of neighboring cells. The modification of LDL by endothelial cells to a form recognized by the macrophage acetyl LDL receptor is an example. Studies along these lines, i.e., of cell-cell interactions in *ad hoc* mixtures, should give valuable insights. Yet, even these are unlikely to be sufficient.

Ultimately, I think we have to engage the problem on its home soil—the artery wall. This almost self-evident statement is, no doubt, eliciting knowing (if not pitying) smiles from the experimental pathologists among us who have been (properly) tilling that soil for some time. I hope they will forgive me since my message is directed not to them, but to biochemists, cell biologists, and molecular biologists, some of whom still nurture the hope that the reconstruction can somehow be effected in its entirety by a synthesis from elements developed at the cellular and molecular level. As indicated above, the wealth of information being developed at the cellular and molecular level will without question inform the attack on the home soil, but the battle must be engaged there. The new experimental pathology will look for ways to assess in the intact artery wall the functioning of the basic processes worked out at the cellular and molecular level. This has already begun, of course. Thymidine-labeling, as used extensively by the group here in Albany and by others, lets us assess effects on cell replication *in vivo.* Using fluorescence-labeled monoclonal antibodies against receptors, we can quantify the expression of receptor activity by individual cells in intact tissues. Using the "trapped ligand" approach and autoradiography, we can now obtain a functional measure of receptor activity in individual cells of the artery wall *in vivo.* Many other examples might be given, and the range of opportunities will predictably expand.

Unfortunately, the methods available to us at this time are such that in most cases the animal must be sacrificed and thus provides only one time point. Perhaps, the time has come to reinvestigate the feasibility of an organ culture system that would maintain vessels long enough to let us see at least the earliest stages in lesion development. In that way, we could explore multiple variables under controlled conditions, and we could possibly evaluate agents that influence atherogenesis at the local level, i.e., other than by regulating lipoprotein levels.

New Directions in Atherosclerosis Research

GARDNER C. McMILLAN

Division of Heart and Vascular Diseases
National Heart, Lung, and Blood Institute
Bethesda, Maryland 20205

In discussion earlier at this meeting, the idea was put forward that the term arteriosclerosis could be applied to any pathological process that took place in the arterial intima. The idea has value in the sense that it keeps us open-minded to mechanisms relevant to atherogenesis, but it goes too far. I would hold that when we know and have defined such entities as luetic aortitis, bacterial arteritis, rheumatic arteritis, specific antigenic vasculitis, and so on, it would be a disservice to lump them with arteriosclerosis, even when we recognize that sclerotic intimal changes occur that share some features with it. Some similar events of proliferative, inflammatory, productive, and degenerative nature may indeed occur, but these speak to the encompassing nature of the injury-repair concept rather than to arteriosclerosis itself. Arteriosclerosis, as we know it today, has well-established epidemiological associations, particular clinical presentations, and pathological developments that strongly emphasize lipid accumulation, thrombotic processes, and the intimal reactions to them.

What of future research? The application of cellular and molecular biology to research on atherogenesis during the past decade has been so successful that one can look forward to another decade of even more successful application of these methods to provide descriptive data, to generate hypotheses, and to test them in the usual cyclic sequence of scientific progress.

What areas seem especially challenging for investigation? We do not know why many plaques are especially rich in proteoglycan matrix, or why cells are stimulated to secrete matrix substances. We have learned much about the platelet in thrombotic and proliferative processes, but we have not explored the roles of the various blood coagulation cascade proteins in much detail. Even fibrin is not extensively studied. In that respect, one should comment that we lack an epidemiology of thrombotic processes and atherosclerotic disease different from lipids and atherosclerosis. At present, the two are confounded, and we have not succeeded in separating them, although one would predict that such a separation is both possible and biologically meaningful.

Several speakers mentioned the possible existence of subsets of lymphocytes and macrophages in plaques. Clearly, this question will be resolved promptly since techniques to do so are at hand. The result should provide a deeper insight into plaque pathogenesis. One issue that arose, although it did not elicit extensive discussion, was the role of the genetic nature of the cells of the vessel wall in modulating the atherogenic process—either through susceptibility to injury or reaction to it. It has been clear for many years that the vascular mesenchyme in animals can modulate atherogenesis. It has been shown by surgical transposition experiments in dogs that the native susceptibility to experimental atherogenesis of a particular aortic segment accompanied the transposed vessel. The Bowman Gray laboratories showed years ago that there was a heritable characteristic of the arteries of the White Carneau pigeon that could be selected to provide birds with more coronary atherosclerosis than aortic atherosclerosis, or vice versa. They are pursuing the matter in nonhuman primates, but, clearly, the genetic makeup of the vascular mesenchyme and its differentiation must be recognized as a risk factor for atherosclerosis. While this research is necessarily in a descriptive stage, it should be susceptible to the methods of cellular and molecular biology in the near future.

Lastly, I would like to return to my own paper, and note again that I think we must restudy human atherosclerosis and plaques with modern methods so that we can better relate the findings to those of modern animal and cellular experiments. In particular, the lesions developing with childhood and before middle age need restudy.

I want to close with the warmest expression of thanks to K.T. Lee for a very instructive and enjoyable conference. I know it will be productive.

Index of Contributors